ARCO DIAGNOSIS SERIES

DIFFERENTIAL DIAGNOSIS

RENAL AND ELECTROLYTE DISORDERS

SAULO KLAHR, M.D.
Professor of Medicine
Director, Renal Division

Washington University
School of Medicine
St. Louis, Missouri

Arco Publishing Company, Inc.
New York

Published by Arco Publishing Company, Inc.
219 Park Avenue South, New York, N.Y. 10003

Library of Congress Cataloging in Publication Data
Main entry under title:

Differential diagnosis of renal and electrolyte disorders.

Includes bibliographical references
1. Kidneys—Diseases—Diagnosis. 2. Water-electrolyte imbalances—Diagnosis. 3. Diagnosis, Differential. I. Klahr, Saulo. [DNLM: 1. Diagnosis, Differential. 2. Kidney diseases—Diagnosis. 3. Water-electrolyte imbalance—Diagnosis. WJ300 D569]
RC904.D53 616.6'1'075 77-10321
ISBN 0-668-04063-7

Printed in the United States of America

Editorial Advisory Board

Contributors

Joan Blondin, M.D.
Assistant Professor of Medicine

John Buerkert, M.D.
Assistant Professor of Medicine

Barbara Cole, M.D.
Assistant Professor of Pediatrics

Herschel Harter, M.D.
Assistant Professor of Medicine
Medical Director
Chromalloy American Dialysis Center

Phillip Hoffsten, M.D.
Assistant Professor of Medicine

Keith Hruska, M.D.
Assistant Professor of Medicine

Saulo Klahr, M.D.
Professor of Medicine
Director, Renal Division

Mabel L. Purkerson, M.D.
Associate Professor of Medicine

Alan Robson, M.D.
Professor of Pediatrics
Associate Professor of Medicine
Director, Pediatric Nephrology Division

W. Ernest Rutherford, M.D.
Assistant Professor of Medicine

Eduardo Slatopolsky, M.D.
Professor of Medicine
Director, Chromalloy American Dialysis Center

Washington University School of Medicine
St. Louis, Missouri

Preface

Prefaces usually have one purpose—to justify the publication of a new book. In the last decade or so the number of books published in the area of nephrology has increased geometrically. The reader may ask, and rightfully so, why another book on renal and electrolyte disorders is needed. Why, indeed! This book is designed not for the specialist in nephrology but for medical students and house officers. Its emphasis is somewhat different from most of the published books in the area of renal and electrolyte abnormalities. It is geared mainly to the interpretation and differential diagnosis of presenting symptoms or signs of renal disease and/or laboratory abnormalities found commonly in the evaluation of hospitalized patients. Each chapter has been contributed by individuals who are or have been, at one time or another, members of the Renal Division at Washington University School of Medicine. All the contributors are on the faculty of either the Department of Medicine or the Department of Pediatrics at Washington University, and most have had a long and close association with the editor. While emphasis has been placed on the differential diagnosis of signs and symptoms of renal disease and electrolyte disorders, the necessary pathophysiologic mechanisms responsible for the alterations observed have also been discussed in each chapter. Hopefully, this will provide the student with a framework to understand mechanisms of disease.

I have tried to organize each chapter in a similar manner. Every chapter includes a representative case problem of each abnormality discussed, followed by questions. The student should utilize the case problems as review material that emphasizes important points made in the different chapters. The questions that follow each case presentation attempt to focus the student's attention on pertinent and important problems exhibited by that patient. Finally, a discussion relative to the different case problems is included after each chapter. Most of the case problems are summaries of the records of patients admitted to either the Medicine or Pediatric services at the Washington University Medical Center during the last 10 to 15 years.

When different authors contribute chapters on sometimes closely related subjects, a certain degree of overlap is unavoidable if each contribution is to be coherent. I have tried, therefore, to avoid duplication of extended accounts of any single topic, but I have not excluded brief accounts of conditions in a special context. Certain duplication is, indeed, necessary for emphasizing points that the authors and myself consider important.

While my main debt is to those who have contributed chapters and therefore written this book, I also want to express my gratitude to Drs. Raymond Bass and Jeffrey Freitag, postdoctoral fellows in the Renal Division, Washington University, who read most of the chapters and provided valuable suggestions and criticisms. The most difficult job of all was done by my secretaries, Patricia Persons, Patricia Verplancke, and Mary Worsdell, who, out of scraps of paper and barely discernible dictations, restored order out of chaos and produced a final manuscript. It is impossible to thank them enough. Lastly, it is a pleasure to acknowledge the authors and publishers who kindly allowed some of their illustrations to be reproduced in this book.

Saulo Klahr, M.D.
St. Louis, Missouri

TO
Carol, James, and Robert

Contents

Chapter 1

Hematuria

General Considerations

Hematuria is the appearance of abnormal amounts of red blood cells in the urine. Normally the daily urinary excretion of red blood cells is less than 1.5 million, the amount contained in a third of a cubic millimeter of blood. Microscopic hematuria may be detected when blood loss in the urine is three times normal, or the equivalent of a cubic millimeter of blood lost in the urine per day. Thus, microscopic hematuria is an exquisitely sensitive manifestation of abnormalities in the urinary tract. The loss of one third of a cubic centimeter of whole blood into the urine per day is usually manifested as gross hematuria.

The significance of hematuria depends upon the clinical setting in which it is seen. Except in cases of trauma or postoperative bleeding, hematuria is not a therapeutic problem so much as a diagnostic one. The objectives of the workup are to localize and characterize the nature of the lesion. Hematuria should always be regarded as a serious symptom deserving thorough investigation in an attempt to establish a definite diagnosis.

The presence in the urine of blood obvious to the unassisted eye is termed gross hematuria. Gross hematuria has a variable appearance depending upon the site and extent of bleeding in addition to the concentration and pH of the urine. If urine has a "bright red blood" appearance, bleeding is relatively recent and usually originates in the lower urinary tract; as blood remains in urine with a pH of 5, hemoglobin is quickly converted to ferritin, which has the rusty brown color expected when the kidney is the site of bleeding. Long cylindrical clots indicate the presence of bleeding in the ureter, while irregular clots favor the bladder as a bleeding site. Patients often seek medical advice because of what they interpret to be gross hematuria; however, it should be remembered that urine may falsely appear to contain blood in many conditions. Examples include food fads such as beets, rhubarb, blackberries, or cold drinks containing red food dyes. A variety of drugs listed in Table 1-1 may give urine a pink-red, red-brown-rust, or orange-red color. Myoglobinuria may be associated with a characteristic wine-red colored urine.

When the amount of blood present in the urine is not obvious to the unassisted eye, the condition is spoken of as microscopic hematuria. By standard technique, 15 ml of fresh urine is centrifuged for 5 minutes at 1000–1500 rpm using a standard laboratory bench-top centrifuge. The supernatant urine is discarded, leaving one quarter to one half milliliter of urine in the tube for resuspension of the sediment. A drop of this suspension is placed on a glass slide, and a coverslip is placed over the drop. The urine is examined with a standard light microscope using subdued illumination. Red blood cells in the urine are best detected using the high-dry objective (43x); more than three cells per high-powered field in many different fields allows one to make the diagnosis of abnormal microscopic hematuria.

Special attention should be paid to the presence of formed elements that may accompany red blood cells in the urinary sediment. If one sees red blood cell casts, the site of bleeding is the kidney. Similarly the presence of casts of other types favors a renal origin of the bleeding. It should be noted that hypotonic urine may result in osmotic lysis of red

Table 1-1

Drugs Giving Urine the Appearance of Hematuria

	Pink-Red	Red-Brown-Rust	Orange-Red
I. Analgesics			
1. Phenacetin	x		
2. Phenazopyridine (pyridium)			x
II. Antibiotic-Antiparasitics			
1. Sulfanilamide	x	x	
2. Rifampin			x
3. Salicylazosulfapyridine	x	x	
4. Thiazolsulfone	x	x	
5. Quinine	x	x	
6. Cinchonine		x	
7. Pamaquin		x	
8. Chloroquine		x	
9. Primaquine		x	
10. Metronidazole		x	
III. Anticoagulants			
1. Anisindione			x
2. Phenindione			x
IV. Antiepileptics			
1. Diphenylhydantoin	x	x	
2. Phensurimide	x	x	
V. Antihypertensives			
1. Methyldopa	x		
VI. Antineoplastics			
1. Adriamycin	x		
2. Daunorubicin	x		
VII. Laxatives			
1. Emodin	x	x	
2. Cascara		x	
3. Phenolphthalein in alkaline urine	x		
VIII. Psychiatric			
1. Phenothiazines	x	x	

blood cells, and thus the osmolality or specific gravity of the urine should be determined on urine specimens examined. Red blood cell casts are difficult to detect in the presence of gross hematuria, and thus their absence in the setting of gross hematuria does not preclude a renal origin for the bleeding. Finally, alkaline urine leads to dissolution of casts; thus the urine pH should be determined and the urine should always be examined as soon after voiding as possible.

The dipstick test (Ames Company) is utilized to detect free hemoglobin in the urine. The test may be negative when small numbers of intact red blood cells are seen. The dipstick is not specific for hemoglobin in that myoglobin will also give a positive test. A positive dipstick test in the absence of microscopic hematuria should alert one to the variety of conditions associated with myoglobinuria.

Clinical Features Important in the Evaluation of Hematuria

When considering hematuria the patient's history is of utmost importance. The occurrence of localized pain or trauma may markedly simplify the diagnostic process. In the absence of localizing symptoms, care should be taken to elicit information on all drugs consumed, such as anticoagulants, quinidine, or cyclophosphamide. The presence of a known associated illness such as hemophilia may shorten the diagnostic workup. As previously noted, dark or red urine may indicate conditions other than hematuria; conditions to keep in mind include myoglobinuria associated with crush injuries, nontraumatic acute rhabdomyolysis, and hemoglobinuria associated with paroxysmal cold hemoglobinuria or paroxysmal nocturnal hemoglobinuria. Rarer conditions include methemoglobinemia, erythropoietic porphyria, and alkaptonuria, all of which may be associated with dark or brown urines.

On physical examination, particular interest should be paid to the flank or costovertebral angle regions and the suprapubic area. A careful and complete examination may lead directly to an appropriate diagnosis. The presence of an abdominal mass may allow one to make the diagnosis of tumor, bladder neck obstruction, or polycystic kidneys in the case of bilateral masses. The presence of dependent petechiae may lead to a diagnosis of abnormal coagulation mechanisms, or if generalized petechiae are present, a diagnosis of Henoch-Schonlein purpura may be suspected. Rare conditions such as the Osler-Weber-Rendu syndrome may be diagnosed by careful examination of the mucocutaneous junctions. Cardiac examination may lead to a diagnosis of bacterial endocarditis with associated glomerulonephritis.

Laboratory Considerations

Appropriate laboratory examinations are pivotal in the evaluation of hematuria. Once the presence of hematuria is established, the physician should perform the so-called three-glass urinalysis. The urethral meatus is thoroughly cleansed and urination initiated into the first container. After a small amount of urine is passed the patient changes containers and collects the midportion of urination in the second container and the last portion in a third container. If blood is noted primarily in the first container, the site of bleeding is usually in the urethra; common causes include a urethral stricture or prostatitis. While initial hematuria is rare in women, terminal hematuria is common and is a sign of urethral or bladder neck lesions. In women the most common cause of terminal hematuria is trigonitis of the bladder secondary to a urinary tract infection. The presence of similar quantities of hematuria in all three containers is of little help in localizing the site of the bleeding.

The significance of other formed elements in the urinary sediment has already been mentioned. The presence of abnormal proteinuria should receive special attention, as this strongly favors the presence of a renal glomerular lesion. While one might be tempted to attribute abnormal proteinuria in the presence of hematuria to the protein that entered with the blood itself, this is rarely a valid consideration. Gross hematuria is evident with the presence of 1 ml of whole blood in the urine; yet 1 ml of blood will contain only 180 mg of protein and only 20 mg of albumin. Thus the amount of protein contributed by 1 ml of blood does not explain the presence of gram quantities of protein in the urine. The presence of abnormal proteinuria can never be explained by the presence of microscopic hematuria.

Routine laboratory examinations including a complete blood count; serum creatinine; serum uric acid, serum electrolytes, serum calcium, and serum phosphorus concentrations; and various clotting parameters should all be obtained. A urine culture should routinely be performed. If renal tuberculosis is suspected, a urine culture for acid-fast bacilli should be performed on three consecutive morning specimens.

Radiological examinations may be very helpful in determining the cause of hematuria, and an intravenous pyelogram should be done routinely. If there is any suspicion that a tumor might be present, nephrotomograms should be obtained. Arteriography of the kidney should be reserved for special situations; this procedure infrequently leads to a definitive diagnosis in cases of hematuria.

In several large series of cases of hematuria, a bladder lesion was found to be responsible for hematuria in 40% of patients. If a firm diagnosis of the cause of the hematuria is not found by the noninvasive procedures delineated above, cystoscopy should be performed.

Finally, definitive diagnosis of glomerular lesions associated with hematuria will require a renal biopsy. There is significant morbidity associated with this procedure, and its performance should be restricted to medical centers providing immunofluorescent and electron microscopic examination in addition to the routine histopathologic examinations.

Differential Diagnosis of Hematuria and Basis for Diagnosis of Specific Conditions

While any structure in the urinary tract may bleed, and many renal diseases are associated with hematuria, the most common causes of hematuria are given in Table 1-2 and discussed below, with pertinent information allowing a definitive diagnosis of the various conditions.

I. Renal Origin

A. Inflammatory Diseases

1. Glomerulonephritis Not Associated with Systemic Disease

a. Acute Glomerulonephritis. This condition is diagnosed by the clinical syndrome of the sudden onset of painless gross hematuria with rusty brown turbid urine. The urinary sediment will contain abnormal quantities of serum proteins in addition to a variety of tubular casts. Constitutional symptoms including malaise, headache, oliguria, and edema are expected, although they are variably present. A preceding upper respiratory tract infection is often noted; proof of pharyngitis with group A beta-hemolytic streptococci is noted in 20% to 40% of the cases in children but in less than 10% of sporadic cases in adults. Renal biopsy is usually not indicated in this condition unless immunosuppressive therapy is contemplated in an attempt to modify a progressive course. The natural history in children is favorable, with complete recovery in more than 90% of cases; the prognosis in adults is more guarded with 40% to 50% of all cases incurring a persistent decrease in renal function.

b. Benign Recurrent Hematuria (Berger's Disease). This recently delineated clinical syndrome is characterized by recurrent episodes of gross hematuria frequently occurring several days after a mild upper respiratory tract infection. In contrast to acute glomerulonephritis, which rarely occurs more than once in any given patient, gross hematuria in this condition may occur many times per year. Gross hematuria persists for several days to a week and then may abate completely, or the patient may have persistent microhematuria. Red blood cell casts are frequently noted. Constitutional symptoms are not expected; hypertension and edema are unusual. Abnormal proteinuria is expected, with daily urinary protein excretions between 1 and 3 gm; the nephrotic syndrome is not expected. Renal function remains stable in 90% of all cases. Because the condition most often follows a very favorable course, no therapy is indicated; in the unusual case associated with progressive renal failure, a trial of immunosuppressive therapy might be attempted on an empirical basis after a renal biopsy. Definitive diagnosis in this condition usually rests upon the clinical findings, and renal biopsy is not routinely indicated.

c. Membranoproliferative Glomerulonephritis. Unlike the two conditions discussed above, this condition is usually not benign. The clinical presentation may simulate acute glomerulonephritis, although presentation as the nephrotic syndrome is equally likely. Hypertension, abnormal proteinuria, and renal failure are very frequent. The serum concentration of the third component of complement is often quite low. Definitive diagnosis rests upon the findings of a renal biopsy. Two pathological types of membranoproliferative glomerulonephritis are known, based upon findings of electron microscopy: (1) type 1 with subendothelial immune complexes and (2) type 2 with intramembranous dense deposits. While the pathogenesis of these two conditions appears to be different, clinically and by light microscopy the two types are not distinguishable. Natural history is variable, with progressive renal failure expected in 1 to 15 years. Immunosuppressive therapy has no predictable effect upon the disease, although sporadic success has been noted.

d. Syndrome of Rapidly Progressive Glomerulonephritis. This condition may be a final common pathway for severe cases of glomerulonephritis, membranoproliferative glomerulonephritis, and various nonclassified cases of chronic glomerulonephritis. Onset is usually acute but may be insidious. Common presenting symptoms include gross hematuria, edema, hypertension, malaise, or oliguria with nausea, vomiting, and central nervous system symptoms. Definitive diagnosis rests upon the dual association of a progressive decrease in glomerular filtration rate and necrotizing glomerulonephritis with crescents noted on renal biopsy. The natural history is unfavorable, with end-stage renal failure usually occurring within 6 months. No predictably effective therapy is known, although sporadic cases respond to immunosuppressive measures.

e. Membranous Glomerulonephritis. This condition most often presents as the nephrotic syndrome; microhematuria occurs rarely, and gross hematuria is not expected. Definitive diagnosis depends upon renal biopsy, which should be performed routinely in the evaluation of nephrotic syndrome in adults. Membranous glomerulonephritis is an unusual cause of the nephrotic syndrome in children; in pediatric cases, renal biopsy is not routinely performed to evaluate the nephrotic syndrome.

f. Nonclassified Chronic Glomerulonephritides. An estimated 30% of all cases of chronic glomerulonephritis are not easily delineated into one of the known clinical syndromes. These unclassified cases may present as renal failure, hypertension, gross or microscopic hematuria, or the nephrotic syndrome. Evaluation usually includes a renal biopsy that does not demonstrate findings definitive for any of the conditions that are discussed above. The condition is most often defined in descriptive pathological terms, although these do not allow the prediction of a frequently associated clinical syndrome.

2. Glomerulonephritis Associated with Systemic Disease

a. Collagen-Vascular Diseases. Among the family of collagen-vascular diseases, systemic lupus erythematosus (LE), polyarteritis nodosa, and scleroderma are each associated with microscopic hematuria. Each of these conditions is associated with a high incidence of renal failure and death due to renal causes in 40% of the cases.

Systemic lupus erythematosus: The diagnosis of this condition is based upon appropriate serological tests (positive LE cell test, positive antinuclear antibody, positive anti-DNA binding) in the setting of a characteristic clinical syndrome of fever (85%), skin rash (75%), and arthritis (90%). Other systems are involved in this disease, which presents in notoriously varied forms. Renal involvement occurs in 60% of cases and may be clinically manifested as an abnormal urinary sediment with microscopic hematuria, marked proteinuria, renal failure, and hypertension. Gross hematuria is not expected. Renal biopsy is often performed to characterize the renal lesion, although it is not required to establish a definitive diagnosis.

Polyarteritis nodosa: This condition is often heralded by nonspecific symptoms such as malaise, weight loss, anorexia, or pulmonary symptoms. Renal manifestations include abnormal urinary sediment, proteinuria, hypertension, and renal failure. Definitive diagnosis is based upon biopsy-proven evidence of inflammatory involvement of arteries or veins. Renal biopsy may be performed for this purpose, although skin or muscle biopsy carry less morbidity and serve equally well if the biopsied areas are involved.

Scleroderma: While the presenting symptoms of scleroderma usually involve the skin or gastrointestinal tract, 50% of the patients die as a result of renal failure with a pathological appearance resembling malignant hypertension. Microhematuria and proteinuria are common. Definitive diagnosis is based upon clinical criteria with a characteristic appearance of skin biopsy.

Table 1-2

Differential Diagnosis of Hematuria

- I. Renal origin
  - A. Inflammatory diseases
    - 1. Glomerulonephritis, not associated with known systemic disease
      - a. Acute glomerulonephritis
      - b. Benign recurrent hematuria (Berger's disease)
      - c. Membranoproliferative glomerulonephritis
        - i. With subendothelial immune complexes (type I)
        - ii. With intramembranous dense deposits (type II)
      - d. Syndrome of rapidly progressive glomerulonephritis
      - e. Membranous glomerulonephritis (hematuria unusual)
      - f. Nonclassified chronic glomerulonephritides (probably 30+% of all cases of chronic glomerulonephritis)
    - 2. Glomerulonephritis associated with systemic disease
      - a. Collagen-vascular diseases
        - i. Systemic lupus erythematosus
        - ii. Polyarteritis nodosa
        - iii. Scleroderma
        - iv. Sjogren's syndrome
        - v. Wegener's granulomatosis
      - b. Infective endocarditis
      - c. Goodpasture's syndrome
      - d. Hemolytic uremic syndrome
      - e. Thrombotic thrombocytopenic purpura
      - f. Henoch-Schonlein purpura
  - B. Infections
    - 1. Renal tuberculosis
    - 2. Pyelonephritis (hematuria is especially common with papillary necrosis)
  - C. Neoplastic diseases
    - 1. Renal cell carcinoma
    - 2. Transitional cell carcinoma of the renal pelvis
    - 3. Others (Wilms tumor, sarcoma, benign adenomas) rarely are associated with hematuria
  - D. Hereditary diseases
    - 1. Alport's syndrome (hereditary glomerulonephritis)
    - 2. Medullary sponge kidney
    - 3. Adult polycystic renal disease
    - 4. Tuberous sclerosis
    - 5. Hemoglobinopathies
      - a. S-S (also S trait only)
      - b. S-thalassemia
      - c. S C
      - d. C C
      - e. D D
    - 6. Osler-Weber-Rendu syndrome
  - E. Trauma and postoperative conditions
  - F. Miscellaneous diseases
    - 1. Acute renal failure
    - 2. Malignant hypertension
    - 3. Amyloidosis
    - 4. Vascular disorders
      - a. Renal infarct
      - b. Renal vein thrombosis in children
    - 5. Coagulation defects
      - a. Hereditary
      - b. Acquired
        - i. Iatrogenic anticoagulation
        - ii. Thrombocytopenia
        - iii. Coagulation defects associated with liver disease

Table 1-2—continued

6. Blood cell dyscrasias
    a. Leukemia
    b. Multiple myeloma

II. Ureteral origin
  A. Malignancy
  B. Nephrolithiasis
  C. Local inflammation 2° to abdominal lesion
    1. Diverticulitis
    2. Appendicitis
    3. Salpingitis
    4. Gastrointestinal neoplasms
  D. Trauma

III. Bladder origin
  A. Infection
    1. Bacterial cystitis
    2. Viral cystitis
    3. Schistosomiasis (most common cause of hematuria in the world)
  B. Neoplasm
  C. Amyloidosis
  D. Foreign body in bladder
    1. Stones
    2. Various foreign objects
  E. Trauma
  F. Drugs
    1. Cyclophosphamide

IV. Urethra and associated structures
  A. Prostate
    1. Benign prostatic hypertrophy
    2. Acute prostatitis
  B. Urethritis
    1. Gonococcal
    2. Reiter's syndrome
    3. Acute or chronic nonspecific
  C. Foreign body or local trauma in urethra

Sjogren's syndrome: This condition results from a lymphocytic infiltrate with resulting inflammation of the lacrimal gland (keratoconjunctivitis sicca) and the salivary gland (xerostomia). Presenting symptoms include difficulty in chewing and swallowing, dental caries, oral ulcers, and irritation of the eyes which, in extreme cases, may present with corneal ulcers that result from inadequate lacrimal secretions. Most patients are women, and most have an associated connective tissue disease syndrome such as lupus erythematosus or chronic rheumatoid arthritis. A significant number of these patients will have interstitial nephritis or immune complex glomerulonephritis with associated abnormal urinary sediment, proteinuria, and varying degrees of renal failure. Definitive diagnosis is based upon the clinical syndrome; usually a renal biopsy is performed to document and characterize renal pathology.

Wegener's granulomatosis: Renal involvement occurs in most patients with this disease, which presents with combinations of rhinorrhea, sinusitis, fever, weight loss, cough, hemoptysis, dyspnea, or malaise. Renal manifestations include abnormal urinary sediment with hematuria, proteinuria, and azotemia, which usually occurs late in the course of the illness. Definitive diagnosis is based upon the clinical syndrome with biopsy of the affected upper respiratory tract, lung, or kidney. Expected pathology includes granulomatous reactions with fibrosis, necrosis, and giant cells; both arteries and veins may be affected. Precise diagnosis of Wegener's granulomatosis carries prognostic importance in that cyclophosphamide provides lifesaving therapy.

b. Infective Endocarditis. Infective endocarditis is associated with circulating immune complexes and the very frequent manifestations of immune complex glomerulonephritis. Definitive diagnosis rests upon a characteristic clinical syndrome with positive blood cultures. Renal considerations are usually not of primary importance unless the infection has been long-standing.

c. Goodpasture's Syndrome. The association of hemoptysis with a rapidly progressive glomerulonephritis was originally described by Goodpasture in the influenza epidemic of 1918. Most commonly the pathogenesis of the glomerulonephritis involves antiglomerular basement membrane antibodies that cross-react with the pulmonary basement membrane. Infrequently, the glomerulonephritis may appear to be an immune complex type. In either case, 90% of all patients progress to end-stage renal failure in 2 years. A severe anemia is characteristic, and in some cases, hemoptysis may be so severe as to threaten exsanguination or death from pulmonary insufficiency. Definitive diagnosis is based upon the clinical syndrome with biopsy-proven glomerulonephritis of either immune complex or antiglomerular basement membrane type.

d. Hemolytic Uremic Syndrome. This is a condition usually of sudden onset with severe hemolytic anemia and renal failure. The disease if often preceded by an episode of gastroenteritis or upper respiratory tract infection, which is followed in 1 to 3 weeks with the onset of oliguria, pallor, gross hematuria, fever, hypertension, and neurological manifestations, including convulsions or coma.

The peripheral blood smear has a microangiopathic appearance with red cell fragments, burr cells, and helmet cells. Urinalysis demonstrates increased numbers of red cells and white cells with cylindruria and abnormal proteinuria. Oliguria or anuria may occur. The condition is most common in childhood but also occurs in adults. Definitive diagnosis depends upon the characteristic clinical syndrome of acute renal failure with microangiopathic hemolytic anemia and usually a normal platelet count. Renal biopsy is usually not helpful in the establishment of a diagnosis.

e. Thrombotic Thrombocytopenic Purpura. Differentiation of this condition from the hemolytic uremic syndrome may be very difficult. Clinical presentations are usually quite similar, except that thrombocytopenia is characteristic of thrombotic purpura and central nervous system symptoms are much more prominent. As in the hemolytic uremic syndrome the diagnosis is based upon clinical considerations, and renal biopsy is usually not required.

f. Henoch-Schonlein Purpura. The triad of acute abdominal pain associated with arthritis and a purpuric skin rash are characteristic of this syndrome. Approximately 20% of these patients will have renal involvement with a focal glomerulonephritis. Renal manifestations include gross or microscopic hematuria, abnormal proteinuria, hypertension, and a decrease in glomerular filtration rate. Because renal failure may occur in the absence of one or more of the characteristic features of the above triad, the diagnosis of Henoch-Schonlein purpura is often established on renal biopsy; characteristically, one sees a necrotizing focal glomerulonephritis with glomerular deposition of immunoglobulins A and G seen by immunofluorescent microscopy.

B. Infections

1. Renal Tuberculosis

This condition most frequently presents as sterile pyuria, which subsequently is demonstrated to have a positive culture for *Mycobacterium tuberculosis.* Microhematuria is common. Definitive diagnosis requires that the urine culture for *Mycobacterium tuberculosis* be positive.

2. Pyelonephritis

The clinical syndrome of pyelonephritis is sometimes associated with microhematuria. Gross hematuria in this setting is frequently a sign of papillary necrosis. Definitive diagnosis requires appropriate urine cultures and radiological demonstration of papillary necrosis.

C. Neoplastic Diseases

1. Renal Cell Carcinoma

Renal cell carcinoma is the most common renal neoplasm, with most cases occurring after age 50. While most patients present with gross hematuria, weight loss, malaise, flank pain, abdominal pain, or fever, this tumor is well known for causing unusual clinical syndromes such as polycythemia, syndrome of inappropriate antidiuretic hormone (ADH) secretion, or fever of unknown origin. Gross or microscopic hematuria occurs in 60% of all cases of renal cell carcinoma, although often not until the tumor is quite large with metastases. Definitive diagnosis requires appropriate radiological demonstration of a tumor, a positive urine cytology, or surgical biopsy.

2. Transitional Cell Carcinoma of the Renal Pelvis

In contrast to renal cell carcinoma, transitional cell carcinoma often presents as gross or microscopic hematuria when the tumor is quite small and still resectable. Definitive diagnosis requires appropriate radiological examination and subsequent surgical intervention. Urine cytology may be quite helpful in establishing this diagnosis.

3. Other Tumors (Wilms Tumors, Renal Sarcoma, Benign Adenomas)

These tumors are rarely associated with hematuria.

D. Hereditary Diseases

1. Alport's Syndrome (Hereditary Glomerulonephritis)

This is a syndrome secondary to any of several different genetic defects. Most commonly, it is transmitted as an autosomal dominant trait, although males are most frequently and more severely affected. The onset of symptoms occurs commonly in the second or third decade of life, with renal failure or proteinuria noted at the time the family members are screened. Many kindreds also have associated deafness or blindness or, less frequently, both. The basis of the association of these sensory defects with the renal disease is not known. Definitive diagnosis relies upon the positive family history and sensory deficits in a patient with abnormal proteinuria and urinary sediment characteristic of glomerulonephritis. Renal biopsy in this condition does not usually allow distinction from several other forms of glomerulonephritis and is therefore not routinely indicated.

2. Medullary Sponge Kidney

This is a relatively rare disorder, the familial nature of which is still disputed. Patients usually present between the ages of 20 and 50 with nephrolithiasis, symptoms of urinary tract infection, or gross or microscopic hematuria. The lesion consists of multiple small cysts in the collecting duct that cause the renal pyramids to have an accentuated fanlike appearance on an intravenous pyelogram. Other congenital conditions exist in approximately 20% of the patients, and half the patients have hypercalciuria. Diagnosis is based upon the findings on an intravenous pyelogram. Renal failure is not expected unless repeated urinary tract infections lead to chronic pyelonephritis.

3. Adult Polycystic Renal Disease

This is an inherited autosomal dominant condition in which both kidneys develop multiple cysts that lead to end-stage renal failure, usually in the fifth decade of life. There are asymptomatic cysts frequently noted in the liver, pancreas, or spleen. Approximately 10% of the patients die from rupture of a cerebral aneurysm. Hypertension is usually a late manifestation of the disease, and anemia is often not as severe as expected for the patient's level of renal function. The diagnosis is based upon the finding of bilaterally enlarged kidneys with multiple cysts (by radiographic examination) in a patient with chronic progressive renal failure.

4. Tuberous Sclerosis

This is a congenital disease that usually presents as epilepsy in the early years of life. Mental retardation is common, although many patients have normal intelligence. A characteristic skin lesion occurs in the malar areas of the face and consists of small lightly pigmented shiny papules that become confluent and deeply pigmented. Benign tumors occur in the brain and often become calcified, having a characteristic appearance on skull films. Multiple benign tumors of both kidneys are characteristic, and some patients present with hypertension, hematuria, or proteinuria. Progressive renal failure is not expected. The diagnosis is based upon the clinical syndrome.

5. Hemoglobinopathies

Either gross or microscopic hematuria is very common in sickle cell anemia. Hematuria also occurs in sickle cell thalassemia, sickle cell hemoglobin C disease, C hemoglobinopathy, and D hemoglobinopathy. Papillary necrosis is very common in sickle cell anemia, although chronic progressive renal disease is unusual. Diagnosis rests upon the finding of the abnormal hemoglobin by electrophoretic techniques.

6. Osler-Weber-Rendu Syndrome

This is a hereditary condition in which telangiectasias occur primarily on mucosal surfaces. Recurrent spontaneous epistaxis is the most common symptom, although gastrointestinal bleeding is clinically the most important problem. Either gross or microscopic hematuria is quite common. The diagnosis is based upon the finding of multiple telangiectasias in the appropriate clinical setting.

E. Trauma and Postoperative Conditions

Microscopic hematuria is expected in the first several specimens passed after participation in a severe contact athletic activity. Gross hematuria in this setting is unexpected. Gross hematuria following severe blows to either flank should be investigated by radiographic techniques to exclude the possibility that the patient has incurred a ruptured kidney. Many surgical procedures in which the kidneys are manipulated may result in either gross or microscopic hematuria for several hours to as long as a week after surgery.

Microscopic hematuria is quite common after renal biopsy, and gross hematuria occurs in 10% of percutaneous renal biopsies. Usually the hematuria ceases spontaneously with several days of bed rest; persistence past four days of bed rest is an indication for further evaluation.

F. Miscellaneous Diseases

1. Acute Renal Failure

Acute renal failure secondary to trauma with shock, toxins, crush injuries, or acute nontraumatic rhabdomyolysis may be associated with hematuria. The diagnosis of acute renal failure rests upon the documentation of a sudden decrease in glomerular filtration rate as measured by appropriate laboratory tests. Hematuria is of little diagnostic importance in acute renal failure, although microscopic hematuria with or without red blood cell casts frequently occurs. Depending upon the inciting trauma, gross hematuria may be present. It should be noted that the presence of red blood cell casts in the urinary sediment is not specific for primary glomerular disease.

2. Malignant Hypertension

When rapidly accelerated end-organ disease develops in response to severe hypertension, microscopic hematuria is an expected finding, and gross hematuria may occur late in the course of the disease. Associated renal failure, proteinuria, and cardiac and cerebral manifestations are expected. Usually the diastolic blood pressure is above 120 mm Hg. It is important to make the diagnosis of malignant hypertension upon clinical grounds alone, because renal biopsies are associated with an unacceptable incidence of bleeding as a result of the surgical procedure.

3. Amyloidosis

The major renal manifestations of amyloidosis are usually renal failure and proteinuria; although microscopic hematuria is sometimes noticed, gross hematuria is unexpected. While the diagnosis is frequently based upon the clinical setting of the nephrotic syndrome with an associated positive biopsy from the rectal mucosa or gingival area, renal biopsy provides the basis for definitive diagnosis. While there is reluctance to biopsy the liver in cases of suspected amyloidosis, renal biopsies are not associated with an inordinate complication rate.

4. Vascular Disorders

a. Renal Infarct. Either embolic or thombotic episodes may result in partial or total renal infarcts. These may present as sudden onset of flank pain and low grade fever in patients liable to generalized vascular accidents. Microscopic hematuria occurs only in 40% of known cases, and gross hematuria is very unusual. The serum concentration of lactic dehydrogenase (LDH) characteristically rises to high levels, greater than 1000 units per milliliter, in cases of renal infarct. Arteriography provides the definitive basis for diagnosis. In patients with a single kidney, renal arterial occlusion may present as anuria; if this diagnosis is suspected, arteriography should be performed within the first 24 hours of the event so that surgical intervention may be helpful. The diagnosis is dependent upon the finding of a normal retrograde pyelogram in the presence of a nonfunctioning kidney by intravenous pyelogram in the appropriate clinical setting.

b. Renal Vein Thrombosis in Children. In contrast to adults, in whom renal vein thrombosis is invariably associated with either immune complex glomerulonephritis or amyloidosis, renal vein thrombosis in infants is usually a catastrophic event resulting from extreme dehydration or an infectious process in some other part of the body. Microscopic hematuria occurs in about two thirds of the cases and gross hematuria in about one third. A flank mass is a common finding.

5. Coagulation Defects

a. Hereditary. Virtually any of the hereditary coagulation defects may be associated with either gross or microscopic hematuria. Gross hematuria may be spontaneous, although it is usually not life-threatening. Definitive diagnosis is based upon appropriate laboratory tests to define the coagulation defect.

b. Acquired

Iatrogenic anticoagulation: Either gross or microscopic hematuria may occur in patients who are excessively anticoagulated with either heparin or the coumadin class of drugs. Hematuria is not an expected finding in patients maintained in the therapeutic range of anticoagulation; several studies have demonstrated that if hematuria occurs when the patient's anticoagulation is in the therapeutic range, an underlying urinary tract lesion may be demonstrated in at least two thirds of the cases. Therefore, judgment based upon the clinical setting and associated findings should dictate the extent of evaluation for anticoagulated patients who manifest hematuria.

Thrombocytopenia: Hematuria is very common in patients who have drug-induced or spontaneous thrombocytopenia. Diagnosis is based upon the appropriate laboratory test.

Coagulation defects associated with liver disease: While microscopic hematuria is very common in patients with end-stage liver disease, these patients are usually so ill that evaluation of microscopic hematuria is of little importance. Hematuria is usually only one manifestation of the spectrum of coagulation defects.

6. Blood Cell Dyscrasias

a. Leukemia. Gross or microscopic hematuria is relatively common in the acute leukemias, especially when blastic crisis results in platelet-associated coagulation defects. Rarely, leukemia will be associated with an immune complex glomerulonephritis or hyperuricemia sufficient to induce uric acid nephropathy or uric acid kidney stones.

b. Multiple Myeloma. Direct tumor involvement of the kidney rarely causes clinical manifestations. However, associated complications such as the hyperviscosity syndrome, amyloidosis, or nephrolithiasis resulting from hypercalciuria may cause either gross or microscopic hematuria.

II. Ureteral Origin

A. Malignancy

Malignancies of the ureter most frequently present as intermittent gross hematuria. Most ureteral tumors are malignant transitional cell carcinomas and are papillary in type. Seeding of the lower urinary tract is very common, and metastases frequently occur in regional lymph nodes, lungs, and liver. Ureteral obstruction is not uncommon and may result in unilateral hydronephrosis with associated flank mass and dull pain. Definitive diagnosis requires histological examination of a specimen after radiological demonstration of the tumor's presence. As a note of caution, malignancies of the ureter may present as gross hematuria, with renal colic secondary to clots in the ureter; these two findings must be carefully evaluated rather than routinely attributed to nephrolithiasis.

B. Nephrolithiasis

As noted above, nephrolithiasis most frequently presents as renal colic with associated gross or microscopic hematuria. The stone responsible for these symptoms may be no larger than 1–2 mm in diameter and therefore very difficult to demonstrate radiographically, although 85% of all renal stones are radiopaque. The evaluation of nephrolithiasis is discussed in Chapter 5.

C. Local Inflammation Secondary to Abdominal Lesion

Inflammation of abdominal structures adjacent to the ureters frequently leads to microscopic hematuria. Examples of such lesions include diverticulitis, appendicitis, salpingitis, and gastrointestinal neoplasms. Evaluation of microscopic hematuria in this setting requires judgment on the part of the physician as to which procedure to perform.

D. Trauma

While external trauma may cause hematuria in either the kidney, bladder, or urethra, it is rarely responsible for hematuria of ureteral origin.

III. Bladder Origin

A. Infection

1. Bacterial Cystitis

This is probably the most common cause of hematuria in women in the United States. The syndrome presents as urinary frequency and urgency, dysuria, and cloudy urine, often without constitutional symptoms or fever. Hematuria may be either gross or microscopic. Extension of the bacterial infection to the kidneys may lead to the syndrome of pyelonephritis with fever, constitutional symptoms and flank pain. The diagnosis of bacterial cystitis requires a positive urine culture in the setting of the appropriate clinical symptoms. In females, further evaluation is usually not indicated with first or second episodes. However, in males the syndrome is unusual enough to warrant further evaluation for possible anatomical abnormalities of the urinary tract after only one episode.

2. Viral Cystitis

Although poorly founded, viral cystitis is the term sometimes applied to cases having the symptoms of cystitis but with a negative urine culture. Urine viral cultures are not routinely available, and therefore, definitive diagnosis is usually not possible.

3. Schistosomiasis

Schistosoma haematobium is characteristically associated with either gross or microscopic hematuria. The condition is epidemic in the Middle Eastern countries about the Mediterranean Sea and, based upon the number of people infected, is probably the most common cause of hematuria in the world. Hematuria results when the venous plexus about the bladder are occluded by parasite eggs. Early symptoms include urinary frequency and dysuria; microscopic hematuria occurs early in the course of the disease and is frequently progressive. Gross hematuria is a late manifestation when severe pathology of the bladder is expected. Definitive diagnosis is based upon finding eggs in the urine when examined under low power in the microscope; the highest concentration of eggs in the urine will occur in the last few drops of the urine specimen.

B. Neoplasm

Bladder—Neoplasms. Intermittent gross hematuria is the most common symptom of tumors of the bladder. Since tumors most commonly arise at the base of the bladder where occlusion of the ureters or the urethra may occur, bladder tumors may present with associated urinary tract obstruction, infection, or renal failure. Most bladder tumors are malignant, with papillary carcinoma or infiltrating transitional cell carcinoma being the most common. Usually physical examination and laboratory findings are not specific unless obstruction of the bladder has led to ureteral obstruction or infection. Appropriate radiographic examinations followed by cystoscopy and biopsy provide the basis for a definitive diagnosis.

C. Amyloidosis

This is a rare cause of hematuria originating in the bladder. The diagnosis is usually made incidentally upon a biopsy obtained at the time of cystoscopy for the evaluation of hematuria.

D. Foreign Body in the Bladder

1. Endogenous

Endogenous bladder stones are relatively rare in the United States, although reportedly more common in the Orient. Because a stone that passes through the ureter will easily pass through the urethra, bladder stones are usually associated with obstruction or other anatomical abnormalities with secondary infection by urea-splitting organisms. Diagnosis is based upon appropriate radiographic procedures and cystoscopy.

2. Exogenous

Because of the short urethra in the female, foreign bodies may be easily introduced into the bladder. The patient's embarrassment often leads to the history being noncontributory in such cases, and thus the foreign body is discovered by radiographic techniques or cystoscopy.

E. Trauma

Severe blows to the lower abdomen or fracture of the pelvis may lead to bladder injury and result in hematuria. The most common site for lesions is the urethral orifice.

F. Drugs

Metabolites of cyclophosphamide are excreted via the urinary tract and concentrated in the urine. A chemical cystitis may occur and is associated with gross or microscopic hematuria.

IV. Urethra and Associated Structures

A. Prostate

1. Benign Prostatic Hypertrophy

This condition is frequently associated with microscopic hematuria, especially if there is associated bladder neck obstruction or urinary tract infection.

2. Acute Prostatitis

Bacterial prostatitis usually presents with symptoms of acute urinary tract infection, fever, and sacral or perineal pain. Gross hematuria is often initial or terminal, although total hematuria does not rule out the diagnosis of acute prostatitis. The basis for a diagnosis rests upon the physical finding of an enlarged, exquisitely tender, firm prostate gland associated with the syndrome of a febrile urinary tract infection.

B. Urethritis

Acute or chronic urethritis may occur as the result of infection from bacteria, *Trichomonas,* or *Chlamydia.* Hematuria is usually overshadowed by the purulent nature of the urethral discharge, although severe cases may be associated with initial gross hematuria. Diagnosis rests upon the clinical syndrome and examination of the urethral discharge for the presence of *Trichomonas* and gonococci.

C. Foreign Body in the Urethra

Almost any item with a relatively small caliber can be introduced into and traumatize the urethra of curious children. The child's embarrassment may prevent the history from being helpful. The diagnosis rests upon a high level of clinical suspicion or the actual finding of a retained foreign body in the urethra.

Results Expected from Evaluation of Hematuria

The relative incidence of various diagnoses in patients with hematuria depends upon whether the hematuria is gross or microscopic. Based upon the study of 1000 cases of gross hematuria, the most common causes were found to be (Lee, 1953):

1. Infection: 37%
2. Tumor: 22%
3. Obstruction: 16%
4. Calculus: 11%
5. Other: 5%
6. No lesion found: 9%

In contrast, patients with asymptomatic microhematuria have a somewhat different distribution of diagnoses (Greene, 1956):

1. Benign prostatic hypertrophy: 24%
2. Urethritis: 21%
3. Renal calculus: 3%

4. Cystitis: 3%
5. Other: 5%
6. No lesion found: 44%

While these two studies were performed prior to the ready availability of renal biopsy and arteriography, they illustrate the point that no diagnosis is obtained in a significant percent of hematuria cases regardless of whether they are gross or microscopic. However, this should not preclude an appropriate evaluation of all cases of hematuria.

While most hematuria cases are associated with a single lesion, the possibility of two or more lesions causing hematuria must not be ignored. The author is aware of a case in which a patient initially had microscopic hematuria subsequently diagnosed as secondary to renal tuberculosis. The condition was appropriately treated, and the patient presented a year later with intermittent gross hematuria frequently following upper respiratory tract infections. On this occasion, renal tuberculosis had apparently been controlled, and urine cultures were negative. A renal biopsy demonstrated focal glomerulonephritis. No therapy was instituted, and the patient continued to have intermittent gross hematuria following upper respiratory tract infections. Two years later, this had ceased, but the patient now had a single episode of gross hematuria not associated with an upper respiratory tract infection. Evaluation on this occasion demonstrated a papillary carcinoma of the bladder!

Clinical Problem

A 17-year-old white male high school student was admitted to the hospital for evaluation of gross hematuria persisting 3 days after trauma to his right flank. The patient had been completely well until 3 days prior to admission when he played in a high school football game. While running at high speed the patient was struck in the right flank by another player's shoulder: the blow was sufficient to knock the patient's feet from under him, and he landed on the right flank. The patient recalls severe pain at the time of this blow and could not continue in the game. Following the game the patient was sore with what he interpreted as routine muscular aches and pains but had no other symptoms.

The following day the patient noted that his urine had a rusty brown turbid appearance, and each urine specimen appeared similar; neither initial nor terminal accentuation of the brown color was noted. There were no constitutional symptoms, and the patient did not seek medical advice until the change persisted for two more days. His physician noted a blood pressure of 150/90, with a pulse rate of 62 beats per minute and respirations of 16 per minute. His weight was 217 pounds, which he stated was 4 pounds heavier than his usual weight. His temperature was 37° C. Physical findings included no flank tenderness and no edema. Examination of the patient's skin revealed no remarkable findings.

The patient's complete blood count was within normal limits with a hematocrit reading of 46%. Urinalysis demonstrated 4+ protein, negative glucose, a urine pH of 5, and a positive dipstick for blood. Examination of the urinary sediment revealed red blood cells too numerous to count, 10 to 30 white blood cells per high-power field, and 1 to 3 granular casts per high-power field. The casts were pigment-stained, but delineation as true red blood cell casts was not possible. No crystals and no bacteria were noted. Other laboratory tests obtained included normal serum electrolytes, a serum creatinine of 1 mg/dl, and a fasting blood glucose of 90 mg/dl.

Questions

1. What further clinical evaluation should be obtained in this patient?
2. How could the role of the trauma to the patient's right flank be delineated?

Discussion

The patient was hospitalized, and a three-glass urine test was obtained upon admission. Each container appeared similar, with sediment unchanged from that found in the physician's office. The patient was placed on bed rest with frequent monitoring of his blood pressure, which was persistently elevated. An intravenous pyelogram was performed the day after admission; there was prompt bilateral excretion of contrast media with a normal pyelogram. No differential excretion of contrast media nor leakage of contrast media from the urinary collecting system was noted. The kidneys measured 17 cm on the right and 18 cm on the left, values at the upper limits of normal for the patient's height and weight. Other pertinent laboratory values obtained included a normal concentration of lactic dehydrogenase and creatine phosphokinase. The patient's platelet count, clot retraction, prothrombin time, and partial thromboplastin time were all within normal limits. The 24-hour excretion of protein in the patient's urine was found to be 6.2 gm.

The finding of casts in the patient's urinary sediment, excessive quantities of protein in the patient's 24-hour urine, and a normal intravenous pyelogram in the absence of localizing physical signs or evidence of rhabdomyolysis all favored the diagnosis of a renal glomerular lesion as the cause of this patient's hematuria. However, because of the hematuria and the clinical history of trauma to the right flank, the patient was cystoscoped and urine selectively collected from each ureteral orifice. Examination of the urinary sediment from each kidney demonstrated casts, red blood cells, and white blood cells, in addition to the presence of abnormal proteinuria. The diagnosis of glomerulonephritis was felt to be firmly established, and the history of renal trauma was not clinically pertinent.

Over the course of the next several weeks the patient's hematuria decreased, although a very abnormal urinary sediment persisted, with many hyalin and granular casts noted. Daily protein excretion in the urine ranged between 6 and 12 gm. The patient's blood pressure remained elevated, with diastolic pressures in the vicinity of 90–100 mm Hg. The patient appeared to be developing a nephrotic syndrome in spite of the fact that the gross hematuria had ceased. After 2 months of observation with limited physical activity, the patient's nephrotic syndrome persisted, although his glomerular filtration rate remained normal with a serum creatinine of 1 mg/dl. In anticipation of a trial of steroid therapy, a renal biopsy was performed, and diffuse proliferative glomerulonephritis was noted. High-dose steroid therapy was administered for a period of 3 months without alteration in the patient's nephrotic syndrome, and the steroids were tapered and stopped. Long-term therapy consisted of salt restriction and diuretics to maintain the patient in an edema-free state. Six years after the onset of his illness, he has spontaneously ceased to have abnormal proteinuria and has a normal glomerular filtration rate.

References

Burkholder, G. V., Rotin, L. N., Thomason, W. B., and Beach, P. D. "Unexplained hematuria." JAMA *210:* 1729–1734, 1969.

Given, G. Z. "Hematuria in children: A guide in differential diagnosis." Urol. Clin. North Am. *1:* 561–572, 1974.

Greene, L. F., O'Shaughnessy, E. J., and Hendricks, E. D. "Study of 500 patients with asymptomatic microhematuria." JAMA *161:* 610–613, 1956.

Kupor, L. R., Mullins, J. D., McPhaul, J. J. "Immunopathologic findings in idiopathic renal hematuria." Arch. Intern. Med. *135:* 1204–1211, 1975.

Labovity, E. D., Steinmuller, S. R., Henderson, L. W., McCurdy, D. K., and Goldberg, M. "Benign hematuria with focal glomerulonephritis in adults." Ann. Intern. Med. *77:* 723–729, 1972.

Lee, L. W., and Davis, E. "Gross urinary hemorrhage: A symptom, not a disease." JAMA *153:* 782–784, 1953.

Stanley, J. A., Jr., and Millinger, G. T. "Urologic evaluation of hematuria occurring during anticoagulant therapy." J. Urol. *101:* 111–113, 1969.

West, C. D. "Asymptomatic hematuria and proteinuria in children: Causes and appropriate diagnostic studies." J. Pediatr. *89:* 173–182, 1976.

Chapter 2

Proteinuria

General Considerations

The normal 24-hour urinary excretion of protein is less than 150 mg; approximately 60% of this protein is similar to serum proteins, and 40% is of renal origin. Serum proteins with molecular weights less than 10,000 are freely filtered by the renal glomerulus, reabsorbed by the renal tubule, degraded, and the products returned to the circulation. As the molecular weight of serum proteins increases to 50,000, progressively decreasing amounts are filtered. Proteins with molecular weights greater than 50,000 are 99.97% retained by the glomerular capillary barrier, although as much as 3 gm/day may enter the glomerular filtrate. These larger molecular weight proteins are reabsorbed by the renal tubules and metabolized, as are the lower molecular weight proteins. Tubular reabsorption appears to be nonspecific for high molecular weight proteins and specific for low molecular weight proteins; thus, large amounts of Bence-Jones proteins (mol wt = 22,000 or 44,000) may appear in the urine in the presence of undetectable amounts of insulin (mol wt = 5000). In contrast, proteins of greater than 50,000 molecular weight appear in the urine at a ratio near that of their glomerular filtration rate.

Two basic types of abnormal proteinuria may occur. The first is glomerular proteinuria in which abnormal quantities of serum proteins pass through the glomerular capillary barrier. Quantitatively, glomerular proteinuria usually results in large amounts of urinary protein loss (3–25 gm/day). Certain glomerular diseases characteristically result in only a slight increase in the molecular weights of the proteins excluded by the glomerular capillary barrier; these diseases have been described as manifesting "selective proteinuria." Urinary protein in cases of selective proteinuria may have large amounts of serum albumin (mol wt = 69,000) with almost undetectable amounts of serum immunoglobulins (mol wt = 160,000). So-called nonselective proteinuria may have, in addition to albumin, large amounts of urinary protein with molecular weights greater than 100,000. Patients with nonselective proteinuria frequently have inflammatory destructive glomerular disease, whereas patients with selective proteinuria most frequently have only fusion of the epithelial foot processes as seen by electron microscopy but lack inflammatory destructive glomerular lesions. The prognosis of the latter is more favorable.

Conceptually, the second pathological lesion that may lead to abnormal proteinuria involves incomplete tubular reabsorption of proteins normally filtered by the glomerulus. Quantitatively, tubular proteinuria usually results in only 1–4 gm of daily urinary protein loss. The incomplete tubular reabsorption may be secondary to a generalized decrease in the tubular reabsorption of protein or to overwhelming the tubular reabsorptive mechanism. An example of the latter case is the increased glomerular filtration of Bence-Jones protein (mol wt = 22,000 or 44,000) that may occur in multiple myeloma. In patients with abnormal proteinuria, both quantitative and qualitative considerations are quite important in arriving at an appropriate diagnosis.

Methods of Detection, Quantification, and Characterization of Abnormal Proteinuria

If a dilute urine is examined, abnormal proteinuria may not be detected because the protein concentration is too low. Thus, urine specimens examined for proteinuria should have a specific gravity of at least 1.010 or more. While first morning specimens are ideal for examination, obtaining these is usually not convenient and certainly not required. Clean voided urine specimens are required in females to assure the absence of secretions from around the vulva.

Because of its convenience and simplicity, the dipstick (Albustix, Ames Company) has become the most common method of detecting proteinuria. However, the dipstick is neither specific for albumin nor quantitatively accurate nor able to detect all the various proteins that might appear in the urine. It is unfortunate that the modern need for speed and simplicity in screening large numbers of urine samples has forced the use of this inadequate method. Use of the Ames dipstick is based upon the ability of a protein to alter the color of an indicator substance (tetrabromophenol) impregnated on the dipstick; the principle of the method is known as the protein error of pH indicators. Tetrabromophenol is yellow at a pH of 3 and normally changes to a blue-green color at a pH of 4. However, the blue-green color will appear at a pH of 3 when protein is present—thus the so-called protein error causing an apparent change in pH. In order to use the dipstick for protein detection, the pH on the indicator stick must be maintained at 3 if a blue-green color is to be attributed to the presence of protein. The paper on the reagent strip contains a citrate buffer that rigidly controls the pH on the paper at 3. Still, a strongly alkaline urine may overcome the citrate buffer and give a false-positive indication of proteinuria by inducing an indicator color change based on an elevated pH. Although albumin is easily detected using the dipstick, several other proteins such as hemoglobin, various globulins, and Bence-Jones protein are inconstantly detected using the Ames dipstick. Thus, a negative result using the Ames dipstick precludes the presence of abnormal albuminuria, although a number of other proteins might be present and not detected. Conversely, trace to 1+ readings on the dipstick are often not confirmed as abnormal on subsequent evaluations. False-positive results may occur from soaking the stick too long or from highly alkaline urine as expected from patients receiving acetazolamide or sodium bicarbonate. Positive results on the urine dipstick should be confirmed by one of the following methods prior to initiating a definitive evaluation for renal disease.

Before the widespread use of the Ames dipstick, abnormal proteinuria was most frequently detected using the so-called heat and acetic acid method. By this method the urine is first filtered or centrifuged for clarification and then boiled. If the heated urine remains clear, no protein is present. However, if cloudiness appears, several drops of acetic acid are added and the urine boiled a second time. Persistent cloudiness is indicative of abnormal proteinuria, with a semiquantitative relationship between the degree of turbidity and the quantity of protein present. Up to 400 mg of albumin per liter of urine may give a falsely negative result using this test; false-positive results occur in the presence of x-ray contrast media, urinary tolbutamide or sulfisoxazole metabolites, cephalothin, or very large doses of penicillin.

A third method used to detect abnormal proteinuria is the sulfosalicylic acid test. The technique involves clarification of the urine by centrifugation and then mixing an aliquot of urine with an aliquot of sulfosalicylic acid solution (3 gm/100 ml). The mixture is allowed to stand at room temperature for 10 minutes before examining for turbidity. Clinical laboratories may have standardized turbidity tubes, which allow a semiquantitative estimation of the amount of protein present in the urine. False-positive results are obtained in the presence of x-ray contrast media, chlorpromazine, promazine, tolbutamide metabolites, massive doses of penicillin, and sulfa drug metabolites. A false-negative result may occur if the urine is very alkaline initially, the added acidifying agent being quantitatively inadequate.

Patients may intermittently have a positive result on one of the tests for urinary protein described above; in the absence of hypertension or an abnormal urine sediment, intermittent positive tests for proteinuria carry no prognostic importance. Clinically significant proteinuria requires a persistently positive result; unless there is other evidence of disease, the isolated observation of abnormal proteinuria should be confirmed on several subsequent urine specimens prior to embarking on an extensive evaluation of the patient's renal status. The first step after the confirmation of persistent abnormal proteinuria is 24-hour quantification of the patient's urinary protein loss. The patient is instructed to collect all urine for 24 hours, and the entire specimen is submitted to a clinical laboratory for quantification. Adult patients may be divided into three groups based upon the quantity of 24-hour urinary protein loss:

1. Less than 1 gm/24 hours—usually these patients have orthostatic proteinuria, fever, or a form of tubular proteinuria. Significant glomerular disease is unusual but does occur in this group.
2. 1–3.5 gm/day—patients in this group may have a diverse group of diseases, and diagnostic workups are often complex. Characteristically, patients with tubular proteinuria, interstitial renal disease, or early glomerular disease are found in this group.
3. Greater than 3.5 gm/day—although some patients with interstitial renal disease or multiple myeloma may have more than 3 gm of urinary protein per day, most patients in this group will have significant glomerular pathology. This observation facilitates the clinical evaluation and often leads to early renal biopsy.

After quantification of daily urinary protein loss, characterization of the protein by electrophoresis may be helpful in those cases having between 1 and 4 gm of urinary protein per day. This is the area in which glomerular proteinuria and tubular proteinuria overlap. When there is greater than 4 gm of urinary protein per day, the major value of urinary protein electrophoresis is in the detection of M components in cases of multiple myeloma or amyloidosis. Many clinical laboratories routinely provide paper electrophoresis of urinary proteins after concentration of the urine. If the patient has glomerular proteinuria, the electrophoretic pattern will have more than 60% albumin, with lesser amounts of alpha, beta, and gamma globulin. If the patient has tubular proteinuria, relatively less albumin will be present, with an increase in the percent of alpha, beta, and gamma globulins.

While paper electrophoresis separates urinary proteins based upon their electrical charge, techniques of separation based upon molecular weights of the urinary protein are relatively new and still available only on a research basis. The technique with the most promise of becoming routinely available in clinical laboratories is called SDS polyacrylamide gel electrophoresis. By this technique the urinary proteins are complexed to a negatively charged detergent (SDS); both the tertiary structure of the protein and its intrinsic electrical charge are lost, and the protein migrates based only upon its molecular weight. An example of the usefulness of this technique is illustrated in Figure 2-1, which shows the findings in several different types of renal disease that have characteristic urinary protein patterns on SDS polyacrylamide gel electrophoresis.

Clinical Features Important in the Evaluation of Proteinuria

Many patients with proteinuria are asymptomatic, or they may have adjusted to and disregarded mild symptoms of insidious onset. Examples include the onset of nocturia over the course of months or the very slow loss of ability to perform daily routines; fatigue and muscular aches associated with a low-grade fever may be treated with aspirin and never reported to a physician. A careful history of the patient's drug consumption may elicit un-

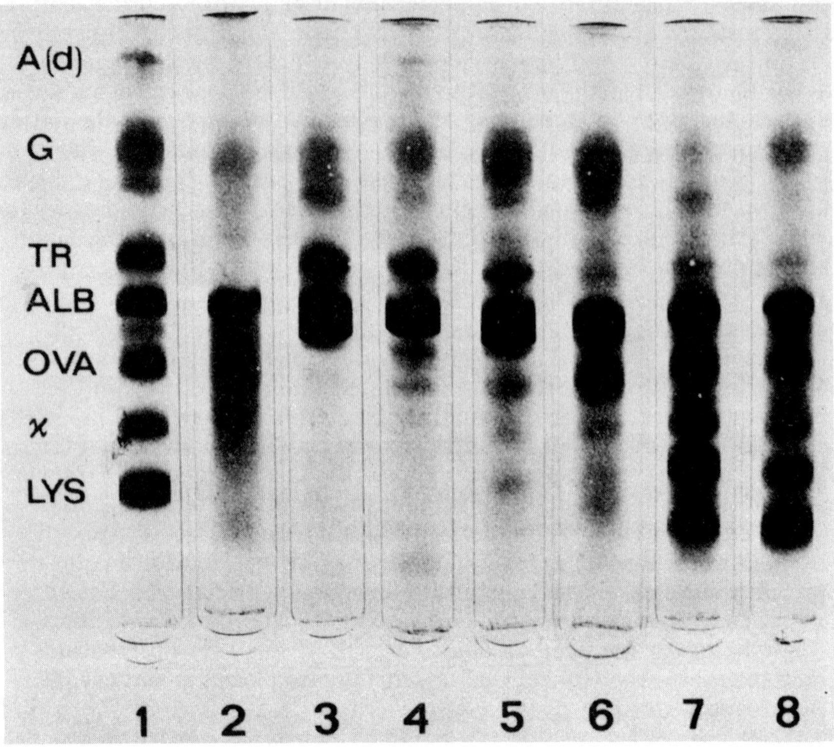

Fig. 2-1.

Disc electrophoresis in SDS polyacrylamide gel of urine from patients with renal disease. (1) A mixture of reference protein including dimeric IgA [A(d)] (mol wt=330,000), normal IgG (G) (mol wt=160,000), transferrin (TR) (mol wt=88,000), human serum albumin (ALB) (mol wt=69,000), egg albumin (OBA) (mol wt=43,000), kappa light chains isolated from a human monoclonal IgG protein (x) (mol wt=22,000), and egg lysozyme (LYS) (mol wt=14,000) were separated on this gel to demonstrate the ability of the technique to resolve various proteins. (2) The small amount of protein in normal human urine has an albumin band, although most of the protein is of smaller molecular weight. Only a trace of high molecular weight protein may be noted. (3) This is the pattern expected from patients with glomerular proteinuria; this patient had membranous glomerulonephritis. Small molecular weight proteins are not present, while there is a marked increase in larger molecular weight proteins such as transferrin and immunoglobulin. (4) This is the urinary protein pattern from a patient who had acute glomerulonephritis with acute renal failure: with a markedly decreased glomerular filtration rate, tubular proteinuria will accompany glomerular proteinuria. (5) This patient's urinary protein demonstrates nonselectivity expected from patients with chronic glomerulonephritis. Note the increased amounts of high molecular weight protein compared to the amount of transferrin and albumin. The patient has a significant decrease in the glomerular filtration rate and therefore has tubular proteinuria in addition. (6) This patient had rapidly progressive glomerulonephritis with severe renal failure; note the marked increase in high molecular weight protein expected with severe proliferative lesions. Tubular proteinuria characteristic of chronic renal failure is also seen. (7) This patient had acute tubular necrosis with a urinary protein pattern that is classical for tubular proteinuria. (8) This is a tubular proteinuria pattern obtained from a patient with malaria induced renal failure. (Reproduced by permission from Nephron *14:* 361, 1975.)

derlying conditions associated with proteinuria or reveal drugs that directly cause proteinuria. In the asymptomatic patient, proteinuria may be associated with activity such as erect posture (orthostatic proteinuria) or unusually strenuous exercise. Past medical history of renal disease, edema, hematuria, urinary tract infections, or abdominal irradiation may be very helpful in delineating the underlying cause for proteinuria. The large number of hereditary conditions associated with proteinuria dictates that a very careful family history be obtained, including information regarding nephrolithiasis, deafness, blindness, arthritis, anemia, or early death from strokes.

While patients with heavy proteinuria may be asymptomatic, more than 3.5 gm of proteinuria per day is often associated with the nephrotic syndrome; its major symptom (edema) is a frequent reason for patients to seek medical advice. Edema of the nephrotic syndrome must be differentiated from edema secondary to liver disease, congestive heart failure, or gastrointestinal disease. A recent history of blood transfusions, drug abuse, jaundice, or alcoholic excess are clues that might indicate liver disease as the cause of edema. A past history of rheumatic fever, undue shortness of breath, or quick fatigue on physical exertion may indicate primary cardiac disease as the cause for edema. While congestive heart failure may be a direct cause of proteinuria, it is very unusual that edema from the nephrotic syndrome may be attributed to this cause alone. Protein-losing enteropathy may present with ascites and edema secondary to severe hypoproteinemia; usually these patients have a history of abdominal pain or diarrhea.

The nephritic syndrome, as distinct from the nephrotic syndrome, is characterized by acute inflammation of the glomeruli. Nephritic patients give a history of acute onset of generalized edema, gross hematuria, headache, and decreased urine output. Severe or recurrent recent upper respiratory tract infections (group A beta-hemolytic streptococcal or other) or a history of skin rashes, arthritis, or fever are helpful historical features in delineating the cause of the nephritic syndrome.

On physical examination of proteinuric patients, a temperature elevation is an important feature to note, because fever alone may cause mild proteinuria. The presence of hypertension is a strong indicator of organic renal disease; life insurance actuarial studies have shown that mild proteinuria ($<$1.0 gm/day) is not associated with increased mortality unless the population is also hypertensive. Incidentally discovered proteinuria may be associated with dependent edema not noted by the patient, a finding requiring careful examination for signs of cardiac or liver disease. Rashes or petechiae associated with proteinuria may be clues to a diagnosis of systemic lupus erythematosus, Henoch-Schönlein purpura, leukemia, drug reactions, or subacute bacterial endocarditis. In elderly males, asymptomatic mild proteinuria may be associated with a suprapubic mass indicative of bladder obstruction secondary to prostatic disease.

Other Laboratory Considerations

Laboratory examinations should always include a complete blood count. Severe anemia may be a cause of abnormal proteinuria (sickle cell anemia) or a manifestation of underlying late-stage renal disease. Alterations in the white blood cell count may be a clue to a diagnosis of leukemia with associated proteinuria.

A major branch point in the evaluation of abnormal proteinuria rests upon the findings of urinalysis. The presence of granular and cellular casts in the urinary sediment is a strong indicator of significant renal disease, and usually the patient is referred for subsequent renal biopsy. The absence of casts or red blood cells in the urinary sediment of proteinuric patients does not rule out significant renal disease, although functional causes are favored if there is less than 1 gm of proteinuria per day.

The serological test for syphilis should be noted in patients with abnormal proteinuria. An elevated value for the serum creatinine or blood urea nitrogen indicates the presence of significant renal disease unless the patient has a decreased cardiac output secondary to hypovolemia or congestive heart failure. Decreased serum bicarbonate concentration or the isolated presence of hyperchloremia may indicate chronic renal failure or a renal tubular disorder such as the Fanconi syndrome, Wilson's disease, or renal tubular acidosis. Evaluation for diabetes mellitus should include a fasting blood glucose and standard 2-hour postprandial blood glucose. Hyperuricemia may indicate primary gout or may be a secondary manifestation of chronic renal disease. Hypocalcemia or hyperphosphatemia is often associated with severe renal failure. Hypercholesterolemia and hypoalbuminuria are two facets of the nephrotic syndrome. Serum protein electophoresis may demonstrate abnormal serum proteins in cases of multiple myeloma. Liver function tests should be obtained routinely in edematous proteinuric patients. A urine culture should always be performed, and proteinuric patients with persistent or unexplained fever must have multiple blood cultures.

Unless functional causes for low levels of proteinuria are clearly demonstrated, proteinuric patients should have an intravenous pyelogram. Renal arteriography is usually not helpful. The performance of other radiographic examinations depends upon the clinician's judgment regarding the possibility of an associated underlying neoplasm; 10% of adults with the nephrotic syndrome have an associated malignancy.

In the absence of specific indications, cystoscopy is not routinely performed in the evaluation of proteinuria.

Usually, definitive diagnosis for the cause of abnormal proteinuria requires a renal biopsy, especially in cases with more than 3.5 gm of proteinuria per day. Renal biopsy is a specialized procedure with significant associated morbidity. The performance of this procedure should be restricted to medical centers providing immunofluorescent and electron microscopic examination in addition to routine histopathology.

Differential Diagnosis of Proteinuria and Basis for Diagnosis of Specific Conditions

Known causes for abnormal proteinuria are listed in Table 2-1 and discussed below. Although conditions are classified according to the usual daily urinary protein loss in the named condition, this classification should be used as a flexible guideline in the evaluation of proteinuria. For example, some patients with nephrosclerosis or chronic bacterial pyelonephritis may have daily urinary protein losses in excess of 3.5 gm; conversely, some with chronic immune complex glomerulonephritis may have only 1 gm of proteinuria per day. Conditions are classified according to their most frequent, although not their only level of proteinuria.

I. Patients with Less than 1 Gram of Proteinuria per Day

The major problem in this group of patients is to differentiate between insignificant functional proteinuria and low levels of proteinuria associated with significant organic renal disease.

A. Strenuous Exercise

Abnormal proteinuria may be noted for a period of 1 to 3 days after an episode of strenuous physical exercise in an unconditioned patient. Individual dipsticks may register 3+, although daily urinary protein losses are usually less than 1 gm. If abnormal proteinuria has ceased by the fifth day after unusual physical exercise and is not noted on subsequent urinalysis, further evaluation is not warranted unless there is associated hypertension, edema, azotemia, or an abnormal urinary sediment.

B. Fever

Patients with any febrile illness may have daily urinary protein losses of 0.5–1.0 gm/day. The proteinuria usually ceases as the patient becomes afebrile. Unless proteinuria persists several days after the cessation of fever, further evaluation is not warranted in the absence of associated abnormal physical findings or laboratory tests indicating the presence of renal disease.

C. Orthostatic Proteinuria

This condition usually occurs in children or young adults and is often associated with a lordotic posture or prolonged standing. Daily urinary protein losses are usually less than 1 gm and are not associated with symptoms. Definitive diagnosis requires the total disappearance of abnormal proteinuria when the patient assumes a recumbent position for 24 hours. It should be noted that diminution *but not disappearance* of abnormal proteinuria in the recumbent position precludes the diagnosis of orthostatic proteinuria.

D. Miscellaneous

1. Thyrotoxicosis

Usually thyrotoxicosis is clinically evident, and mild proteinuria is noted during routine evaluation. Unless proteinuria persists after appropriate treatment of thyrotoxicosis, further evaluation is not warranted.

2. Severe Anemia

Patients with severe anemia (hematocrit reading of less than 25%) may have associated mild proteinuria not indicative of intrinsic renal disease. The cause is not known, although it has been suggested that the proteinuria results from anoxia. Attention should be directed to the patient's anemia and the proteinuria evaluated only if it persists after the anemia is adequately treated.

3. Central Nervous System Lesions

Mild proteinuria is often associated with head trauma or with conditions that elevate cerebrospinal fluid pressure. Normal renal function with a normal urinary sediment and persistent mild proteinuria should alert the physician to the possibility of a central nervous system lesion with consideration of skull films and lumbar puncture.

II. Patients with 0.5 to 3.5 Grams of Proteinuria per Day

A. Berger's Disease (Benign Recurrent Hematuria)

See discussion in Chapter 1 on hematuria.

B. Acute Interstitial Nephritis

This is usually a drug-associated renal disease in patients taking sulfa or penicillin analogs. Rare cases are idiopathic. Nonoliguric renal failure progressing over 1 to 2 weeks in association with an abnormal urinary sediment and proteinuria comprise the characteristic clinical triad. Definitive diagnosis requires a renal biopsy with predominant lymphocytic or eosinophilic interstitial renal infiltrates. Glomerular changes are usually not remarkable. Differentiation from acute tubular necrosis may be difficult; acute tubular necrosis usually manifests more severe renal failure and is usually more acute in onset than drug-induced acute interstitial nephritis. If the inciting drug is discontinued, acute interstitial nephritis usually has a favorable outcome; occasional cases have been reported in which a beneficial effect of glucocorticoids has been noted.

Table 2-1

Differential Diagnosis of Proteinuria

I. Patients with less than 1 gm of proteinuria per day
  A. Strenuous exercise
  B. Fever
  C. Orthostatic proteinuria
  D. Miscellaneous
    1. Thyrotoxicosis
    2. Severe anemia
    3. Central nervous system lesions
II. Patients with 0.5–3.5 gm of proteinuria per day
  A. Berger's disease (benign recurrent hematuria)
  B. Acute interstitial nephritis
  C. Chronic interstitial nephritis
    1. Nephrosclerosis
    2. Bacterial pyelonephritis
    3. Gouty nephropathy
    4. Analgesic abuse
    5. Obstruction
    6. Nephrolithiasis
    7. Sickle cell anemia
    8. Renal tuberculosis
    9. Hypokalemic nephropathy
    10. Radiation nephritis
  D. Tubular proteinurias
    1. Fanconi syndrome
    2. Wilson's disease
    3. Galactosemia
    4. Renal tubular acidosis
    5. Balkan nephropathy
    6. Renal transplants
    7. Leukemia
    8. Bence-Jones proteinuria
      a. With multiple myeloma
      b. With amyloidosis
    9. Cadmium poisoning
    10. Lead poisoning
    11. All cases of severe chronic renal failure
    12. Acute renal failure
  E. Crisis states of selected conditions
    1. Sickle cell crisis
    2. Tabes dorsalis crisis
    3. Thyroid storm
  F. Hereditary conditions
    1. Polycystic renal disease
    2. Medullary cystic disease
    3. Tuberous sclerosis
    4. Fabry's disease (angiokeratoma corporis diffusum)
    5. Nail patella syndrome
III. Patients with more than 3.5 gm of proteinuria per day
  A. Primary renal glomerular disease
    1. Minimal change nephrotic syndrome
    2. Focal glomerulosclerosis
    3. Acute glomerulonephritis
    4. Immune complex glomerulonephritis
      a. Membranous glomerulonephritis
      b. Membranoproliferative glomerulonephritis
        i. Type I—subendothelial deposits
        ii. Type II—intramembranous dense deposits
      c. Unclassified (probably accounts for 30% of all chronic glomerulonephritis)

Table 2-1—continued

5. Rapidly progressive glomerulonephritis
6. Antiglomerular basement membrane antibody-mediated disease
7. Hereditary nephritis (Alport's syndrome)
8. Infantile nephrosis

B. Infection
  1. Viral
    a. Viral hepatitis
    b. Measles infections with subacute sclerosing panencephalitis
  2. Bacterial
    a. *Treponema pallidum,* congenital or secondary stage
    b. Infective endocarditis
    c. Tuberculosis
    d. Leprosy
  3. Parasitic
    a. Malaria
    b. *Schistosoma mansoni* infection
    c. Kala-azar

C. Neoplastic diseases
  1. Any carcinoma
  2. Multiple myeloma
  3. Hodgkin's disease

D. Diabetes mellitus

E. Collagen-vascular disorders
  1. Systemic lupus erythematosus
  2. Polyarteritis nodosa
  3. Scleroderma
  4. Sjogren's syndrome
  5. Wegener's granulomatosis

F. Vascular disorders
  1. Renal vein thrombosis
  2. Constrictive pericarditis
  3. Severe congestive heart failure
  4. Tricuspid insufficiency
  5. Inferior vena cava obstruction

G. Allergic or toxic causes
  1. Pollen hypersensitivity
  2. Bee sting
  3. Poison oak
  4. Snake bite

H. Drug-associated disorders
  1. Heavy metal poisoning
    a. Mercury (injected diuretics or topical ointments)
    b. Bismuth
    c. Gold (injected antirheumatic agents)
  2. Penicillamine
  3. Probenecid
  4. Paramethadione and trimethadione
  5. Serum sickness

I. Miscellaneous causes
  1. Sarcoidosis
  2. Amyloidosis
  3. Massive obesity
  4. Toxemia of pregnancy
  5. Hemolytic uremic syndrome—thrombotic thrombocytopenic purpura
  6. Malignant hypertension

C. Chronic Interstitial Nephritis

A diverse group of primarily interstitial renal diseases leads to moderate proteinuria. Although characteristic glomerular pathology is not expected, the proteinuria is usually a mixture of glomerular and tubular types.

1. Nephrosclerosis

Long-standing hypertension with arteriolar nephrosclerosis is often associated with moderate proteinuria. Other evidence of end-organ disease, such as retinopathy or cardiac manifestations, is expected. Abnormal urinary sediment is common, although glomerular filtration rates may be near normal. Definitive diagnosis requires a renal biopsy lacking significant glomerular disease but with arteriolar and interstitial changes consistent with the diagnosis of nephrosclerosis in a patient with long-standing hypertension.

2. Bacterial Pyelonephritis

This condition is only occasionally associated with proteinuria. When present the proteinuria is usually moderate in amount and consists of a mixture of tubular and glomerular types. In the clinical setting of acute urinary tract infection, moderate proteinuria may be disregarded unless it persists after the urinary tract infection is adequately treated. Patients with persistent proteinuria in the setting of recurrent symptomatic urinary tract infection or chronic asymptomatic bacteriuria present a dilemma; localized infection of hematomas that may lead to septicemia are an unacceptable complication of percutaneous renal biopsy in such patients. Therefore, a diagnosis of bacterial pyelonephritis as the cause for moderate proteinuria rests primarily on the clinical setting with an associated positive urine culture.

3. Gouty Nephropathy

Patients with long-standing hyperuricemia and associated gouty arthritis frequently develop mild renal insufficiency with moderate proteinuria. The proteinuria is not expected to result in the nephrotic syndrome. Definitive diagnosis is based upon the presence of long-standing hyperuricemia, mild azotemia, and moderate proteinuria in a patient believed to have gout. Renal biopsy is not required but when done for incidental reasons, it demonstrates chronic interstitial infiltrates with interstitial uric acid crystals and areas of tubular atrophy. Glomerular changes are usually not prominent.

4. Analgesic Abuse

Excessive intake of phenacetin and nonprescription analgesics has become a major health problem in Europe and, to a lesser extent, in the United States. Typical patients may consume as many as 20 analgesic tablets per day for symptoms of stress, headache, or nonspecific muscular aches and pains. This level of analgesic consumption is equivalent to approximately 3 gm/day of phenacetin. Several clinical studies have related the onset of renal disease to a total ingested dose of 2 kg of phenacetin. Typical clinical manifestations include mild azotemia with moderate proteinuria and papillary necrosis as seen on an intravenous pyelogram. Definitive diagnosis rests upon the clinical history with appropriate findings on intravenous pyelography. Renal biopsy is not routinely performed; expected pathology includes chronic interstitial infiltrates, tubular atrophy, and an increase in interstitial matrix.

5. Obstruction

Urinary tract obstruction is not usually associated with proteinuria; however, in patients who develop chronic renal failure or secondary chronic urinary tract infections, the loss of 1–3.5 gm of protein in the urine per day may occur. In occasional patients, moderate proteinuria may be an incidental finding that alerts the physician to the presence of renal abnormalities and the discovery of urinary tract obstruction.

6. Nephrolithiasis

Abnormal proteinuria in renal stone disease is usually a manifestation of secondary complications such as obstruction or urinary tract infection.

7. Sickle Cell Anemia

Patients who are homozygous for the sickle cell trait frequently develop chronic progressive renal disease with papillary necrosis and chronic interstitial nephritis secondary to multiple microemboli and thrombosis of vessels in the renal medulla. Definitive diagnosis of the papillary necrosis is based upon radiographic examination. Occasional patients with sickle cell anemia may develop heavy proteinuria with the nephrotic syndrome. These patients have frequently been found to have membranous glomerulonephritis on a renal biopsy.

8. Renal Tuberculosis

The common clinical manifestations of renal tuberculosis include pyuria, which is sterile on routine bacterial culture, weight loss, fever, and occasionally gross hematuria. A positive skin test for tuberculosis is expected. Definitive diagnosis requires a positive urine culture for *Mycobacterium tuberculosis.*

9. Hypokalemic Nephropathy

Long-standing severe potassium deficiency from gastrointestinal loss, adrenal overactivity, or certain intrinsic renal diseases may be associated with a renal concentrating defect manifest as polyuria, nocturia, and polydipsia. Associated symptoms include muscular weakness, anorexia, and palpitations. Usually the glomerular filtration rate is near normal, and there is no associated azotemia. Mild to moderate proteinuria may be present. Definitive diagnosis requires documentation of the potassium-deficient state, with reversal of the concentrating defect and proteinuria after potassium repletion. characteristic hydropic degeneration of proximal tubular cells may be seen on a renal biopsy, although this is not a routinely required examination.

10. Radiation Nephritis

Patients undergoing radiation therapy for the treatment of abdominal neoplasms may develop severe hypertension, edema, and azotemia or uremia in response to as little as 2500 roentgens of irradiation to the kidneys. The insidious onset of edema, decreased stamina, and headaches may begin months to years after the irradiation has been administered. Hypertension may be quite severe and difficult to control. The diagnosis is usually based upon clinical criteria with a history of previous abdominal irradiation. Although renal biopsy is not routinely performed, expected pathology includes fibrinoid necrosis of interlobular arteries, tubular atrophy, chronic interstitial infiltrates, and glomeruli that show increased lobulation and mesangial matrix.

D. Tubular Proteinuria

1. *Fanconi Syndrome*

This syndrome refers to a constellation of proximal tubular reabsorptive defects that result in excessive urinary loss of potassium, phosphorus, amino acids, bicarbonate, uric acid, and calcium. There is decreased tubular reabsorption of filtered proteins, with a resulting pattern of tubular proteinuria. Common clinical manifestations include bone pain from osteodystrophy and muscle cramps or weakness from electrolyte abnormalities. Definitive diagnosis requires delineation of several of the tubular reabsorptive defects mentioned. A common underlying condition is Bence-Jones proteinuria in which the Bence-Jones protein appears to act as a specific tubular toxin. Findings on renal biopsy are nonspecific, ranging from normal tissue architecture to interstitial nephritis with tubular atrophy.

In childhood, a hereditary condition called cystinosis is associated with all the features described above, as well as tissue deposition of cystine. This condition is usually recognized at 6 months to 2 years of age when the child fails to thrive or develops clinical evidence of rickets. A defect in the metabolism of cystine results in massive deposition of this amino acid in cells of the reticuloendothelial system, in fibroblasts, in the epithelium of various organs, and in the eye. Definitive diagnosis is based upon the finding of cystine crystals in lymph nodes, bone marrow, or circulating leukocytes. The prognosis is poor, with survival past the second decade not expected.

2. *Wilson's Disease*

This is a hereditary disease that results from the absence of the serum copper transporting protein (ceruloplasmin). Symptoms are usually attributable to cirrhosis of the liver or central nervous sytem lesions; the renal lesion is usually asymptomatic and manifested only as the Fanconi syndrome described above and tubular proteinuria. Definitive diagnosis is based upon the absence of the serum copper transporting protein.

3. *Galactosemia*

This is a rare inborn error of metabolism with an enzyme deficiency that prevents normal metabolism of galactose. The condition is usually discovered in infancy when the child fails to thrive on a normal diet. Major clinical manifestations are attributable to cirrhosis of the liver, cataracts, and mental retardation. Renal abnormalities include the Fanconi syndrome and tubular proteinuria. The renal manifestations are completely reversible if galactose is excluded from the child's diet at an early age.

4. *Renal Tubular Acidosis*

A decrease in serum bicarbonate concentration may result from either a proximal tubular defect in bicarbonate reabsorption or a distal tubular defect with abnormal de novo bicarbonate generation. The proximal form of renal tubular acidosis may occur in an isolated form or in association with tubular proteinuria and other manifestations of the Fanconi syndrome. The distal form of renal tubular acidosis is not associated with abnormal proteinuria unless there is associated secondary renal damage from hypokalemia, nephrocalcinosis, or chronic urinary tract infection. Criteria for the diagnosis of proximal or distal renal tubular acidosis are given in the chapter on metabolic acidosis.

5. Balkan Nephropathy

This is an endemic acquired renal disease occurring in selected river valleys of Yugoslavia and Bulgaria and affecting adults of both sexes between the ages of 20 and 50. Neither the pathogenesis nor the cause are understood. The onset is usually insidious, with weakness, anorexia, weight loss, and vague pain being the most frequently reported symptoms. Renal manifestations include azotemia, abnormal urinary sediment, and abnormal urinary protein loss with a tubular proteinuria pattern. Definitive diagnosis is based upon the appropriate clinical history and abnormal renal function tests. When performed, renal biopsy shows nonspecific abnormalities including tubular atrophy, interstitial fibrosis, and hyalinization of glomeruli.

6. Renal Transplants

Chronic rejection in renal transplants is frequently associated with tubular proteinuria.

7. Leukemia

Tubular proteinuria is frequently associated with various forms of leukemia. The nature of the association is not clear, although in the myelogenous forms of leukemia, abnormal quantities of lysozyme, a leukocyte enzyme, are found in the urine. The lysozymuria is believed to result from high serum concentrations of this enzyme and increased filtered loads, which overwhelm the tubular reabsorptive capacity. Rarely, patients with leukemia may develop an immune complex type of glomerulonephritis and an associated nephrotic syndrome.

8. Bence-Jones Proteinuria

Either multiple myeloma or light-chain associated amyloidosis may result in Bence-Jones proteinuria. The abnormal proteinuria may be the only abnormality noted, although in selected cases the abnormal protein is associated with manifestations of the Fanconi syndrome. Definitive diagnosis of multiple myeloma requires appropriate examination of the bone marrow, serum protein electrophoresis, or radiographic evidence of osteolytic lesions. Diagnosis of amyloidosis requires biopsy of an appropriate site, such as the rectal mucosa or the kidney.

9. Cadmium Poisoning

This is an occupational disease associated with the refining of ores rich in cadmium, which is ingested via inhalation of dusts. Renal manifestations include tubular proteinuria, mild hypertension, and rarely, progressive renal failure. Biopsy findings are nonspecific. Diagnosis is based upon a clinical history of cadmium exposure with associated renal abnormalities.

10. Lead Poisoning

Lead poisoning may occur from industrial exposure, the consumption of contaminated "moonshine whisky," or from domestic exposure to lead-containing paint. Domestic exposure in adults may result from drinking rainwater drained from painted roofs; in young children, it may result from oral contact with lead-painted surfaces or from eating lead paint. Renal manifestations of lead poisoning include the Fanconi syndrome, tubular proteinuria, hypertension, and mild azotemia. Definitive diagnosis requires the demonstration of abnormal quantities of urinary lead.

11. Severe Chronic Renal Failure

As the glomerular filtration rate falls in chronic progressive renal disease, there is usually an increased glomerular filtration rate per nephron. Many small molecular weight proteins are metabolized by glomerular filtration with subsequent tubular reabsorption and degradation. As the glomerular filtration rate falls, the serum concentration of these small molecular weight proteins rises, leading to an increase in their filtered load per nephron that may exceed the tubular reabsorptive capacity. Therefore, tubular proteinuria is expected in all late-stage renal disease regardless of the underlying cause.

12. Acute Renal Failure

Either toxic or hemodynamically induced acute renal failure is associated with tubular proteinuria. This carries no diagnostic or clinical significance. It is important to note that 1–3 gm of daily urinary protein loss does not necessarily indicate a glomerular cause for the acute failure.

E. Crisis States of Selected Conditions

Patients acutely ill with sickle cell crisis, tabes dorsalis crisis, thyroid storm, or other such catastrophic conditions may have abnormal proteinuria of 1–3 gm/day. This usually subsides as the crisis abates, and clinical judgment must be exercised in the further evaluation of this abnormal proteinuria.

F. Hereditary Conditions

1. Adult Polycystic Renal Disease

See Chapter 1 on hematuria. Mild proteinuria is frequently noted as the disease progresses.

2. Medullary Cystic Disease

In this condition, multiple small cysts occur in the renal medulla, with resultant progressive renal failure and severe anemia in the second and third decades of life. The kidney is characteristically unable to reabsorb sodium normally, and the condition is often referred to as "salt-wasting nephritis." The urinary sediment is usually normal, and mild proteinuria is frequently noted. Premortem diagnosis is based upon clinical criteria; interstitial nephritis with tubular atrophy is usually noted on renal biopsy, the findings being nonspecific. Definitive diagnosis is based upon examination of whole kidneys from autopsy or nephrectomies.

3. Tuberous Sclerosis

See Chapter 1 on hematuria. Mild proteinuria frequently occurs in this condition and may be the presenting symptom in adults not having mental retardation or epilepsy.

4. Fabry's Disease

This is an X-linked "incompletely recessive" disease usually presenting in male children as intermittent fevers, paresthesias, and intermittent pain in the extremities and abdomen. Affected males develop purple-red slightly elevated papules about the lower trunk and thighs. When brought to medical attention these children usually have mild proteinuria and azotemia. Through the third and fourth decades, renal function slowly deteriorates with associated hypertension, and death usually occurs by the fifth decade. Seizures and cerebral hemorrhage are frequent central nervous system manifestations of the disease. These patients have a hereditary lack of the enzyme ceramidetrihexosidase, which results in abnormal tissue deposition of the glycolipid ceramide trihexoside. Definitive diagnosis is based upon the clinical syndrome.

5. Nail Patella Syndrome

This is a rare autosomal dominant hereditary disease manifest as dysplasia of the fingernails, aplasia or hypoplasia of the patella, and characteristic posterior iliac horns. Mild proteinuria occurs in 40% of affected individuals, and the nephrotic syndrome occurs in 10%. Twenty-five percent of patients with this disease develop chronic progressive renal failure usually manifested in childhood as mild proteinuria, although terminal renal failure usually does not occur until the third to the fifth decades. Definitive diagnosis is based upon the clinical syndrome. Renal biopsies are not required; electron microscopy has demonstrated abnormal cross-striated fibrils that may represent abnormal collagen deposition in the glomerular basement membrane. There is no known therapy.

III. Patients with More than 3.5 Grams of Proteinuria per Day

A. Primary Renal Glomerular Disease

1. Minimal Change Nephrotic Syndrome

These patients usually present with edema, hypoalbuminemia, and hypercholesterolemia associated with severe proteinuria. They are usually not hypertensive, and dependent edema is the only expected physical finding. The urinary sediment and glomerular filtration rate are usually normal. Definitive diagnosis is based upon the renal biopsy finding of normal glomerular architecture by light and immunofluorescent microscopy; fusion of the epithelial foot processes may be seen by electron microscopy. This condition occurs in 75% of children and 10% of adults who develop the nephrotic syndrome; occasional patients with Hodgkin's disease develop the nephrotic syndrome with no glomerular histopathology. Neither the cause nor the pathogenesis of minimal change nephrotic syndrome is known. The condition usually abates in response to glucocorticoid or cyclophosphamide therapy.

2. Focal Glomerulosclerosis

This condition usually presents as the nephrotic syndrome and is frequently associated with hypertension. Patients are often azotemic and mildly anemic in addition to being nephrotic. The basis for this diagnosis is the finding of focal sclerotic areas in the glomeruli examined by light microscopy; immunoglobulin M (IgM) and the third component of complement may be deposited in glomeruli examined by immunofluorescent microscopy. Electron microscopy is nonspecific. Focal glomerulosclerosis is frequently a chronic progressive renal disease unresponsive to drug therapy. This condition is responsible for approximately 10% of adult cases of nephrotic syndrome.

3. Acute Glomerulonephritis

See Chapter 1 on hematuria.

4. Immune Complex Glomerulonephritis

a. Membranous Glomerulonephritis. This condition is responsible for approximately 10% of adult nephrotic syndrome cases. Most patients first seek medical advice because of edema, which is the only consistent historical or physical finding. The urinary sediment may have hyaline and granular casts; red blood cells or red blood cell casts are not prominent. Laboratory studies are usually not remarkable except for the manifestations of the nephrotic syndrome or azotemia. The definitive diagnosis is based upon the finding of subepithelial glomerular deposits of immune complex material in a renal biopsy examined by light, immunofluorescent, and electron microscopy. The clinical course is highly variable, with no predictable response to drug therapy. Renal function often remains stable over prolonged periods of time.

b. Membranoproliferative Glomerulonephritis. See Chapter 1 on hematuria.

c. Unclassified Immune Complex Glomerulonephritides. See Chapter 1 on hematuria.

5. Rapidly Progressive Glomerulonephritis

See Chapter 1 on hematuria.

6. Antiglomerular Basement Membrane Antibody-Mediated Disease

See Chapter 1 on hematuria.

7. Hereditary Nephritis (Alport's Syndrome)

See Chapter 1 on hematuria.

8. Infantile Nephrosis

This is a familial condition that presents as the nephrotic syndrome in the first few days or weeks of life and is uniformly fatal within 1½ years. There are no remarkable physical or laboratory findings except those characteristic of the nephrotic syndrome. The diagnosis is based upon the occurrence of the nephrotic syndrome in a young infant; at autopsy, histological changes include glomerular fibrosis, tubular dilatation with microcysts, and fibrosis of the interstitium. There is no known therapy.

B. Infection

1. Viral

a. Viral Hepatitis. The anorexia, jaundice, and malaise in the acute stage of viral hepatitis is associated with mild proteinuria that abates as the liver function abnormalities return to normal. Rarely, patients with viral hepatitis may develop an associated immune complex glomerulonephritis or polyarteritis nodosa, both of which may cause heavy proteinuria and progressive renal failure. The glomerulonephritis has been noted to be of the membranous or the type I (subendothelial deposits) membranoproliferative variety. Definitive diagnosis requires renal biopsy in a patient with laboratory or biopsy evidence of viral hepatitis.

b. Measles Infection with Subacute Sclerosing Panencephalitis. While mild proteinuria is frequently associated with the acute stage of measles infection, rare patients not immunologically capable of eliminating the measles virus develop a chronically infected state. The primary manifestations of this condition involve the central nervous system, although immune complex glomerulonephritis also may occur. Definitive diagnosis requires biopsy-proven immune complex glomerulonephritis in a patient with massive elevation in the measles antibody titer and panencephalitis manifested as slow mental deterioration or ataxia.

2. Bacterial

a. Treponema pallidum, *Congenital or Secondary Stage.* This form of syphilis has been associated with a membranous form of glomerulonephritis manifested as the nephrotic syndrome. Definitive diagnosis requires renal biopsy with appropriate histopathology in a patient with serological evidence of syphylitic disease. Eradication of the infection reverses the renal disease.

b. Infective Endocarditis. Fever, weight loss, fatigue and embolic phenomenon are the usual symptoms of this condition. Occasional patients present with the nephrotic syndrome secondary to an immune complex type of glomerulonephritis presumably induced by the infecting agent. Most patients with endocarditis have abnormal urinary sediments and mild proteinuria although a near-normal glomerular filtration rate; rarely, endocarditis patients develop chronic progressive renal disease. Diagnosis and treatment of the cardiac disease assumes primary importance because glomerulonephritis in this condition is reversed by appropriate therapy of the endocarditis. Renal biopsy is contraindicated while the patient is septicemic. The rickettsia of Q fever should be suspected in the rare patient with sterile blood cultures and the endocarditis-glomerulonephritis complex.

c. Tuberculosis. Prior to the development of antibiotic therapy, chronic tuberculous infection occasionally resulted in amyloidosis with renal involvement. This was manifested as severe proteinuria with chronic progressive renal failure. Tuberculosis-induced amyloidosis is exceedingly rare today except in areas where untreated tuberculosis is prevalent. Definitive diagnosis requires culture-proven tuberculosis with proteinuria and biopsy-proven amyloidosis.

d. Leprosy. Amyloidosis is a frequent complication of the lepromatous form of leprosy. Renal involvement is manifested as proteinuria, often with the nephrotic syndrome and chronic progressive renal failure. Whereas leprosy-induced amyloidosis formerly presented a hopeless situation, there are indications that modern therapy may be able to arrest the underlying leprosy infection and the complicating amyloidosis as well.

Renal involvement also occurs in the so-called erythema nodosum leprosum reaction occurring in lepromatous patients after months of drug therapy. This complication is characterized by the appearance of tender erythematous subcutaneous nodules developing in crops and lasting 1 to 2 weeks. These have been related to drug-induced release of bacterial antigen, which then forms circulating immune complexes. The development of a proliferative glomerulonephritis is manifested as proteinuria, abnormal urinary sediment, and rarely as progressive renal failure. Definitive diagnosis should be based upon the abnormal urinary findings in a patient with erythema nodosum leprosum. Glucocorticoid therapy may be helpful for severe reactions.

3. Parasitic

a. Malaria. In certain endemic areas of equatorial Africa and South America, chronic infection with *Plasmodium malariae* may cause an immune complex glomerulonephritis with associated nephrotic syndrome. The condition is most common in 4- to 10-year-old children, although adults are also affected. Definitive diagnosis requires demonstration of *P. malariae* in the blood of a patient with the clinical manifestations of proteinuria and the nephrotic syndrome. Renal biopsy may be helpful in demonstrating the immune complex nature of the disease.

b. Schistosoma *Infection.* It has recently been shown in endemic areas of South America that infection with *Schistosoma mansoni* may be associated with mild proteinuria and urinary sediment abnormalities. Renal biopsy studies have demonstrated the presence of immune complex glomerulonephritis in these patients. Diagnosis depends upon the finding of parasite ova in the stools or rectal mucosa.

c. Kala-azar. This disease, which is endemic in several Mediterranean countries, the Middle East, northeastern Africa, and the Orient, is initially manifested as fever with chronic progressive weakness, pallor, weight loss, and hepatosplenomegaly. An abnormal urinary sediment and proteinuria frequently occur secondary to amyloidosis or immune complex glomerulonephritis. Definitive diagnosis requires demonstration of the *Leishmania* organisms from blood or splenic puncture.

C. Neoplastic Diseases

As previously noted, 10% of all cases of the nephrotic syndrome in adults are associated with various malignancies. Appropriate screening for neoplastic conditions should be carried out routinely in adult nephrotics over the age of 40. Carcinomas most frequently induce a membranous form of glomerulonephritis; multiple myeloma may induce renal amyloidosis or more rarely an immune complex nephritis secondary to cryoglobulins. Hodgkin's disease may induce a minimal change nephrotic syndrome or immune complex glomerulonephritis. Diagnosis in each case requires a renal biopsy to define the histopathology and appropriate clinical evaluation to define the malignancy.

D. Diabetes Mellitus

Renal involvement in diabetes mellitus is common in both juvenile and maturity onset types. Proteinuria with the nephrotic syndrome and chronic progressive renal failure are late diabetic complications occurring after 10 to 15 years of glucose intolerence. The pathogenesis of the glomerular disease remains controversial; control of hyperglycemia has not been shown to predictably affect the progression of the glomerular disease. Usually, renal involvement occurs in association with multiple other diabetic complications such as peripheral vascular disease, coronary artery disease, retinopathy, and neuropathy. The diagnosis of diabetic glomerular sclerosis is usually based upon the occurrence of heavy proteinuria and progressive renal failure in a patient with long-standing diabetes. Renal biopsy is not routinely performed; diffuse membranous glomerulosclerosis is expected in patients who develop the nephrotic syndrome and renal failure.

E. Collagen-Vascular Disorders

See Chapter 1 on hematuria.

F. Vascular Disorders

A variety of conditions associated with elevated renal venous pressure may cause severe proteinuria and the nephrotic syndrome. The most common of these is renal vein thrombosis, which occurs as a complication of immune complex glomerulonephritis or amyloidosis. Flank pain, severe edema accumulating over a short period of time, and nonspecific malaise are the most prominent symptoms of renal vein thrombosis. Physical findings and laboratory tests characteristic of the nephrotic syndrome may be the only abnormalities noted. The presence of markedly enlarged kidneys seen on intravenous pyelogram is a helpful, although inconstant, sign of renal vein thrombosis. Definitive diagnosis requires venographic demonstration of filling defects in a renal vein. It should be noted that thrombi in only one renal vein may be associated with abnormal proteinuria from both kidneys and the nephrotic syndrome. Renal biopsy will invariably show immune complex glomerulonephritis or amyloidosis.

The pathogenesis of the nephrotic syndrome in other causes of elevated renal venous pressure remains obscure. Constrictive pericarditis, severe congestive heart failure, tricuspid insufficiency or inferior vena cava obstruction have all been associated with the presence of severe edema, heavy proteinuria, and the hypoalbuminemia-hypocholesterolemia expected in the nephrotic syndrome. These causes of the nephrotic syndrome are remarkably rare, and conclusive information regarding renal histopathology is not available.

G. Allergic or Toxic Causes

The medical literature is replete with case reports and letters to editors purporting to show a cause-effect relationship between a variety of allergens and the occurrence of proteinuria or the nephrotic syndrome. The majority of these reports lack credibility. However, selected items are worthy of comment:

1. Pollen Hypersensitivity

Some patients with seasonal attacks of hayfever or asthma develop proteinuria during the pollen season. Pollen hypersensitivity has usually been documented by appropriate skin tests. The associated proteinuria is usually mild but has been reported to result in the nephrotic syndrome. Physical examination shows evidence of mucous membrane inflammation or asthma; laboratory examinations are usually not remarkable. The urinary sediment is usually normal, and hypertension or renal failure is unexpected. When performed, renal biopsy has demonstrated normal glomerular histology without immunofluorescent microscopic evidence of immune complex deposition. The patient's proteinuria usually abates when the pollen season ends and may or may not recur in subsequent seasons. Children are most frequently involved. The diagnosis must be presumptive based upon the clinical syndrome and the absence of demonstrable renal pathology.

2. Bee Sting

A dramatic syndrome of the sudden onset of the nephrotic syndrome 1 to 4 days after a single or multiple bee stings has been reported many times. Usually the patient has had prior bee stings with minor allergic reactions such as asthma or undue wheal and urticaria. The patient usually has a benign urine sediment, no hypertension, and no renal failure. The condition is benign and resolves in a period of weeks to months.

3. Poison Oak

A single series of cases in the older medical literature reports the occurrence of proteinuria, the nephrotic syndrome, and even acute renal failure in association with a dermatitis from poison oak exposure. Proteinuria and the nephrotic syndrome usually begin several days to a week after exposure to the toxic plant. The pathogenesis of the proteinuria or renal failure is unknown.

4. Snake Bite

The severe rhabdomyolysis resulting from viper poisoning is frequently associated with acute renal failure and proteinuria. There is a single credible report of the occurrence of the nephrotic syndrome after poisoning by an unknown brown snake in Australia.

H. Drug-Associated Disorders

1. Heavy Metal Poisoning

Repeated injections of mercurial diuretics or topical application of ammoniated mercury to treat skin disorders has been associated with the occurrence of the nephrotic syndrome. Discontinuing the mercury-containing medication leads to resolution of the nephrotic syndrome. Bismuth-containing medications are able to induce heavy proteinuria and the nephrotic syndrome, although the mechanism is unknown. Discontinuance of the drug results in resolution of the nephrotic syndrome. Heavy proteinuria with the nephrotic syndrome is a known complication of gold injections used to treat rheumatoid arthritis. The renal disease usually occurs only after repeated injections with an accumulated dose of 1–2 gm of gold salt. Renal biopsy most frequently demonstrates a membranous form of glomerulonephritis; electron-dense deposits believed to represent the gold salts themselves have been noted on the glomerular basement membrane and in renal tubular epithelium. Cessation of gold injections usually results in resolution of the renal disease in several months.

2. Penicillamine

Repeated injections of penicillamine are used to treat a variety of conditions. The onset of severe proteinuria and the nephrotic syndrome may occur within the first few months of drug injection. Renal biopsy demonstrates a membranous glomerulonephritis. Resolution of the condition is expected with cessation of the drug.

3. Probenecid

The nephrotic syndrome has been reported to occur in some patients after long exposure to probenecid. Renal biopsies demonstrate no remarkable glomerular pathology. Resolution follows cessation of the drug.

4. Paramethadione and Trimethadione

Paramethadione and trimethadione are used to treat petit mal epilepsy. The onset of the nephrotic syndrome has been reported to occur after prolonged exposure to these drugs. Pathogenesis is unknown. Resolution of the proteinuria occurs with discontinuation of the drug.

5. Serum Sickness

Injections of heterologous sera often result in an acute illness 7 to 20 days later, manifested as inflammation of serous surfaces, carditis, and glomerulonephritis. Certain drugs such as penicillin may act as a haptene attached to a protein in a patient's serum and result in a similar syndrome. The severity of the reaction is highly variable but may be fatal. Residual renal impairment is not expected if the patient survives. The diagnosis is based upon the clinical history of drug or serum injection followed by the appropriate clinical syndrome.

I. Miscellaneous Causes

1. Sarcoidosis

Renal involvement in sarcoidosis is a rare complication. The occurrence of the nephrotic syndrome has been reported associated with a membranous form of glomerulonephritis. Very rarely granulomatous involvement of the renal interstitium may result in moderate proteinuria without the nephrotic syndrome.

2. Amyloidosis

Heavy proteinuria with the nephrotic syndrome is a common manifestation of amyloidosis. Recent findings have resulted in the classification of amyloidosis into cases secondary to immunoglobulin light-chain deposition (some primary cases and B cell dyscrasias), amyloid A protein deposition (chronic infections and rheumatoid arthritis), and hereditary causes the nature of which is poorly understood (familial Mediterranean fever and others). The clinical manifestations of renal involvement are common to all types and consist of heavy proteinuria, abnormal urinary sediment, and progressive renal failure. Definitive diagnosis requires a renal biopsy with the demonstration of glomerular amyloid deposition.

3. Massive Obesity

Recently the occurrence of heavy proteinuria with the nephrotic syndrome has been noted in several cases of massive obesity. Renal pathology has been nonspecific, and in certain cases there has been resolution of the proteinuria as the patients lost weight.

4. Toxemia of Pregnancy

The triad of hypertension, edema, and proteinuria occurring in the third trimester of pregnancy is a well-known entity with characteristic glomerular pathology. On renal biopsy, these patients are found to have swelling of the capillary endothelial cells and massive fibrin deposition in the glomerular capillary loops. Proteinuria is severe, and renal failure may occur. Definitive diagnosis usually rests upon the recognition of the clinical triad in a previously healthy person. Renal biopsies are not routinely performed. Postpartum resolution of the renal manifestations is expected within 4 weeks. Persistence of proteinuria past 1 month postpartum is an indication for further evaluation.

5. Hemolytic Uremic Syndrome—Thrombotic Thrombocytopenic Purpura

See Chapter 1 on hematuria.

6. Malignant Hypertension

See Chapter 1 on hematuria.

Results Expected from Evaluation of Proteinuria

The group of patients with less than 3.5 gm of proteinuria per day is composed of such diverse conditions as to preclude a meaningful estimation of the relative incidence of the various conditions. Frequently the extent of the patient's evaluation is dictated by nonrenal considerations. Based upon the results of several series, it may be predicted that less than 1 gm of proteinuria per day will not be associated with intrinsic renal disease in 66% of the evaluated cases. In contrast, most cases of proteinuria with 1–3.5 gm of urinary protein loss per day will be found to have some form of renal disease.

The relative incidence of the causes of the nephrotic syndrome has been tabulated in many series. The most common associated renal histopathology, based on renal biopsies, is given in Table 2-2 based on data compiled from 10 reports involving 939 biopsies.

The data in Table 2-2 were collected prior to the clinical pathological correlations on which the diagnosis of membranoproliferative glomerulonephritis and focal glomerulosclerosis are based; also, diabetics are not routinely biopsied. Thus, these three entities are probably underrepresented and occur much more frequently than the data in the table would indicate.

The relative incidence of the causes of the nephrotic syndrome in children is quite different from that in adults. A compilation of histopathologic diagnoses from 859 cases in four series is shown in Table 2-3.

The clinical syndrome associated with minimal change nephrotic syndrome in children is clinically well recognized, and a trial of glucocorticoid therapy is often administered without renal biopsy. Therefore, this entity is underrepresented in Table 2-3.

Table 2-2

Relative Incidence of Histopathologic Diagnoses in Adults

1. Glomerulonephritis	
Proliferative	14.5%
Membranous	22.7%
Membranoproliferative	5.7%
Other	13.3%
2. Minimal change nephrotic syndrome	19.8%
3. Increased renal vein pressure	1.3%
4. Diabetes mellitus	7.7%
5. Amyloidosis	4.5%
6. Systemic lupus erythematosus	6.8%
7. Nephrosclerosis	0.7%
8. All others	2.9%

Table 2-3

Relative Incidence of Histopathologic Diagnoses in Children

1. Minimal change nephrotic syndrome	61.1%
2. Focal glomerulosclerosis	11.0%
3. Membranous glomerulonephritis	5.0%
4. Membranoproliferative glomerulonephritis	8.0%
5. Other glomerulonephritides	14.8%
6. Infantile nephrotic syndrome	1.5%
7. All others	1.5%

Clinical Problem

A 52-year-old white male was admitted to the hospital for evaluation of disabling dependent edema of 4 weeks' duration. The patient had been well all of his life with no history of medication requirement. Four weeks prior to admission, he noted that his feet were swollen and marked by his shoes at the end of the day. In the next several weeks the swelling became more pronounced with aching, cramps, and weakness of his legs. He consulted his personal physician who elicited no other remarkable symptoms; specifically there was no suggestion of cardiac or liver disease. On physical examination, his blood pressure was 100/60 with a pulse of 92 beats per minute, and he had soft pitting edema below the knees. No other remarkable physical findings were noted. The physician strongly suspected that the patient had the nephrotic syndrome, and this was quickly confirmed with a 4+ urinary protein dipstick. The patient was hospitalized for further evaluation.

On admission to the hospital, the following laboratory data were obtained: hematocrit reading, 36%; white blood cell count, 6200 cells/mm^3 with a normal differential; urinalysis showed 3+ glucose, pH 6.5, 4+ protein, hemitest for blood negative, no ketones, and only an occasional hyaline cast in the urine. Serum electrolytes showed a sodium content of 134 mEq/liter. The serum creatinine was 1.3 mg%, and the blood urea nitrogen was 36 mg%. The fasting blood glucose was 82 mg%, and 2-hour postprandial blood glucose was 102 mg%. Serum calcium concentration was 9.2 mg%; serum phosphorus, 2.3 mg%; serum uric acid, 2.6 mg%; total serum protein, 5 gm%; serum albumin, 2.3 gm%. Liver function tests were within normal limits; daily urinary protein loss was measured at 14 gm. Chest film was within normal limits, and electrocardiogram was noted to have low voltage. A serum protein electrophoresis showed that the patient had hypogammaglobulinemia with 0.6 gm% of gamma globulin and a very small spike of questionable significance in the gamma region.

Questions

1. Is this patient's proteinuria secondary to glomerular abnormalities or tubular abnormalities or both?
2. Based upon the data available, what items should be considered in the differential diagnosis of this patient's proteinuria?
3. What further diagnostic procedures should be performed to arrive at a definitive diagnosis?

Discussion

The large daily urinary protein loss indicates that the patient has significant glomerular pathology. Other data in the patient's workup strongly suggest that he also has the Fanconi syndrome; clues to this diagnosis are the low serum concentrations for potassium, phosphorus, uric acid, and bicarbonate in addition to the high urine pH and glycosuria with a normal blood glucose. This provides strong presumptive evidence that the patient has tubular proteinuria, although data for a definitive diagnosis were not provided.

The differential diagnosis for this patient's renal disease must include entities that may be associated with both glomerular and tubular proteinuria. Reference to the conditions associated with tubular proteinuria yields two different diagnoses that could simultaneously cause both tubular and glomerular proteinuria with the nephrotic syndrome. The first is Bence-Jones proteinuria with associated amyloidosis or multiple myeloma, and the second is leukemia with an associated immune complex glomerulonephritis and excessive lysozymuria. Alternatively the Fanconi syndrome and the glomerular proteinuria might be caused by two independent conditions occurring simultaneously. Possible diagnoses could include acquired primary renal glomerular disease, a neoplasm, constrictive pericarditis, or possibly an inferior vena cava obstruction. Further evaluation should include investigation of the patient's anemia with reticulocyte counts, red blood cell indices, stool guaiacs, and a bone marrow examination. The patient's small, questionably abnormal spike in the serum protein electrophoresis should be investigated further by serum immunoelectrophoresis and quantification of the serum concentration of IgG, IgA, and IgM. Because of the strong possibility that the patient may have multiple myeloma, a radiographic survey of the patient's bones should be performed. Urinary protein electrophoresis will probably be of little help because of the large amount of high molecular weight protein in the urine. Finally, a renal biopsy should be performed to define the pathology in the kidney.

The patient had normal red blood cell indices, and the reticulocyte count was 1%. Stool guaiacs were negative, and the bone marrow revealed abnormal numbers of small lymphocytes consistent with chronic lymphocytic leukemia. The skeletal survey was unrevealing. Serum immunoelectrophoresis demonstrated IgM myeloma protein, which by radial immunodiffusion was found to be present in a concentration of 0.3 gm%, a value nearly three times the normal serum concentration for IgM. Serum concentrations for IgG and IgA were abnormally low. Urinary protein electrophoresis demonstrated the expected glomerular pattern of proteinuria and also an abnormal component in the gamma region but with a different mobility than the IgM spike seen on serum electrophoresis.

Examination of the patient's renal biopsy demonstrated extensive amyloid deposition in all glomeruli. There was no remarkable interstitial infiltrate or tubular atrophy.

This patient's illness was apparently a composite of multiple diagnoses, including chronic lymphocytic leukemia, amyloidosis, the Fanconi syndrome, and an abnormal IgM myeloma-like protein. Yet, this patient actually had only one disease process.

It is now known that chronic lymphocytic leukemia is most frequently a massive proliferation of B cells; in addition it is known that B cells normally have IgM on their surface and secrete this protein in small quantities. Finally it is known that B cells differentiate to become plasma cells that secrete the various immunoglobulins in serum. This patient had a form of multiple myeloma in which the malignant cell was a B cell at an early stage in differentiation toward the plasma cell series. The amyloidosis in the patient's glomeruli was of the light-chain myeloma-related type, and the patient had Bence-Jones proteinuria as demonstrated on the urinary protein electrophoresis. SDS polyacrylamide gel electrophoresis of the patient's urine demonstrated an abnormal quantity of urinary protein with molecular weight of 22,000. By Ouchterlony double-diffusion analysis of the urinary protein, lambda light chains, but not kappa chains, were identified. The patient's clinical picture could now be explained by one disease as follows: (1) The patient has a malignancy of a late B cell prior to its assuming the morphology of a plasma cell. (2) These malignant cells were producing a myeloma IgM protein that was without pathological consequence. (3) These cells were producing large amounts of lambda light chains, which were depositing in glomeruli as amyloidosis, causing the nephrotic syndrome. (4) The lambda light chains were entering the glomerular filtrate and acted as proximal tubular toxins with the resulting Fanconi syndrome.

References

Bienenstock, J., and Poortmans, J. "Renal clearance of 15 plasma proteins in renal disease." J. Lab. Clin. Med. *75:* 297, 1970.

Cameron, J. S. "Histology and protein clearance in response to treatment in the nephrotic syndrome." Br. Med. J. *4:* 352, 1968.

Doch, W. "Proteinuria; the story of 280 years of trials, errors, and rectifications." Bull. N.Y. Acad. Med. *50:* 659–666, 1974.

Dodge, W. F., West, E. F., Smith, E. H., and Bunce, H. "Proteinuria and hematuria in school children; epidemiology and early natural history." J. Pediatr. *88:* 327–347, 1976.

Maack, T. "Renal handling of low molecular weight proteins." Am. J. Med. *58:* 57–63, 1975.

Peterson, P. A., Evrin, P., and Berggard, I. "Differentiation of glomerular, tubular, and normal proteinuria; determinations of urinary excretion of b_2 microglobulin, albumin, and total protein." J. Clin. Invest. *48:* 1189, 1969.

Pires, M. T., Cunha, A. S., Virella, G., and Simoes, J. "Analytical characterization of urinary proteins by sodium dodecyl sulphate-PAGEP in renal disease." Nephron *14:* 321, 1975.

Rennie, I. D. "Proteinuria." Med. Clin. North Am. *55:* 213–230, 1971.

Stober, W., and Waldman, T. A. "The role of the kidney in the metabolism of plasma proteins." Nephron *13:* 35–66, 1974.

West, C. B. "Asymptomatic hematuria and proteinuria in children; causes and appropriate diagnostic studies." J. Pediatr. *89:* 173–182, 1976.

White, R. H. R., Glasgow, E. R., and Mills, R. J. "Clinical pathological study of nephrotic syndrome in childhood." Lancet *1:* 1353, 1970.

Chapter 3

Pyuria

General Considerations

Pyuria is the appearance of abnormal numbers of white blood cells in the urine. Thomas Addis performed quantitative urinalyses of timed urine specimens in the 1920s, and his studies stimulated other research on the subject. Based on these studies, pyuria may be defined as more than 3 million white blood cells excreted in the urine per day. As will be discussed, translation of this number into commonly used laboratory examinations is imprecise and not standardized; in this chapter two methods of quantification of pyuria will be described. Those clinical conditions in which pyuria is the presenting or predominant feature will be considered in the differential diagnosis. Pyuria is an incidental accompanying laboratory finding in a myriad of diseases; no attempt will be made in this chapter to exhaustively include all conditions in which an abnormal number of white blood cells may appear in the urine.

Laboratory Considerations in the Detection, Quantification, and Characterization of Pyuria

Pyuria is usually a sign of disease found by examining the urinary sediment from a patient who seeks medical advice for other reasons. Rarely is pyuria an isolated presenting symptom. The method of urine collection is pivotal in the interpretation of microscopic urinary sediment findings. Only urine obtained by the clean-catch method or by catheterization of the bladder should be examined, and special care must be exercised to avoid contamination. It is sometimes advisable to use the three-glass urine test as described in Chapter 1 to obtain urine for microscopic examination. Urine in the first fraction contains sediment washed from the urethra; urine in the second fraction represents findings characteristic of urine itelf; and urine in the third fraction reflects abnormalities of the bladder. Thus, urinary sediment abnormalities seen in only the first or the third fraction of urine may help localize disease states to either the urethra or bladder, respectively.

The most commonly used method for the examination of the urinary sediment employs concentration of the sediment from 10 ml of urine by centrifugation. The clarified supernatant urine is decanted, leaving a "small amount of urine" for resuspension of the sediment; a drop of suspension is placed upon a glass slide and a coverslip applied. The preparation is examined using a standard bright field microscope with subdued light and 430x magnification. Because of the normal variation of urine flow rate, the number of white blood cells seen per high-power field (WBC/hpf) varies. Normal urine has less than 5 white blood cells per high-power field. Once an abnormal number of white blood cells is noted in the urinary sediment, no significance should be attached to their further quantification; that is, 10 WBC/hpf or 100 WBC/hpf do not denote the "extent" or "severity" of the disease process.

The second and preferred method for detection of pyuria is simpler, more rapid, and ideal for office practices. The urine specimen is thoroughly mixed and a drop placed in the counting chamber of a standard hemacytometer. The number of white blood cells per cubic millimeter of urine is quantified by standard counting practice. More than 10 WBC/mm^3 of uncentrifuged urine is abnormal. No significance regarding "severity" or "extent" of disease should be attached to the number of white blood cells per cubic millimeter once the sediment is diagnosed as abnormal. Technical competence to differentiate red and white blood cells in the counting chamber is required. Urinary white blood cells lyse rapidly at a urine pH above 6.8 or in hypotonic urine; urine may be kept for hours without a decrease in the number of white blood cells present provided it has an acid pH, is at least isotonic, and is cool.

Use of the standard light microscope does not permit the differentiation of white blood cells from renal tubular epithelial cells. Phase contrast microscopy provides an effective means of differentiating polymorphonuclear leukocytes, mononuclear lymphocytes, and renal tubular epithelial cells. Examples of the advantages of phase contrast microscopy are shown in Figure 3-1. Recent studies indicate that in bacterial urinary tract infections, more than 60% of the white blood cells in the urine are polymorphonuclear leukocytes. While such information may be helpful in selected cases, the general clinical usefulness of phase contrast microscopy for examination of urinary sediments is not established.

In selected cases, examination of urine that has not passed through the urethra may be desirable. For this purpose, suprapubic needle aspiration of bladder urine may be performed using a sterile 21-gauge spinal needle. Such urine should normally have no more than 2 WBC/mm^3 of unspun urine or an average of 1 or less WBC per high-powered field when centrifuged urine is examined.

Clinical Features Important in the Evaluation of Pyuria

The most common cause of pyuria is contamination of a normal urine collected by improper technique. Thus the physician should always ascertain the conditions under which the urine was collected. Interpretation of findings in urine specimens collected by other than clean-catch techniques, aspiration, or catheterization is meaningless.

The most common pathology associated with pyuria is that induced by bacterial infection of the urinary tract. Acute cystitis most frequently presents with dysuria, urinary frequency and urgency, gross hematuria, or cloudy urine. If the infection is confined to the bladder, constitutional symptoms such as fever, malaise, or prostration may be absent. When a patient has acute bacterial pyelonephritis, constitutional symptoms are expected. Flank pain may be caused directly by the bacterial infection or obstruction of the urinary tract by tumor or stones. Alternatively, chronic urinary tract infection may be discovered incidentally and may have no associated symptoms. History of contact with tuberculosis should be sought in patients with chronic symptoms of fever, weight loss, malaise, and vague flank pains.

Urethritis secondary to gonococcal infection is usually symptomatic in males with white blood cells entering the urine at the level of the urethra. In females, gonococcal infection may be silent, with pyuria resulting from urine being contaminated with vaginal discharge. Recently, a syndrome clinically indistinguishable from gonococcal infection has been shown to be secondary to a rickettsia-like organism, chlamydia. Pyuria occurs in the urethritis associated with Reiter's syndrome; the urethritis, arthritis, and conjunctivitis that comprise the characteristic triad of Reiter's syndrome need not occur simultaneously, and the condition may be difficult to recognize if an isolated urethritis is the presenting symptom.

In males, bacterial infection of the sexual organs may be manifested as pyuria with

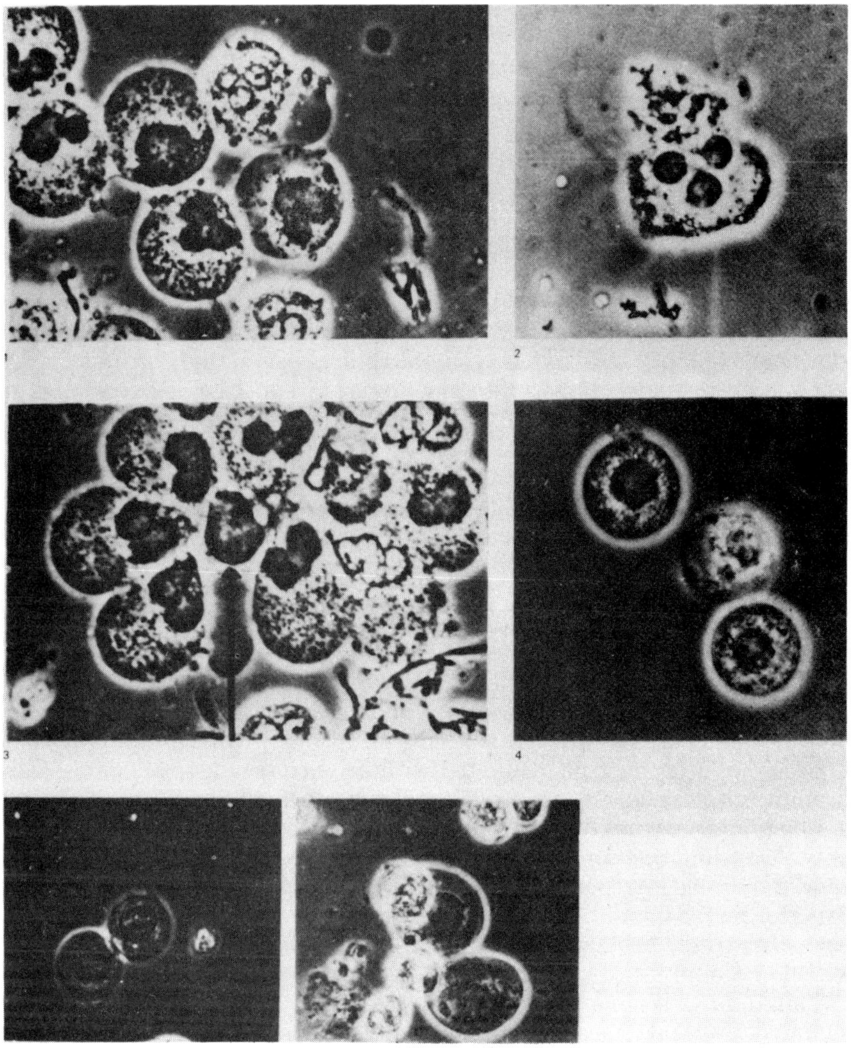

Fig. 3-1.

Phase contrast microscopy of urinary sediment. Photographs were taken with a phase contrast microscope at magnification of 1000x. As can be seen from the figure, nucleated cells may be differentiated into polymorphonuclear granulocytes (1,2), mononuclear leukocytes (3,4), and renal epithelial cells (5,6). The polymorphonuclear granulocytes are seen to have two or more dark coupled nuclei and cytoplasm with highly motile granules. The mononuclear leukocytes are similar in size to polymorphonuclear granulocytes, although their nuclei were rounded or kidney shaped. Renal epithelial cells were round and contained eccentrically located light grey nuclei in which nucleoli were clearly visible. (Reprinted with permission from Acta Med. Scand. *198:* 505–509, 1975.)

either initial or terminal accentuation of the number of white cells in the urine. Orchitis, epididymitis, or acute prostatitis are usually symptomatic with localized pain and fever. Chronic prostatitis may be silent with only a subclinical symptom of pain in the perineal area.

Neoplasms anywhere in the urinary tract may be associated with pyuria and present with localized or constitutional symptoms. Disease in organs contiguous to the urinary tract may cause pyuria and present with symptoms referrable to the large bowel, the small bowel, or the female reproductive tract. A history of introduction of foreign bodies into the urethra should be sought in cases of asymptomatic pyuria, although a negative history should be regarded as inconclusive.

A tabulation of medications consumed is useful. Aspirin and glucocorticoids are known to induce abnormal pyuria.

On physical examination the patient's temperature and blood pressure should be noted. Evidence for local tenderness over the flanks, abdomen, external genitalia, and rectal examination should be sought, and pelvic examination should be routine. The abdomen should be examined for the presence of masses that might represent neoplasms, a distended bladder, or a horseshoe kidney.

Formed elements accompanying pyuria in the urinary sediment should receive special attention. The presence of casts localizes the pathology to the kidney, while the presence of crystals may provide information allowing a diagnosis of gout, urinary tract infection, cystinuria, or nephrolithiasis. Any patient with pyuria should have a quantitative urine culture. The role of urine cultures for L-forms (protoplasts) or viruses is controversial; they are not routinely available and have no general clinical use. Urine cultures for tuberculosis should be reserved for patients with "sterile" pyuria, a positive tuberculin skin test, and clinical features suggestive of renal tuberculosis. Similarly, urine cytology should be reserved for special situations with a high index of suspicion for neoplastic disease. Other laboratory examinations may be helpful in the evaluation of pyuria, although a physician's acumen should be employed in regard to which tests are necessary. A first case of bacterial cystitis in a young female may require nothing more than a urinalysis and routine urine culture. In contrast, sterile pyuria with an abdominal mass may require an exploratory laparotomy.

An intravenous pyelogram should be performed on any male with pyuria unless the pathology can be localized to the urethra or genitalia. In females the short urethra permits frequent bacterial contamination of the bladder, with resulting acute cystitis; single or very infrequent episodes of acute cystitis do not require an intravenous pyelogram for adequate evaluation. Recurrent urinary tract infections, infections with symptomatic renal involvement, or chronic pyuria must be evaluated with an intravenous pyelogram. Care must be exercised in interpreting intravenous pyelograms performed in the setting of acute pyelonephritis; functionally reversible hydronephrosis may occur with no associated anatomical abnormality. A voiding cystourethrogram may be very helpful in evaluating bladder abnormalities and detecting vesicoureteral reflux. Radiographic examination of other systems should be performed, depending upon the clinical situation and the physician's judgment.

Males with a single urinary tract infection or females with recurrent urinary tract infections should be referred to a urologist to be considered for cystoscopy. Some potentially correctable anatomical lesions in the bladder are detectable only by cystoscopy. Occasionally, collection of ureteral urine at cystoscopy may localize an infection to one kidney.

Renal biopsy should be an infrequent consideration in the evaluation of pyuria. Specifically, percutaneous renal biopsy should never be performed in a patient with suspected or proven renal parenchymal infection.

Differential Diagnosis of Pyuria and Basis for Diagnosis of Specific Conditions

I. Contamination of Urine by Improper Methods of Collection

By far the most common cause of pyuria is contamination caused by incorrect methods of collection of urine specimens. In one series of 2000 consecutive urine specimens, pyuria was detected in 285; of these, 225 occurred secondary to contamination of the urine specimen. The incidence of contamination can be markedly reduced if the patient receives proper instruction on methods of collection of the urine specimen. Collection of urine by the clean-catch method is preferred over catheterization. Males should thoroughly cleanse and dry the urethral meatus before collecting urine in three containers (see Chapter 1 on hematuria). If this is not possible, a single, clean-catch, midvoided urine sample is the best alternative. In females, instruction and assistance from a nurse or medical assist-

Table 3-1

Differential Diagnosis of Pyuria

I. Contamination of urine by improper methods of collection
II. Microbial or idiopathic inflammation of the urinary tract
 A. Acute cystitis syndrome in females
  1. Bacterial cystitis or pyelonephritis
  2. Vaginitis
   a. Monilial or other fungal infections
   b. Trichomonal
  3. Gonococcal infection
  4. Negative urine culture (?)
  5. Interstitial cystitis
 B. Chronic or recurrent urinary tract infection in females
  1. With normal anatomy of the urinary tract
  2. With abnormal anatomy of the urinary tract
 C. Urinary tract infection in males
  1. Cystitis
  2. Pyelonephritis
  3. Prostatitis
 D. Granulomatous infection of the urinary tract
  1. Tuberculosis
  2. Brucellosis
  3. Fungal infections
 E. Urethritis
  1. Gonococcal infection
  2. Nongonococcal urethritis
  3. Reiter's syndrome
III. Neoplasms of the urinary tract
IV. Disease in organs contiguous to the urinary tract
 A. Involving the colon
  1. Diverticulitis
  2. Crohn's disease—ulcerative colitis
  3. Appendicitis
 B. Involving the small intestine—regional ileitis
 C. Involving the female genital organs
  1. Tubal pregnancy
  2. Pelvic inflammatory disease
V. Congenital anomalies of the urinary tract (Common entities include urethral stricture, bladder neck obstruction, congenital urethral valves, ureteral stricture, double-collecting system, horseshoe kidney, or vascular obstruction to drainage of the renal pelvis)
VI. Foreign bodies in the urinary tract
 A. Endogenous stones present in the renal pelvis, ureters, bladder, or urethra
 B. Foreign bodies in the urethra or bladder
VII. Drug-induced pyuria
 A. Glucocorticoid or aspirin administration
 B. Phenacetin-induced chronic interstitial nephritis
 C. Drug-induced acute interstitial nephritis (penicillin analogs, sulfa analogs, and rarely other drugs)

ant may be very helpful in adequately cleansing the urethral meatus and retracting the labia to allow a clean-catch specimen.

II. Microbial or Idiopathic Inflammation of the Urinary Tract

A. Acute Cystitis Syndrome in Females

In women, ascending infection of the bladder occurs frequently, presumably as a result of the short urethra. Acute cystitis presents with dysuria, urinary urgency and frequency, gross hematuria, or turbid urine with the subsequent finding of pyuria. It must be noted that only half of the women presenting with this syndrome will subsequently be found to have a positive urine culture; these patients may be firmly diagnosed as having a bacterial urinary tract infection. Localization of the infection to the bladder based upon symptomatology is tenuous, and more sophisticated techniques are required for a firm conclusion (see Thomas, Shelokov, and Forland, 1974, for discussion). The absence of constitutional symptoms, flank pain, or fever does not rule out renal involvement.

Female patients with symptoms consistent with acute bacterial cystitis, but with negative urine cultures, comprise a heterogeneous group. Some may have monilial or trichomonal vaginitis; pyuria in such patients is almost always due to contamination of the urine with vaginal discharge. The patient taking unprescribed antibiotics for dysuria induced by bacterial urinary tract infection may present with a negative urine culture and fungal vaginitis. Gonococcal infection can mimic acute bacterial cystitis with true pyuria that does not result simply from contamination; diagnosis in such patients requires appropriate culture for gonococci. After removal of the above groups, there still remains a large group of female patients with pyuria and acute cystitis and negative urine cultures. Most frequently, these patients are presumed to have a bacterial urinary tract infection and are treated with antibiotics; the syndrome is self-limiting, and the true cause for the symptoms and the pyuria is not known.

If the acute cystitis syndrome occurs for the first time, very infrequently, or in association with increased sexual activity, the patient's evaluation may be terminated with a urine culture and sensitivity with appropriate antibiotic therapy. Further evaluation with various blood tests, intravenous pyelogram, or cystoscopy is probably not warranted.

Interstitial cystitis (Hunner's ulcer) is a chronic inflammatory disease usually affecting the vertex of the bladder in middle-aged women; the occurrence in men is rare. Symptoms are usually chronic, with dysuria and urgency being very common, although exacerbations of the condition may present as the acute cystitis syndrome. Sterile pyuria is the only remarkable laboratory finding. Definitive diagnosis requires cystoscopy to demonstrate characteristic inflammation of the bladder. Patients suffering from interstitial cystitis may mistakenly be diagnosed as neurotic until appropriate evaluation leads to the correct diagnosis.

B. Chronic or Recurrent Urinary Tract Infection in Females

When the acute cystitis syndrome occurs recurrently or when pyuria-bacilluria persists after a course of adequate treatment for an acute urinary tract infection, further evaluation of the patient is in order. Repeated cultures of the urine should be performed to determine if the same organism is isolated each time. Multiple different organisms favor reinfection of the bladder, whereas culturing the same organism each time favors relapse of a persistent infection, usually of renal origin. An intravenous pyelogram and cystoscopy are indicated to rule out anatomical abnormalities of the urinary tract. Recurrent cystitis secondary to different organisms may be treated with urinary antiseptics such as mandelamine-methionine or sulfa-trimethoprim. Chronic persistent infection of a normal urinary tract with the same organism favors the diagnosis of chronic pyelonephritis, and prolonged therapy with specific antibiotics is indicated.

When intravenous pyelography or cystoscopy demonstrates an anatomically abnormal urinary tract, eradication of an associated bacterial infection is extremely difficult. The anatomical abnormality (stone, tumor, diverticulum, papillary necrosis, etc.) should be recorded as part of the diagnosis with the associated microbial infection and attention directed to correction of the abnormal anatomy if possible. Chronic antibacterial therapy is usually required.

C. Urinary Tract Infection in Males

Urinary tract infection is infrequent in males, and a single symptomatic episode should be evaluated thoroughly. The most common cause of pyuria in males is prostatitis which may be acute or chronic. Acute prostatitis may present as urgency, frequency, dysuria, perineal or low back pain, fever, and turbid urine. Urinary retention is not uncommon. Diagnosis is based upon the finding of an exquisitely tender prostatic gland in the clinical setting described above. Cultures of prostatic secretions are not routinely performed.

Chronic prostatitis may be asymptomatic or present with pain in the perineum or low back and a low-grade fever. On rectal examination the prostatic gland may be normal or enlarged and turgid. The degree of tenderness of an asymptomatic prostatic gland carries no clinical significance. An inflamed prostate should not be massaged until antibiotic therapy has been in effect for at least a week; secretions with large numbers of white blood cells then provide a firm basis for the diagnosis of chronic prostatitis. Radiographic or cystoscopic examination is not necessary. Acute epididymitis rarely occurs in the absence of prostatitis and may result from undue massage of a chronically inflamed prostate.

In males, pyelonephritis or cystitis is rare in the absence of an anatomical abnormality of the urinary tract or an associated systemic illness. Presenting symptoms include dysuria, urgency, frequency, fever, or flank pain with pyuria and a positive urine culture. Noninvasive examinations such as blood tests and radiographic examinations should be followed by cystoscopy if indicated.

D. Granulomatous Infection of the Urinary Tract

Chronic pyuria with negative routine urine cultures in a patient with a past history of tuberculosis infection or exposure strongly suggests the possibility of renal tuberculosis. Hematogenous spread of the tuberculosis infection to the kidney is followed by the appearance of *Mycobacterium tuberculosis* in the urine; untreated, this is followed by tuberculous infection of the ureter, bladder, and, in the male, the prostate, epididymis, and testis. Pyuria is an early sign of genitourinary tuberculosis, and hematuria occurs later. Symptoms are nonspecific, with low-grade fever, malaise, and weight loss frequently being noted. Definitive diagnosis requires culture of *Mycobacterium tuberculosis* from a urine specimen.

Infection of the kidney with *Brucella* organisms is quite rare but should be considered in patients with sterile pyuria who clinically appear to have renal tuberculosis but lack positive skin test or cultures for *Mycobacterium tuberculosis. Brucella* infection is acquired through contact with infected cattle and is an occupational disease of farmers and meat-processing workers. Definitive diagnosis requires serological demonstration of an increase in the serum *Brucella*-agglutinating titer in a patient with the appropriate clinical syndrome.

Fungal pyelonephritis is a rare disease except in patients with immunological deficiency states. Opportunistic fungal infections may occur in patients on immunosuppressive therapy for malignancies, lupus erythematosus, or renal transplant recipients. Fungal pyelonephritis is characteristically an indolent disease with nonspecific symptoms and pyuria sterile to routine culture. Fungi that might grow on routine bacterial culture are often not reported. Definitive diagnosis requires appropriate fungal culture of the urine or demonstration of the fungi in tissue obtained at the time of abcess drainage.

E. Urethritis in Males

Isolated urethritis is a male disease. Gonorrheal infection presents as a purulent urethral discharge with dysuria 4 to 10 days after sexual exposure. Local inflammation of the meatus, tenderness of the urethra, purulent urethral discharge, and pyuria with initial accentuation are expected. Definitive diagnosis requires culture of the gonococcal organism.

Many male cases of urethritis acquired by sexual contact are not associated with gonococcal infection. Recently, a mycoplasma (*Chlamydia trachomatis*) has been cultured from approximately 40% of men who have sexually contacted nongonococcal urethritis. Culture techniques for this organism are not routinely available, and thus definitive diagnosis is available only in certain laboratories. Approximately 60% of all males with nongonococcal urethritis are not infected with a culturable mycoplasma; the cause of the syndrome in these individuals is unknown. *Chlamydia trachomatis* is effectively treated with tetracycline, which should be routine therapy for a nongonococcal urethritis.

Reiter's syndrome is a rare disease manifested as conjunctivitis, arthritis, and urethritis. Each of the features of the triad may present as an isolated symptom, making diagnosis extremely difficult until the entire syndrome is manifested. Most commonly, urethritis is the first symptom to appear and is associated with diarrhea. In a minority of patients characteristic dermatological lesions, termed balanitis circinatea and keratoderma blennorrhagica, may occur and leave no question regarding the diagnosis. There are no other pathognomonic or distinctive features, and definitive diagnosis requires recognition of the clinical syndrome.

III. Neoplasms of the Urinary Tract

While most neoplasms of the urinary tract present with hematuria, pyuria may be an isolated finding in some patients who seek medical attention because of fever, malaise, weight loss, anorexia, or localized pain. Such patients should have careful examination of the prostate, an intravenous pyelogram, and cystoscopy; in highly suspect cases, nephrotomograms should be performed. The three most common neoplasms of the urinary tract in males are carcinoma of the prostate (61%), bladder (24%), kidney (10%), with others (5%) occurring much less frequently. The incidence of urinary tract carcinoma is less in females, with carcinoma of the bladder and kidney occurring about equally frequent.

IV. Disease in Contiguous Organs

Pyuria may occur secondary to inflammatory disease in organs contiguous to the urinary tract. Diverticulitis, appendicitis, Crohn's disease, or ulcerative colitis may each occur in direct contact with the ureters or bladder. Usually, signs and symptoms of the underlying disease lead directly to an appropriate diagnosis, although occasionally the occurrence of pyuria may misdirect the physician's attention to the urinary tract. Similar problems may arise with diseases of the genital tract, such as female pelvic inflammatory disease or tubal pregnancy.

V. Congenital Anomalies of the Urinary Tract

Urinary tract infections in children under the age of 10 years involve the kidney much more frequently than do urinary tract infections in the adult. Potential renal failure or death from symptomatic or asymptomatic infection of the urinary tract is primarily dependent upon the presence of congenital anomalies of the urinary tract. Based upon results of several series, an average of 15% of children under the age of 10 with culture-proven urinary tract infection will have anatomical congenital anomalies of the urinary tract. An additional one third of all children with urinary tract infection will be found to have vesicoureteral reflux with an otherwise anatomically normal urinary tract.

Pyuria is expected in symptomatic urinary tract infections in children; however, only 25% of childhood asymptomatic urinary tract infections manifest pyuria, making this an insensitive screening index of infection. The extent of the diagnostic evaluation to be pursued in children with urinary tract infections depends upon:

1. *Age of the child:* Younger children are more likely to have anatomical abnormalities; all children under the age of two should

be thoroughly evaluated at the time a urinary tract infection is first documented.

2. *Sex of the patient:* All males should be evaluated at the time a urinary tract infection is first documented. Older females with isolated or infrequent urinary tract infections may be treated and observed without extensive evaluation.
3. *Presenting signs and symptoms:* Severe acute illness is an indication for more thorough evaluation than asymptomatic bacteria.
4. *Nature of the infecting microorganism:* Infections with unexpected microorganisms such as *Pseudomonas* or *Proteus* are an indication for more thorough evaluation.
5. *Number of infections:* Several infections in a short period of time should be more thoroughly evaluated especially if the same microorganism is cultured each time.

After urinalysis and urine culture the next step in evaluation is an intravenous pyelogram and a voiding cystourethrogram. The most common abnormalities encountered involve various duplications of the ureter and malrotation of the kidney. Less commonly encountered abnormalities include horseshoe kidney, "cake" kidney at the bifurcation of the aorta, vascular obstruction of the ureter, stricture of the ureter, ureterocele, diverticuli, bladder neck obstruction, and strictures of the urethra. These conditions can usually be adequately evaluated by radiographic procedures; in the evaluation for vesicoureteral reflux, cystoscopy may be helpful in characterizing the bladder mucosa or the site of ureteral entry into the bladder.

Controversy regarding the significance of versicoureteral reflux in children persists, although certain tenets seem to be well accepted. Mild to moderate reflux is known to accompany acute urinary tract infection and usually resolves in the course of several months, being of no significance in predisposition to urinary tract infection or its subsequent recurrence. So-called heavy or severe reflux may predispose to chronic or recurrent urinary tract infections and should be evaluated by a urologist when first detected.

VI. Foreign Bodies in the Urinary Tract

Calculi lodged in the renal pelvis, the ureter, the bladder, or the urethra may predispose to chronic urinary tract infections or may be associated with sterile pyuria, presumably secondary to local irritation. Definitive diagnosis requires radiographic demonstration of the calculus; in the case of radiolucent uric acid stones that may lodge in the ureter, the diagnosis may be missed unless hydronephrosis or other local signs are present.

A variety of exogenous foreign bodies may be introduced into the urethra and may enter the bladder in females. Embarrassment may make histories unreliable, and diagnosis requires a high index of suspicion. Hematuria is expected in addition to pyuria if the trauma is acute. Chronic local irritation from a retained foreign body may present as pyuria with or without urinary tract infection.

VII. Drug-Induced Pyuria

Certain drugs such as aspirin or glucocorticoids may induce an abnormal number of white blood cells in the urine in normal individuals. Phenacetin-induced analgesic nephropathy may present as sterile pyuria in a patient consuming excessive quantities of analgesics. Sulfa analogs or penicillin analogs may induce acute interstitial nephritis with pyuria as the predominant sign in the urinary sediment. Any of a variety of heavy metals or toxic compounds may induce pyuria secondary to a chronic interstitial nephritis. Definitive diagnosis requires documentation of drug or toxin consumption with the associated appropriate laboratory findings.

Results Expected from Evaluation of Pyuria

Little information is available regarding the relative incidence of the causes of pyuria. As previously noted, pyuria occurs secondary to contamination of the urine specimen in the majority of cases; the incidence of contamination may be reduced if the patient receives proper instruction on the method of urine collection.

If a clean-voided midstream urine specimen has an abnormal number of white blood cells present, the most likely associated condition is infection of the urinary tract, with all other causes comprising a small fraction of the causes of pyuria. Thus the first step in the evaluation of pyuria is a routine urine culture which, when positive, requires the physician to consider further evaluation based upon the clinical setting. Malignancy, unusual infections, toxic or drug-induced nephropathies, or idiopathic inflammatory conditions are responsible for pyuria in those cases with negative routine urine cultures.

Clinical Problem

A 48-year-old white male executive sought medical attention because of chronic low back and perineal pain not associated with activity. The patient was aware of a recent 4 pound weight loss (3% of body weight) associated with mild anorexia and malaise which he often treated with aspirin. He had not noted chills or fever and had no remarkable gastrointestinal symptoms. He was a moderate smoker with a 25 pack a year history of cigarette consumption and a chronic cough with increased purulent sputum production on arising in the morning. Fifteen years previously the patient had culture-proven pulmonary tuberculosis with apical infiltrates that completely cleared on streptomycin and isoniazid therapy. Yearly reexaminations had not demonstrated evidence of recurrent tuberculosis.

On physical examination the patient's blood pressure was 140/90 and his temperature was 37.8° C. Other pertinent physical findings included an enlarged soft prostate gland, gentle palpation of which accentuated the patient's complaint of perineal pain.

The patient was instructed regarding the method of cleansing the urethral meatus and collecting a three-glass urine specimen. The specific gravity on the middle fraction was 1.018, pH 5.5, glucose 2+, protein 1+, and the urinary sediment contained an abnormal number of white blood cells but no red cells or casts. The complete blood count was within normal limits, as was the patient's serum creatinine. A random blood glucose was 152 mg%. A urine specimen was submitted for quantitative culture.

The patient was advised that he probably had chronic prostatitis, and antibiotic therapy with a sulfa antimicrobial agent was started. The urine culture was subsequently reported as "no significant growth." On a return visit 1 week later the patient reported that the perineal and low back pain had improved, and he was found to be afebrile. Repeat urinalysis demonstrated persistent pyuria.

Questions

1. What conditions should be considered in the differential diagnosis of this patient's pyuria?
2. What further diagnostic evaluation is indicated?

Discussion

Based upon the presence of perineal pain and the physical finding of an enlarged prostate gland, a diagnosis of chronic prostatitis is compatible with the patient's pyuria; the patient's fever, anorexia, and mild weight loss are also compatible with this diagnosis.

However, these latter features may be manifestations of other systemic illnesses and require further evaluation. From this patient's clinical history, an obvious possibility is the diagnosis of renal tuberculosis with subsequent involvement of the prostatic gland. If the patient's glycosuria and single elevated blood glucose are shown to be manifestations of diabetes mellitus, the possibility of an associated bacterial urinary tract infection or renal tuberculosis is markedly enhanced. The possibility of a primary or metastatic malignancy involving the urinary tract must be considered.

This patient's further evaluation should include a roentgenogram of the chest to evaluate the status of the patient's tuberculosis and to rule out malignancies involving the lung. A roentgenogram of the abdomen should be performed to detect abnormal calcifications involving the kidneys or ureters. A fasting blood glucose and 2-hour postprandial blood glucose should be obtained after a standard 100 gm glucose ingestion. The consumption of aspirin should be discouraged, and the patient should chart his temperature three times daily while continuing sulfa therapy for his diagnosed prostatitis. Because the patient's condition is stable, there is no urgency to hospitalize and evaluate this patient.

This patient was subsequently found to have a normal chest roentgenogram and a normal roentgenogram of the abdomen. A fasting blood glucose was found to be 103 mg% with a 2-hour postprandial level of 220 mg%. Two weeks after initial evaluation the patient's prostate gland was found to be less tender, and his complaints of perineal and low back pain had ceased, although pyuria persisted. Under the protection of sulfa therapy, a course of twice weekly prostatic massage was instituted; initially, the expressed prostatic secretions had large numbers of white blood cells present with clearing after 1 month of massage therapy, which was then discontinued. A urine specimen examined 2 weeks later was normal, and his temperature record for the previous week demonstrated that he was afebrile. Because of the patient's history, an intravenous pyelogram and urine culture for acid-fast bacilli were obtained during the month of massage therapy. Neither of these demonstrated abnormalities, and the patient's final diagnoses were (1) chronic prostatitis, (2) diabetes mellitus, (3) history of treated pulmonary tuberculosis, and (4) mild chronic bronchitis.

References

Dans, P. E., and Klaus, B. "Dysuria in women." Johns Hopkins Med. J. *138:* 13–18, 1976.

Govan, B. E. "Investigation and management of urinary tract infections in female children." Urol. Clin. North Am. *1:* 397–412, 1974.

Gower, P. E. "A prospective study of patients with radiological pyelonephritis, papillary necrosis, and obstructive atrophy." Q. J. Med. *XLV:* 315–349, 1976.

Guinan, P. V., Neter, E., and Murphy, G. P. "The significance of L-forms in human renal disease." J. Urol. *108:* 50–53, 1972.

Holmes, K. K., Hansfield, H. H., Wang, S. P., Wentworth, B. B., Turck, M., Anderson, J. B., and Alexander, E. R. "Etiology of non-gonococcal urethritis." N. Engl. J. Med. *292:* 1199–1205, 1975.

Kraft, J. K., and Stamey, T. A. "The natural history of symptomatic recurrent bacturia in women." Medicine *56:* 55–61, 1977.

Lindberg, U., Claesson, I., Hanson, L. A., and Jodal, U. "Asymptomatic bacturia in school girls." Acta Paediatr. Scand. *64:* 425–431, 1975.

Lindqueist, B., and Wahlin, A. "Differential count of urinary leukocytes and renal epithelial cells by phase contrast microscopy." Acta Med. Scand. *198:* 505–509, 1975.

Lyttle, J. B. "The Addis sediment count in normal children." J. Clin. Invest. *12:* 87–93, 1933.

Musher, D. M., Thorsteinsson, S. B., and Airola, V. M. "Quantitative urinalysis; diagnosing urinary tract infection in men." JAMA *236:* 2069–2072, 1976.

Stansfeld, J. M. "The measurement and meaning of pyuria." Arch. Dis. Child. *37:* 257–262, 1962.

Thomas, V., Shelokov, A., and Forland, M. "Antibody coated bacteria in urine and site of urinary tract infection." N. Engl. J. Med. *290:* 588–591, 1974.

Chapter 4

Glycosuria

General Considerations

Glycosuria is the excretion of glucose in the urine in detectable amounts. Its presence may be suspected by the finding of reducing substances in the urine. Glucose specific tests provide positive identification of the reducing substance as glucose.

Renal Handling of Glucose

Normally, the concentration of glucose in the glomerular filtrate is the same as that in the plasma water. Glucose is reabsorbed in the proximal tubules chiefly in the convoluted portion. The reabsorption occurs by a carrier-mediated system that exhibits saturation kinetics. As the concentration of glucose in plasma increases, the amount of glucose reabsorbed by the tubules reaches a transfer maximum (transfer maximum of glucose or TmG) which in the normal adult is about 300–375 mg/min. When the arterial blood glucose exceeds a certain level (usually about 150–180 mg/100 ml) and the amount of glucose presented to the tubules for reabsorption is greater than the TmG, glucose appears in the urine. However, this concentration of glucose, often called the renal threshold, is not rigidly fixed and is not the sole factor concerned. Changes in the glomerular filtration rate (GFR) may alter the total quantity of glucose reaching the proximal tubule per unit time, and variations in the activity of tubules of individual nephrons influence the composite effect. Glucose titration curves can be determined by measuring the amount of glucose that is reabsorbed at increasing plasma glucose concentrations. At a constant GFR, when the plasma concentration of glucose is increased, there will be a progressive rise in the filtered load of glucose (GFR × plasma glucose). This results in an increase in the amount of glucose presented to the proximal tubules for reabsorption. The system is "titrated" to determine the plasma concentration at which the carrier for glucose becomes saturated and glucose starts to spill out in the urine. A representative glucose titration curve in humans is presented in Figure 4-1. From the shape of the curve, it can be appreciated that it has the characteristics of a Tm-limited active transport. Usually, all the filtered glucose is reabsorbed, and .1% or less of the amount filtered is excreted. This is the case at normal plasma glucose concentrations. As the maximal capacity of the tubules for reabsorbing glucose is reached, much more glucose is excreted in the urine. It should be noted from the curve that the TmG is reached somewhat gradually along the curve rather than abruptly with a sharp deflection. This gradual deflection is known as the splay, and it probably has at least two explanations. The first involves the kinetics of the chemical reaction between glucose and a postulated carrier. Since the carrier may have a finite affinity for glucose, a "supersaturating" concentration of glucose in tubular fluid may be needed to saturate the carrier. Hence, glucose may appear in the urine before Tm is reached and some splay will result. The second explanation involves the concept of morphological diversity of nephron

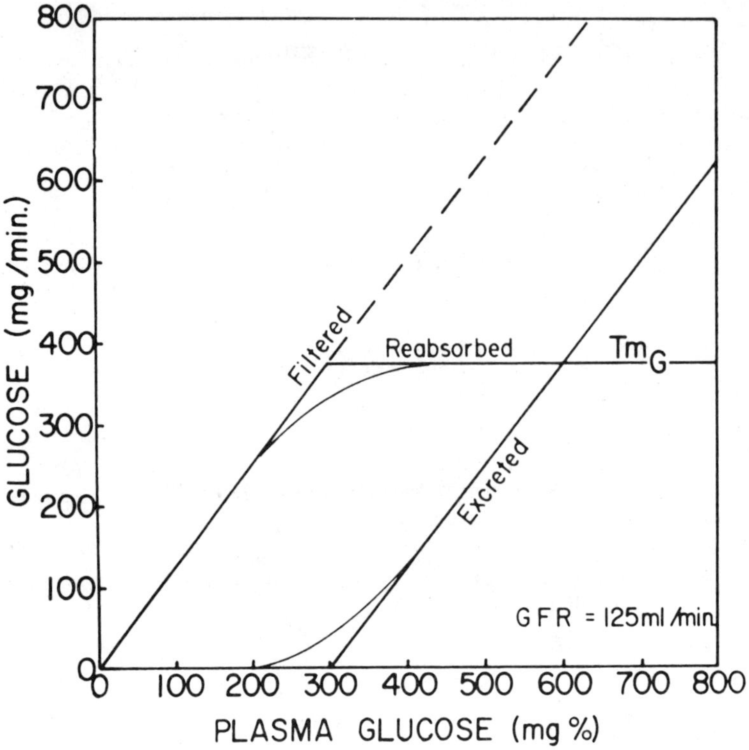

Fig. 4-1.

Normal glucose titration in humans. (Reproduced by permission from Pitts, R.F., The Physiology of the Kidney and Body Fluids, 3rd ed., 1974, Yearbook Medical Publishers, Chicago.)

populations, including both cortical and juxtamedullary nephrons. The capacity of these two populations to reabsorb glucose may be quite different. One population of nephrons may saturate at an earlier time and start to spill glucose before the other population reaches saturation. Hence, some nephrons may excrete glucose before the TmG for other nephrons is reached. Thus the degree of splay in the glucose titration curve may, in part, reflect the extent of an anatomical glomerulotubular balance in both cortical and juxtamedullary nephrons. Glycosuria may result when the filtered load of glucose markedly exceeds the ability of the tubules to reabsorb glucose. In this case, hyperglycemia or a marked increase in glomerular filtration rate is usually present. The most common cause of glycosuria of this type is diabetes mellitus. Glycosuria can also occur when the filtered load of glucose is normal, but there is a decreased ability of the renal tubules to reabsorb glucose or a displacement in the threshold for glucose.

Regulation of Blood Glucose Concentration

Under normal conditions the concentration of glucose in blood is held within narrow limits. Human subjects when fasted or fed a diet free of carbohydrates maintain blood glucose concentrations between 65 and 95 mg/100 ml. The lowest point during the day occurs about 3 P.M. and the highest point about 4 A.M. When carbohydrate is fed, the blood glucose rises but seldom exceeds 160 mg/100 ml in normal subjects. A major factor in the ability of the body to dispose of a glucose load is the capacity of the liver for taking up glucose and storing it as glycogen or fatty acids. Direct measurement of the ability of the splanchnic system (intestine plus liver) to remove glucose from the circulation indicates that the rate of absorption is sufficient to account entirely for the disappearance of glucose from the blood after a 100 gm glucose load. However, under normal circumstances, only about half the glucose load is taken up by the liver, the remainder being removed by peripheral tissues. If the liver is unable to cope with the flow of glucose into the blood, the plasma concentration may rise high enough that sugar is filtered by the renal glomeruli faster than it can be reabsorbed by the renal tubules. Under these circumstances, as discussed before, glucose appears in the urine.

In the fasting subject, the blood glucose is maintained by secretion of glucose from the liver. The stimulus to glucose secretion is, in part, the rate of fall of the arterial glucose, since evidence of hepatic glucose secretion may be obtained even when the arterial level is quite high if the concentration is falling rapidly. There is secretion of growth hormone, ACTH, epinephrine, and glucagon, which helps to prevent further hypoglycemia. These antihypoglycemic adjustments, however, are used only to combat moderate to marked depressions of blood glucose. The minor fluctuations associated with fasting, exercise, or physiological secretion of insulin are apparently compensated by adjustments within the liver, chiefly by alterations of the activity of glucokinase, glucose-6-phosphatase, and the gluconeogenic enzymes without mediation of the other hormonal systems. The anti-insulin effects of increased plasma-free fatty acids also play a protective role.

Laboratory Considerations

A screening procedure for the presence of glucose in urine is through use of nonspecific tests using Benedict's reagent to detect reducing substances. The reactive element in Benedict's reagent is soluble copper-carbonate-citrate ion, which is blue in color. Heating this solution with compounds containing one or more free aldehyde or ketone groups reduces soluble cupric ions to the cuprous form and they are precipitated as yellow or red cuprous oxide. Clinitest (Ames Company) is a convenient, commercially available tablet preparation that incorporates a modification of the ingredients used in Benedict's reagent. The initial screening test done with these nonspecific reagents will give a positive reaction for a number of reducing agents besides glucose. Maltose, fructose, lactose, pentose, and galactose are reducing sugars that may appear in the urine in addition to glucose. Nonsugar reducing substances that may appear in the urine include ascorbic acid, chloroform and formaldehyde (used as preservatives), increased concentrations of creatinine, increased amounts of protein, homogentisic acid, penicillin, and streptomycin. Glucuronic acid also has reducing properties and may be found in the urine after administration of salicylates, cephalosporin, acetanilid, and chloral hydrate.

Identification of sugars in the urine should be systematically approached once a reducing substance has been detected (see Table 4-1). It should be pointed out that false-positive reactions for copper reduction in urine may occur under the conditions listed in Table 4-2. However, false-negative copper reduction tests may occur when outdated reagents are used.

Commercial availability of the glucose oxidase impregnated dipstick for urine has significantly reduced the effort required for positive identification of glucose. Detection of urinary glucose by the commercially available glucose-specific (glucose oxidase) dipstick (Clinistix, Combistix, Tes-Tape or Labstix) usually indicates concentrations exceeding 10–20 mg/100 ml and is considered significant. This finding must be interpreted relative to simultaneous plasma glucose concentrations. Precaution must be taken to ensure preservation of the test material for reliable results.

It should be pointed out that false-positive results with glucose oxidase enzyme strips may be obtained when unclean glassware (contaminated with cleaners or detergents) is used. False-negative (or delayed positive) glucose oxidase strip tests may be observed in patients receiving L-dopa therapy, patients with alkaptonuria, and when urine contains certain reducing substances such as salicylates, ascorbic acid, and the like. In addition, patients with carcinoid (caused by 5-hydroxyindolacetic acid), hepatic disease (caused by bilirubin glucuronide) or uremia (caused by indols) may have negative (or delayed positive) glucose oxidase tests.

When urine shows a positive test with either Benedict's reagent or Clinitest tablets, this only indicates the presence of a reducing substance. Before attributing this to

Table 4-1

Identification of Reducing Substances in Urine

Urinary Constituent	Glucose Oxidase Test	Copper Reduction Tests (Benedict's or Clinitest)	Specific Test for Identification of Sugar
Sugars (nonglucose)			
Maltose	0	+	Paper chromatography*
Pentoses	0	+	Bial's test
Galactose	0	+	Occurs in young infants on milk feedings Tollen's test and galactokinase reaction
Lactose	0	+	Occurs in late pregnancy or lactating women Chromatography*
Fructose	0	+	Rare metabolic defect Selinwanoff's test and fructokinase reaction

*Only indicates presence of disaccharide; further chemical tests are necessary for identification.

Table 4-2

Conditions in Which False-Positive Reactions for Copper Reduction in Urine may Occur

Condition	Substances Responsible
Contaminated glassware	Cleaners, bleaches
Antibiotic therapy	Penicillin, cephalosporins, nalidixic acid, chloramphenicol, tetracyclines, streptomycin
Blockers of tubular transport	Para-aminosalicylic acid, carinamide, probenecid
L-dopa therapy	3,4-dihydroxyphenylacetic acid
Alkaptonuria	Homogentisic acid
Miscellaneous drugs	Salicylates, ascorbic acid, chloral hydrate, chloroform, hippuric acid, amino acids, formaldehyde, oxalic acid, phenols, morphine, isoniazid, synthetic estrogens
Certain x-ray contrast materials	Sodium diatrizoate (Hypaque), diatrizoate meglucamine (Renovist), meglumine iothalamate (Conray)
Substances normally present in the urine	Creatinine, uric acid (large quantities)

glycosuria the urine should be tested with one of the enzyme-impregnated strips (Tes-Tape, Diastix, Combistix, Clinistix). A positive result indicates the reducing substance to be glucose. This is the most important reducing substance found in urine, and at this point in the workup, if no symptoms are present, the most straightforward approach is to proceed to the glucose tolerance test.

Glucose Tolerance Test

Proper interpretation of this test depends upon an adequate carbohydrate intake (300 gm/day for at least 3 days prior to testing) by the patient. The patient is fasted overnight.

In the morning, a fasting blood glucose is obtained, and the patient empties the bladder. Either 1.00 gm or 1.75 gm/kg body weight of glucose is administered. Blood and urine samples are obtained at ½, 1, 1½, 2, and 3 hours after the administration of the glucose load. Normally, for the "true blood sugar method," using venous blood, the range of concentration is from 70–100 mg/100 ml. The peak glucose level (occurring at 30 minutes or 1 hour) should be below 160 mg/100 ml, and at the end of 2 hours, it should have fallen to its fasting level.

If the peak is greater than 160 mg/100 ml and the 2-hour value is above 120 mg/100 ml in a properly performed test, the diagnosis of diabetes may be made. (These values are for blood; values for measurements made on serum are approximately 15% higher.)

The glucose tolerance test is often used in the diagnosis of diabetes mellitus. For the test to be valid in helping to make this diagnosis, it is essential for the patient to have ingested adequate amounts of carbohydrate in the diet for at least a week prior to the test. Unless this precaution is taken, normal subjects who have received low amounts of carbohydrate for prolonged periods may demonstrate abnormal blood glucose levels similar to those seen in mild diabetes.

Severe cases of diabetes mellitus can usually be recognized from history, fasting, and 2-hour postprandial blood glucose and urine examination. If fasting values above 120 mg/100 ml are obtained on several occasions, the diagnosis of diabetes can be made without the performance of a glucose tolerance test. On the patient who demonstrates only hyperglycemia and who is otherwise asymptomatic, a glucose tolerance test performed will reveal a fasting level above 120 mg/100 ml (and it may even be 200–300 mg/100 ml). Following the test, in these patients, blood glucose rises, and at the end of 2 hours, it will not have returned to normal levels.

One of the most useful functions served by the glucose tolerance test, however, is not the diagnosis of diabetes mellitus but rather the exclusion of this diagnosis in persons with symptomless glycosuria. A normal glucose tolerance test with the constant finding of glucose in the urine indicates a diagnosis of renal glycosuria. Further information concerning the nature of the defect resulting in glucose in the urine will be available through performance of the glucose titration studies (see below).

Differential Diagnosis of Glycosuria

The possible cause of glycosuria should be approached based on the concomitant presence or absence of hyperglycemia. Diabetes mellitus is the most common cause of glycosuria. Less commonly, glycosuria may occur in a number of more benign conditions. The differential diagnosis of glycosuria is listed in Table 4-3.

I. Glycosuria Occurring as a Consequence of Hyperglycemia

Glycosuria occurs as a consequence of hyperglycemia when the blood glucose concentration exceeds the renal tubular capacity to reabsorb it from the glomerular filtrate. This usually occurs when the blood glucose concentration exceeds 180 mg/100 ml.

A. Diabetes Mellitus

Diabetes mellitus is the most common of the endocrine disorders and is caused by a deficiency or a decreased effectiveness of insulin. It is characterized clinically by hyperglycemia and glycosuria with consequent polyuria and polydipsia. Episodes of ketoacidosis may occur. Two types of diabetes are recognized on the basis of etiology.

Table 4-3

Differential Diagnosis of Glycosuria

- I. Usually associated with hyperglycemia
  - A. Diabetes mellitus
    1. Primary (idiopathic)
    2. Secondary to destruction of islets of Langerhans
       - a. Surgical removal of the pancreas
       - b. Pancreatitis (acute or chronic)
       - c. Carcinoma of the pancreas
       - d. Hemochromatosis
       - e. Cystic fibrosis
  - B. Endocrine hyperfunction
    1. Acromegaly
    2. Hyperthyroidism
    3. Hyperadrenocorticism
    4. Pheochromocytoma
    5. Functional α-cell tumors
  - C. Nervous system disease
    1. Severe emotional stress
    2. Cerebral hemorrhage
    3. Brain tumors; brain trauma
    4. Hypothalamic damage
  - D. Hepatic or gastrointestinal disease
    1. Severe liver disease
    2. Glycogen storage disease
    3. Alimentary glycosuria
  - E. Metabolic alterations
    1. Poststarvation feeding
    2. Potassium deficiency
    3. Burns
  - F. Drugs
    1. Certain diuretics (thiazides, ethacrynic acid?)
    2. Diazoxide
    3. Adrenal steroids, ACTH
    4. Salicylates
    5. Infusion of glucose-containing solutions
- II. Relation to hyperglycemia uncertain or variable
  - A. Pregnancy
  - B. Renal disease
    1. Nephrotic syndrome, chronic renal disease
    2. Acute tubular necrosis (ischemic)
  - C. Malignancy
  - D. Drugs (curare, morphine, strychnine, chloroform)
- III. Usually occurring without hyperglycemia
  - A. Renal
    1. Renal glycosuria (idiopathic)
    2. Fanconi syndrome
    3. Lowe's syndrome
    4. Cystinosis
    5. Wilson's disease
    6. Hereditary tyrosinemia
    7. Fanconi syndrome and glycogen storage disease
  - B. Due to chemicals or poisons that affect renal glucose reabsorption
    1. Phlorizine
    2. Heavy metal salts (chromium, mercury, uranium, ferric compounds, lead, cadmium)

1. Primary (Idiopathic) Diabetes

Primary diabetes occurs in those genetically susceptible; environment and other factors may be important in determining when it is manifested.

2. Secondary Diabetes

Secondary diabetes usually results from insulin deficiency as a consequence of ablation of the islets of Langerhans. It is seen following *surgical removal of the pancreas* or following destruction of the islets during *pancreatitis,* either *acute* or *chronic. Carcinoma of the pancreas* may also result in destruction of the islets. *Hemochromatosis* is a rare disorder of iron metabolism characterized by the gradual accumulation of excessive tissue iron associated with parenchymal damage and fibrosis. The principal organs involved are the liver, pancreas, heart, and gonads. The majority of patients with hemochromatosis are males (80%), two thirds of whom manifest the disease between the ages of 40 and 60. Hyperglycemia occurs in the majority of patients, and insulin therapy is required. *Cystic fibrosis* is a generalized disorder of exocrine and sweat glands. It is inherited as an autosomal recessive and probably always makes its presence known in the first decade of life. Malabsorption from deficiency of pancreatic enzymes is the leading problem of childhood. Chronic pulmonary infection, emphysema, bronchiectasis, pulmonary fibrosis, and cor pulmonale represent the other major problems of later childhood and adolescence. Involvement of the pancreas may result in the destruction of islets of Langerhans with the production of secondary diabetes.

B. Endocrine Hyperfunction

1. Acromegaly

Acidophil tumors and some chromophobe tumors of the pituitary are characterized by an excessive and inappropriate secretion of human growth hormone, which produces acromegaly in adults and gigantism in children. The symptoms in acromegalics are those resulting from the space-occupying mass and the overproduction of growth hormone. Since growth hormone is diabetogenic, excessive secretion may result in mild diabetes mellitus, polyuria, polydipsia, and polyphagia. The typical changes in somatic appearance help in making the diagnosis.

2. Hyperthyroidism

Thyrotoxicosis (excess thyroid hormone) may result in impaired glucose tolerance. The diagnosis of hyperthyroidism can be made readily when the hypermetabolic and epinephrine-like effects of the excess thyroid hormone are prominent. The combination of weight loss and a vigorous appetite is a strong clue pointing to hyperthyroidism. Catabolic and hypermetabolic effects of excessive thyroid hormone include increased oxygen consumption, loss of muscle mass with negative nitrogen balance, and increased dissolution of adipose tissue. An increased sensitivity to endogenous catecholamines may account for at least some of the central nervous system manifestations. Increased irritability and nervousness may bring the patient to the attention of the physician. A more detailed description of clinical symptoms and physical findings of hyperthyroidism may be found in a standard textbook of medicine.

3. Hyperadrenocorticism

The constellation of clinical and metabolic abnormalities that result from excessive and inappropriate cortisol production defines Cushing's syndrome. This may result from adrenal hyperplasia, either idiopathic or secondary to increased pituitary activity and elevated plasma levels of ACTH. It also may result from adrenal tumors. In addition, certain malignancies, such as carcinoma of the lung, ovary, testes, thymus, and exocrine and endocrine pancreas, have been associated with Cushing's syndrome. The main physical findings are obesity, centripetal redistribution of fat, and the induction of carbohydrate metabolism abnormalities with the development of hyperglycemia by increasing the hepatic glucose output and by inhibiting insulin's effect on peripheral tissues. While ketosis and diabetic coma are rare, a difficulty in controlling hyperglycemia and insulin resistance may be noted.

4. Pheochromocytomas

These are uncommon tumors of chromaffin tissue of the sympathetic chain. The majority of lesions are located in the adrenal medulla. The tumors secrete catecholamines, predominantly norepinephrine but also epinephrine. These agents produce hyperglycemia by increasing liver glycogen breakdown and suppression of insulin secretion.

5. Functional α-Cell Tumors

Increased production of glucagon may result in increased hepatic gluconeogenesis and increased glucose output from the liver with resulting hyperglycemia.

C. Nervous System Diseases

Severe *emotional stress* may result in hyperglycemia. The mechanism presumably relates to increased levels of catecholamines. Epinephrine has been shown to block glucose-induced insulin release from the pancreas and to prevent an appropriate response in the secretion of the hormone as hyperglycemia develops. *Other central nervous system abnormalities:* Hyperglycemia with glycosuria may occur as a result of increased glycogen breakdown in patients with any cerebral catastrophe that may result in increased intracranial pressure *(brain tumors, cerebral hemorrhage, head trauma).*

D. Hepatic or Gastrointestinal Disease

Severe liver disease may result in hyperglycemia following carbohydrate ingestion due to decreased ability of hepatic cells to store glycogen. Hyperglycemia may also occur in certain *glycogen storage diseases,* presumably through the same mechanism. However, hypoglycemia occurs much more commonly in these conditions. Also, hypoglycemia may occur in patients with hepatic disease following alcohol ingestion. The occasional hyperglycemia that is observed in patients with hepatic disease usually follows the ingestion of large amounts of carbohydrate in the diet. It presumably is related to the inability of the patient to store a rather large load of glucose as glycogen in the liver.

Alterations in the mechanics of the upper gastrointestinal tract, such as that seen following gastrectomy, hyperthyroidism, or with liver disease, may produce *alimentary glycosuria* as a result of a lag-storage effect. This effect is produced by extremely rapid absorption of sugar from the small intestine with a transitory increase in blood glucose after a meal, so that glycosuria is produced because the blood concentration of glucose exceeds the renal threshold. This entity may also occur in healthy individuals who have rapid absorption of glucose from the small intestine.

E. Metabolic Alterations

1. Poststarvation Feeding

Persons whose carbohydrate intake has been insufficient (less than 100 gm/day) for protracted periods, either because of diet or decreased intake resulting from illness, develop a condition in which a diabetic glucose curve associated with glycosuria may occur. Administration of 250 gm of glucose per day for 3 days is sufficient to correct this and to restore the glucose curve to normal. The real difficulty in starvation diabetes is that it may be thought to be true diabetes mellitus if the glucose tolerance test is performed without considering previous glucose intake.

2. Potassium Deficiency

Hypokalemia may result in decreased peripheral glucose utilization and entry of glucose into cells, particularly muscle and liver. This may result in hyperglycemia and subsequent glycosuria. It should be remembered that glucose administration and hyperglycemia per se may result in hypokalemia due to transfer of potassium from the extracellular to the intracellular compartment and to an osmotic effect of glucose that promotes the urinary excretion and loss of potassium.

3. Burns

Extensive burns may result in the development of hyperglycemia. Presumably, increased protein breakdown with increased gluconeogenesis at the level of liver and simultaneously increased levels of catecholamines due to stress may play a role in the hyperglycemia seen in this condition.

F. Drugs

1. Certain Diuretics

Administration of thiazide diuretics, in particular, have been reported to be associated with hyperglycemia. The mechanism of this hyperglycemic effect of thiazide diuretics is not completely clarified and it may be multifactorial in nature. Proposed mechanisms include inhibition of pancreatic release of insulin and blockage of peripheral insulin action by the thiazides.

2. Diazoxide

Diazoxide is a rapidly acting antihypertensive agent that has been shown to produce hyperglycemia, increased serum free-fatty acids, and decreased plasma insulin levels by a mechanism thought to involve both suppression of insulin release and enhanced catecholamine action.

3. Adrenal Steroids, ACTH

These drugs presumably interfere with the effects of insulin peripherally. Patients treated with glucocorticoids (cortisol, prednisone) will develop glucose intolerance. Glucose tolerance may remain normal only if sufficient insulin is secreted to maintain effective circulating concentrations.

4. Salicylates

Some cases have been reported in which hyperglycemia and glycosuria occur during salicylate intoxication. The proposed mechanism involves inhibition of liver and muscle glycogen synthesis, perhaps due to epinephrine release via central sympathetic centers. Other factors that may play a role include a decrease of aerobic glucose metabolism with increased glucose-6-phosphatase activity, thereby increasing blood glucose concentrations and adrenal cortical activity that may produce sustained hyperglycemia.

5. Infusion of Glucose-containing Solutions

Infusion at relatively fast rates may exceed the capacity of the pancreas to secrete insulin, and hyperglycemia may develop. Discontinuation of the intravenous glucose-containing solutions may result in rapid normalization of blood glucose.

II. Conditions in which Glycosuria and Its Relation to Hyperglycemia Are Uncertain or Variable

A. Pregnancy

Glycosuria may occur in 20% to 25% of pregnant women. This may be seen in women who are genetically predisposed to diabetes mellitus. Glycosuria usually disappears following delivery. Its presence has been variously attributed to (1) an increased production of hormonal antagonists to insulin, which in turn demands an increased rate of insulin secretion and release; in such genetically predisposed individuals, this demand may not be met, and hyperglycemia may result; (2) an increased glomerular filtration rate, which usually occurs in the first two trimesters of pregnancy. Under these conditions the filtered load of glucose and the delivery of glucose to the proximal tubules may be increased in the absence of marked or detectable hyperglycemia.

B. Renal Disease

As kidney mass decreases, certain renal diseases characterized by a progressive decrement in the nephron population may exhibit an increased glomerular filtration rate per nephron. This may result in an increased filtered load of glucose. Despite presumably an increased reabsorption of glucose per nephron as renal mass decreases, the increment is less than the rise in filtered load of glucose and may result in modest glycosuria. Elevations in blood glucose, which sometimes occur in advanced renal failure, may also contribute to the development of glycosuria.

There are numerous causes of the Fanconi syndrome (see below). These are related either to hereditary disorders (see below) or to acquired disorders such as:

1. Human kidney transplant
2. Multiple myeloma or Bence-Jones proteinuria
3. Amyloidosis
4. Sjogren's syndrome
5. Nephrotic syndrome
6. Pancreatic carcinoma
7. Hyperparathyroidism
8. Heavy metals (see below) as exogenous toxins
9. Exogenous toxins such as lysol, maleic acid, methyl-3-chromone, outdated tetracycline, streptozotocin, vitamin D

In all of the above-listed entities, glycosuria may be a prominent finding.

In acute tubular necrosis, presumably due to decreased glucose reabsorption, glycosuria may sometimes be present.

C. Malignancy

Patients with multiple myeloma or malignancies accompanied by the nephrotic syndrome or amyloidosis may develop the Fanconi syndrome with glycosuria and other proximal tubular transport defects (see below).

D. Drugs

Morphine-induced hyperglycemia is clinically insignificant in humans but is prominent in other species. The hyperglycemia may involve secretion of epinephrine from the adrenal medulla and may require an intact pathway from the central nervous system to the adrenal gland. The mechanisms by which some of the other drugs listed in Table 4-3 produce glycosuria have not yet been determined.

III. Glycosuria Occurring Without Hyperglycemia

A. Renal (Predominantly Hereditary Entities)

1. Renal Glycosuria

This entity may be defined as a state in which the "appearance threshold" for glucose in urine is abnormally low; that is, glycosuria occurs at levels of the blood glucose that would not cause glycosuria in normal subjects. The condition is inherited as a typical Mendelian dominant trait and has been recognized in one family in seven successive generations. When strict criteria for the diagnosis of the entity are applied, it is found to be a rare disease occurring in about .2% of approximately 50,000 cases of glycosuria presenting at the Joslin Clinic. The criteria for diagnosis include (1) glycosuria without hyperglycemia; (2) glycosuria independent of diet; (3) levels of blood glucose influenced only slightly by dietary carbohydrate—glucose tolerance test is normal or slightly flat; (4) glucose is the sugar excreted; (5) subjects are able to store and utilize carbohydrate normally; (6) there are no other discernible renal tubular defects.

Utilizing glucose titration techniques, Elsas and Rosenberg (1969) conducted a genetic analysis of familial renal glycosuria. Based on their data of glucose titrations, they described two types of abnormal curves (see Fig. 4-2): (1) type A patients (true glycosuria), characterized by a low threshold and low TmG, and (2) type B patients (pseudoglycosuria), characterized by a low threshold, an exaggerated splay, and a normal TmG. Most cases of isolated renal glycosuria are a harmless anomaly of renal function and there is no evidence of disease elsewhere. Whether diabetes mellitus may appear in later life in young persons diagnosed initially as having renal glycosuria is a debatable issue. Marble (1932) does not believe that diabetes mellitus does develop in patients with renal glycosuria when his criteria are applied to the diagnosis. Isolated reported cases of diabetes mellitus appearing at a later date in renal glycosuria patients suggest, however, that on rare occasions the conditions may be associated. The tubular transport mechanisms responsible for the defect in renal glycosuria remain uncharacterized. Monasterio et al. (1964) claim there are pathological changes in the proximal tubular cells consisting of vacuolization, accumulation of abnormal periodic acid-Schiff positive material, and abnormalities in the brush border.

In *glucose-galactose malabsorption,* a rare autosomal recessive condition, there is a dual defect of glucose and galactose transport in both the jejunum and proximal renal tubule. The jejunal transport defect causes severe fermentative diarrhea and failure to thrive immediately after birth unless the infant is fed a diet containing fructose as the sole carbohydrate. By contrast, the renal glycosuria, although severe, is of no clinical significance except as an aid to diagnosis. Although galactose transport in the proximal tubule can be shown to be impaired, there is no galactosuria, as plasma galactose concentrations are virtually zero.

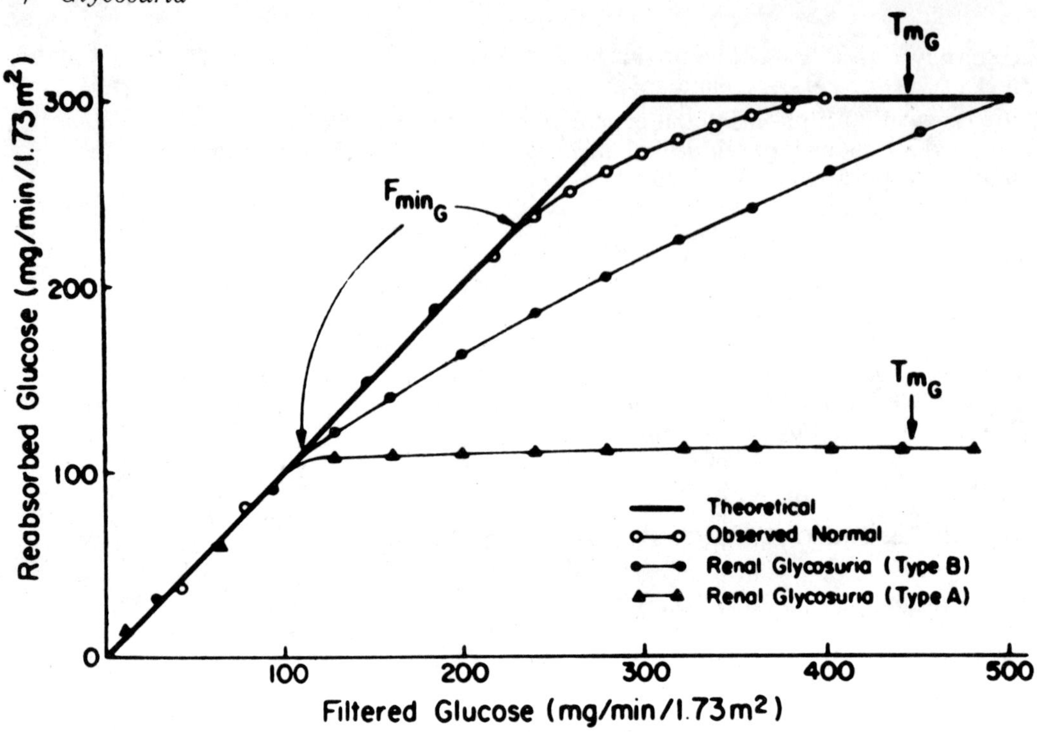

Fig. 4-2.

Renal glucose titration curves. F_{minG}, minimal threshold for filtered glucose (filtered glucose load in which significant amounts of glucose—greater than 1 mg/min—first appear in the urine); TmG, tubular maximal for glucose reabsorption. (Reproduced by permission from J. Clin. Invest. *48:* 1845, 1969.)

Käser et al. have described a unique family in which there was a dual proximal tubular reabsorption defect for glucose and glycine transmitted as an autosomal dominant character. This combination is somewhat remarkable, as there is no other indication that transport of these two compounds is in any way related.

The age at which detection of renal glycosuria occurs is quite variable and, once diagnosed, persists throughout life. Individuals in whom the diagnosis is made are generally asymptomatic, the finding being an incidental one frequently picked up during the second or third decade during a routine physical examination. It has been noted as early as one month of life, and it may be noted in older individuals.

2. Fanconi syndrome

Fanconi syndrome is a generic name for a variety of diseases characterized by hypophosphatemic rickets or osteomalacia, generalized amino aciduria involving all amino acid transport groups, renal glycosuria, and usually systemic acidosis. It results from generalized, nonspecific proximal tubular damage from either hereditary or acquired noxious agents. Causes of the Fanconi syndrome of hereditary origin include cystinosis, Wilson's disease, tyrosinemia, galactosemia, fructose intolerance, and, very occasionally, glycogen storage disease. Other cases that are clearly genetically determined are of unknown origin and are generally termed the adult Fanconi syndrome or "de Toni-Debre-Fanconi" syndrome. Lowe's syndrome is a separate hereditary disease and includes the Fanconi-type renal tubular defect in addition to severe ocular and cerebral damage.

a. Adult Fanconi Syndrome. More than 30 cases of idiopathic Fanconi syndrome without cystinosis or other known causes have been reported, but only a proportion of these are of genetic origin. The term "adult Fanconi syndrome" is strictly a misnomer, as many cases are recognized in childhood. The prognosis of this condition, especially when treated with vitamin D, is relatively good, and many patients survive into adult life. The syndrome probably is a heterogenous group with apparently identical phenotypes but with different hereditary abnormalities. In two families there was, in addition to the syndrome, retinitis pigmentosa. Unlike the specific tubular defects, the generalized tubular abnormalities of the Fanconi syndrome may not necessarily be present at birth, and there is clear evidence of progression of the disease in many case reports. In one family (Luder and Sheldon) when first described, there was only defective tubular reabsorption of glucose and amino acids, but 6 years later the disease had progressed with clear-cut abnormalities of phosphate reabsorption and the development of hypophosphatemic rickets and acidosis.

3. Lowe's Syndrome (Oculocerebrorenal Syndrome)

Close to 100 cases have been described. The syndrome is characterized by dwarfism and rickets, mental deficiency, and hypotonia of muscle. Ocular changes include bilateral cataracts and glaucoma. In the first year, there is nystagmus and impaired vision, and blindness is usually complete by the age of 1 or 2 years. There is cerebral and cerebellar atrophy with ventricular dilatation, neuronal atrophy, and sometimes demyelination. Proteinuria is always present but is variable in amount; early in the disease, it is of the tubular type, with a beta globulin as the main electrophoretic fraction. Renal glycosuria may occur but is relatively infrequent. All described cases have been males except for a single family in which there were two affected females.

4. Cystinosis (Lignac-Fanconi Syndrome)

Cystinosis is an autosomal recessive disease in which the main abnormality is a deposition of cystine crystals in the cornea and reticuloendothelial cells. It occurs in two distinct forms, a benign adult type in which the kidney is unaffected and a serious infantile type, which causes progressive renal failure and death from uremia in late childhood or adolescence. Affected homozygotes of the severe type of the disease can be clinically divided into two groups. About half of the cases present within the first 2 years of life with polyuria, polydipsia, profound anorexia, photophobia, vomiting, dehydration, pyrexia, and failure to thrive. The other half has a less severe clinical course and are in fair health up until early school age, when they suffer from vitamin D-resistant rickets and proximal renal tubular defects consisting of a generalized aminoaciduria, renal glycosuria, phosphaturia, and acidosis. Later, there is progressive contraction of the kidneys with deterioration of renal function leading to terminal uremia at the age of 8 to 15 years.

5. Wilson's Disease (Hepatolenticular Degeneration)

In this entity, there is accumulation of copper, particularly in the liver, brain, kidneys, and cornea. The main symptoms of the disease are due to either degenerative changes in the basal nuclei or to hepatic cirrhosis, but abnormalities of renal function can be shown to occur in most established cases. There is a tubular type of proteinuria, a generalized renal aminoaciduria, renal glycosuria, a high clearance of phosphate and urate, and renal tubular acidosis of the proximal tubular type. Hypercalciuria is frequent and may lead to the formation of calcium phosphate calculi. The renal abnormalities are probably secondary to the presence of copper, particularly in the proximal tubular epithelial cells. The presence of the Kayser-Fleischer ring on ocular examination, increased serum copper or ceruloplasmin levels, and urinary copper excretion help in establishing the diagnosis.

6. Hereditary Tyrosinemia

This is a rare disorder of amino acid metabolism causing secondary renal damage. There is a lack of p-hydroxyphenyl pyruvate oxidase with a high plasma concentration of tyrosine but not of phenylalanine and increased urinary excretion of p-hydroxyphenyllactic acid. There is severe renal damage with generalized aminoaciduria, glycosuria, and phosphaturia with tubular dilatation at necropsy. The clinical picture resembles the Fanconi syndrome with hypophosphatemic rickets. A generalized aminoaciduria occurs similar to that of cystinosis or the adult Fanconi syndrome except that there is a greater output of tyrosine. In addition, there is often hyperplasia of the islets of Langerhans, which may possibly cause the hypoglycemia that occurs in many cases of the disease.

7. Fanconi Syndrome and Glycogen Storage Disease

Three unrelated patients have been described with aminoaciduria, renal glycosuria, and phosphaturia in association with glycogen storage disease type I (hepatic glucose-6-phosphatase deficiency). Glycogen deposits occur in the kidney in this type of glycogenosis, but in almost all described cases, this does not cause any renal functional abnormality. Therefore, the Fanconi syndrome is probably not secondary to the glycogenosis, but the occurrence of the two diseases in three individuals suggests the possibility of genetic linkage, both conditions being the result of a recessive trait.

B. Glycosuria Due to Chemicals or Poisons that Affect Renal Glucose Reabsorption

Phlorizin, when administered to experimental animals, produces a specific defect in glucose reabsorption. Intoxication with heavy metals, particularly chromium, mercury, uranium, ferric compounds, lead, and cadmium, can cause a syndrome resembling the Fanconi syndrome. There is a multiplicity of renal proximal tubular defects characterized by glycosuria, hypophosphatemia, acidosis, aminoaciduria, and some degree of tubular proteinuria. History of previous occupation, accidental or voluntary ingestion of heavy metals for suicidal purposes, and so forth may help in establishing the diagnosis. Measurements of the excretion of heavy metals in the urine may lend support in establishing a definitive diagnosis.

Clinical Problem

L. W. was born in June 1967, weighing 3.7 kg. She was the product of an uneventful pregnancy and delivery. The infant gained weight poorly from birth, and vomiting was frequent. Polydipsia and polyuria were noted at 1 year of age, and there were symptoms of photophobia. She sat at 7 months and started to speak at 12 months, but she did not walk until 3 years of age. At that time, a diagnosis of rickets was made but not specifically investigated. The child was referred to Children's Hospital at the age of 4½ years because of her poor progress. She was alert, pale, and irritable. She was extremely short (82 cm), with a height corresponding to an age of 1.5 years. Although she weighed only 12.6 kg, she was markedly obese for her height. She had a striking body configuration, consisting of a round fat face, short neck, fat shoulders, but thin legs and arms. Roentgenograms revealed the presence of rickets, and there was dental hypoplasia. Bone age was 1 year. Urinalysis showed 2+ proteinuria and 1+ glycosuria. The specific gravity was 1007–1012. Serum calcium concentration was 10.9 mg/dl, inorganic phosphorus, 5.5 mg/dl. The BUN was 50 mg/dl, and her serum creatinine was 1.9 mg/dl. Blood glucose was 125 mg/dl on a random sample. A subsequent fasting blood glucose was 85 mg/dl. Repeated urinalysis revealed 1 to 2+ glycosuria.

Questions

1. What is the most likely cause for the glycosuria in this girl?
2. What additional diagnostic procedures and laboratory data should be obtained?
3. The patient has one sibling, age 15 months. Should he be studied as well?

Discussion

The findings of glycosuria, polyuria, and polydipsia suggest the diagnosis of diabetes mellitus. While diabetes mellitus can occur at an early age, there was no demonstrable family history of diabetes in this case. In addition, glycosuria occurred at a time when blood glucose levels were within normal limits and probably did not exceed the normal renal capacity for glucose reabsorption.

Renal glycosuria is an entity that should be considered in the differential diagnosis. In general, however, patients with renal glycosuria would not have a marked failure to thrive and do not show the degree of growth impairment that this patient demonstrated. While some calories are lost in the urine, in the form of glucose, these losses are presumably not of a significant nature as to markedly impair growth and development. In addition, the presence of renal insufficiency, as evidenced by the plasma creatinine of 1.9 mg/dl and the BUN of 50 mg/dl, would be unusual in renal glycosuria. The association of rickets also points to a diagnosis other than renal glycosuria in the present case. The findings of proteinuria, glycosuria, and renal insufficiency, in addition to rickets, suggest the possibility of multiple renal tubular defects. Analysis of urinary amino acids and measurement of urinary phosphorus and uric acid excretion seem indicated in the present case. The presence of a serum phosphorus concentration of 5.5 mg/dl may suggest that the Fanconi syndrome is probably not responsible for the findings observed. However, the renal insufficiency may have masked the presence of hypophosphatemia. Careful examination of the eyes revealed typical crystalline deposits in the cornea, which were consistent with the diagnosis of cystinosis. Similar deposits were also seen in the bone marrow. In addition, analysis of her urine revealed general aminoaciduria.

The child's rickets was treated initially with 10,000 international units (IU) of vitamin D_2 per day and the rickets healed. However, within 6 months, mild hypercalcemia (12.5 mg/100 ml) developed, which required reduction of the dose to 5000 IU of vitamin D_2 per day. Hyponatremia, acidosis, and eventually hypocalcemia developed, at first responding well to sodium and potassium citrate supplementation. However, renal insufficiency progressed rather rapidly. Despite some negligence on the part of the parents regarding her treatment, the rickets remained well controlled for several years. Growth both in stature and weight was extremely poor and genu valgum gradually developed. During the subsequent 4 years the patient was admitted on four separate occasions to the hospital. Each one of these admissions was prompted by the development of severe acute metabolic acidosis. The final admission to the hospital was when the patient was almost 8½ years, at which time height age was only 2½ years and genu valgum was prominent. Roentgenographic signs of rickets had returned. Hypocalcemia and extreme hyperphosphatemia (11.2 mg/dl) were present, and acidosis and uremia were severe. Terminally, the child lapsed into coma, and death was attributed to uremia.

The diagnosis of cystinosis was confirmed at postmortem. Cystine crystals were present in the bone marrow, spleen, lymph nodes, cornea, and kidney. Typical crystals were also seen in alcohol-fixed sections of the anterior pituitary gland. The kidneys were extremely small. The glomeruli were reduced in number, sclerosed, and hyalinized. Tubules were reduced in number and the remaining tubules were dilated. The liver showed evidence of acute passive congestion but was otherwise found to be normal. Rickets was present histologically.

This case represents a childhood form of cystinosis, a heritable metabolic disorder in which many tissues are affected. Deposits of cystine, as described in this case, are typical of those described in other subjects affected by this entity. Abnormal cystine metabolism has been demonstrated in leukocytes and fibroblasts. From the clinical standpoint the kidney is severely affected, leading to renal impairment and death from uremia, as in this case.

References

Elsas, L. J., and Rosenberg, L. E. "Familial renal glycosuria: A genetic reappraisal of hexose transport by kidney and intestine." J. Clin Invest. *48:* 1845–1854, 1969.

Krane, S. M. "Renal glycosuria." *In:* Metabolic Basis of Inherited Disease, 3rd ed., J. B. Stanbury, J. B. Wyngaarden, and D. S. Fredrickson (eds.). McGraw-Hill, New York, pp. 1536–1547, 1972.

Lawrence, R. D. "Symptomless glycosurias: Sugar tolerance tests." Med. Clin. North Am. *31:* 289, 1947.

Marble, A. "Renal glycosuria." Am. J. Med. Sci. *183:* 811, 1932.

Milne, M. B. "Renal tubular dysfunction." *In:* Diseases of the Kidney, 2nd ed., M. B. Strauss and L. G. Welt (eds.). Little, Brown, Boston, pp. 1104–1107, 1971.

Milne, M. D. Genetic Aspects of Renal Disease in Progress in Medical Genetics, Vol. VII, Steinberg, A. G. and Bearn, A. G., (eds.). Grune & Stratton, New York, 1970.

Monasterio, G., Oliver, J., Muiesan, G., Pardelli, G., Marinezz, W., and McDowell, M. "Renal diabetes as a congenital tubular dysplasia." Am. J. Med. *37:* 44, 1964.

Mudge, G. H., Berndt, W. O., and Valtin, H. "Tubular transport of urea, glucose, phosphate, uric acid, sulfate and thiosulfate." *In:* Handbook of Physiology—Renal Physiology (Section 8). American Physiological Society, Washington, D.C., pp. 598–600, 1973.

Chapter 5

Renal Stones

General Considerations

The severe flank pain associated with acute ureteric obstruction, referred to inappropriately as renal colic, is one of the most severe pains experienced by human beings and one of the oldest recognized maladies, dating back to the age of the Greeks (200–300 B.C.) as a known diagnosis. This pain does not technically qualify as a "colic," since it is not intermittent. Rather, the pain is steady, continuous, and crescendo in character, with only minor fluctuations in intensity. The pain may last 30 minutes to 24 hours, and its onset may be insidious or sudden. It characteristically radiates to the genitalia and thighs. A brief differential diagnostic list of causes of acute urinary retention and renal colic is presented in Table 5-1. This chapter will discuss renal calculi. The other diagnoses in Table 5-1 are discussed in their appropriate chapters, but since calculi often present as renal colic, the differential diagnosis of this acute pain will be considered here.

The description of the pain itself, given above, is not helpful in determining its cause. In addition, the history frequently reveals associated dysuria and abnormalities of urinary volume, such as polyuria, anuria, or alternations between the two. A past history of one of the diseases in the differential diagnosis is the most helpful diagnostic point in the history.

The physical examination is usually negative except for excruciating costovertebral angle tenderness caused by movement of the stretched renal capsule or pelvis. Again, the

Table 5-1

Most Common Causes of Acute Urinary Obstruction and Renal Colic

Acute obstruction
Causing obstruction at all levels of urinary tract:
Calculi
Papillary tissue
Trauma or clots
Renal tubule and infundibulum
Polycystic kidneys
Renal pelvis
Tumors
UPJ* strictures
Ureter
Bladder
Benign prostatic hypertrophy
Nonobstructive causes of renal colic
Trauma
Acute pyelonephritis

*UPJ, ureteropelvic junction.

physical examination is usually not helpful in the differential diagnosis, except in occasional cases of trauma where other injuries may lead to the suspicion of the correct diagnosis.

The urinalysis in patients with renal colic often reveals hematuria, pyuria, proteinuria, and crystalluria. The latter may be helpful, if it is severe, in establishing the cause of the pain as calculi and also in pointing to the type of stone present for purposes of later evaluation. Bacteriologic examination of the urine is essential to establish the presence of infection. This may be primary, as in acute pyelonephritis, or superimposed on any of the other diagnoses. Fever and leukocytosis also suggest infection associated with the cause of pain. Abnormalities of renal function may be present if the obstruction has been present for a sufficient period of time or if the process is a chronic one.

Radiographic analysis begins with a flat film of the abdomen and proceeds through intravenous pyelography. The latter reveals not only the site of the obstructing lesion but also the morphological details of an enlarged kidney, the calyceal system, on the obstructed side and the lower urinary tract. The correct diagnosis is usually suggested by pyelography, and this procedure is, therefore, the cornerstone of the evaluation for renal colic. The vast majority of renal stones are radiopaque, since they contain calcium. Uric acid and matrix stones are radiolucent. Cystine stones are weakly radiopaque as a result of their sulfur content.

When satisfactory visualization of the urinary conduit system cannot be obtained by intravenous pyelography, retrograde pyelography can be of value. However, it must be used judiciously because of the risk of disseminating bacteria from an infected urinary tract. A new technique, computer-assisted tomography, is an extremely useful noninvasive technique for evaluating obstruction of the urinary tract and has replaced some of the indications for retrograde pyelography. The exact role of this new technique in the evaluation of acute urinary obstruction will be established as greater familiarity with it is gained.

Once the cause of the renal colic is established, treatment proceeds toward relief of pain with removal of the obstruction. Renal stones are either allowed to pass spontaneously or approached by various urologic techniques. The evaluation of the cause of the stone-forming disorder must wait until the patient is stable and eating a regular diet, until renal function has stabilized, and until collections of 24-hour urine samples will not be interrupted by recurrent obstruction.

Differential Diagnosis of Renal Calculi

The second phase of the differential diagnosis begins following the identification of a renal stone-forming disorder and the return to stability following treatment of acute renal colic or obstruction. This has often been documented and known for several years prior to an adequate pathogenetic evaluation. In the past, delays in the evaluation of stone-forming processes have reflected the frustration of many physicians in their inability to diagnose the cause and undertake a successful treatment program for most stone formers. Advances in the understanding of the pathogenesis of stone-forming diseases now allow the vast majority of individuals to be much better categorized as to the pathogenetic mechanisms involved in their stone-forming process, and more successful treatment programs have resulted.

A list of the most common diagnostic possibilities in patients with renal calculi is given in Table 5-2 according to the major stone constituents. This approach to the differential diagnosis of stone-forming processes ascribes a central role to the analysis of crystal composition. By crystallography the differential diagnosis is narrowed to the consideration of disease states involved in the precipitation of the known crystal. Analysis of renal stones can yield information beyond basic qualitative determination of crystal type. Techniques such as x-ray diffraction and polarizing microscopy yield a topographic analysis of stone architecture that describes the time sequence involved in the development of stones with a mixed crystal composition. For instance, a calcium apatite core in a largely calcium oxalate stone indicates urinary supersaturation with calcium phosphates rather than calcium oxalate as the pathogenesis of the stone nidus. A more simple example is a shell of triple phosphates on a calcium oxalate stone indicating urinary tract infection, with urea-splitting bacteria complicating the underlying calcium oxalate stone-forming disorder.

I. Calcium-containing Stones

Approximately 90% of all renal calculi contain calcium. Of those patients known to form calcium-containing stones, 40% to 60% will have hypercalciuria. An incidence higher than 60% has been reported in more recent series. Thus, 24-hour excretion rates of calcium are important parts of any stone evaluation. The definition of hypercalciuria, however, is not as simple as the 300 mg/day upper limit of normal excretion for men and 250 mg/day for women often referred to in textbooks.

Normal individuals absorb sufficient calcium from their diet to be in slight positive calcium balance. Thus, between 200 and 400 mg are absorbed from the intestine each day, with 50–150 mg appearing in the urine and the remainder being secreted back into the intestine as endogenous fecal calcium (100–200 mg) or incorporated into the exchangeable calcium pool largely in bone. Thus, from dietary calcium intakes of 400–2000 mg/day, intestinal calcium absorption will not vary greatly, and subsequently urinary calcium excretion varies little compared to changes in dietary calcium intake. However, patients with idiopathic hypercalciuria all manifest intestinal hyperabsorption of calcium either primary or secondary in nature. At low calcium intakes the degree of hyperabsorption may be such that urinary calcium is in the textbook normal range, that is, a patient who may excrete 220 mg/day of calcium on a 400 mg/day intake. This patient, when given a diet containing 1 gm/day of calcium, may manifest urinary excretion rates of 300–500 mg/day, which is definitely hypercalciuric. Thus, it is important to define hypercalciuria in terms of calcium intake. This is a difficult task on a general medical hospital floor because of inaccuracies inherent in diet histories and the inconstancy of hospital diets.

A rough estimate of dietary calcium intake can be gained from simultaneous determination of calcium and phosphorus excretion, since the major dietary sources of calcium in the United States—dairy products—are also high in phosphorus content. A phosphorus excretion rate of 600 mg/day indicates a maximum dietary calcium intake of 680 mg if all the phosphorus was of dairy product origin, and a 70% absorption rate for phosphorus is assumed. Urinary excretion of 1–1.5 gm of phosphorus per day usually indicates adequate calcium intakes for the detection of hypercalciuric states. Patients with hypercalciuria will excrete greater than 4 mg/kg body weight of calcium per day with dietary intakes of 1 gm/day of calcium (phosphorus excretion 1–1.5 gm/day) or 200 mg/day on calcium intake of 400 mg/day according to more accurate balance type data.

A. Hypercalciuria

1. Resorptive

As listed in Table 5-2, there are three general pathogenetic mechanisms that produce hypercalciuria. The first is an increased rate of bone resorption resulting in the release of calcium-containing bone salts into the circulation. The most common entity that causes renal stones in this category is primary hyperparathyroidism.

Primary hyperparathyroidism is characterized typically by elevated levels of circulating parathyroid hormone, hypercalcemia (especially high ionized plasma calcium), hypophosphatemia, and elevated alkaline phosphatase. The diagnosis should be suspected in asymptomatic individuals who are found to be hypercalcemic on chemical screening profiles. The disease accounts for 10% to 15% of all renal stone formers, and prior to large-scale chemistry screening tests, nephrolithiasis was the most common presenting complication of primary hyperparathyroidism.

Table 5-2

Differential Diagnosis of Stone-forming Diseases by Stone Constituents

I. Calcium-containing stones
  A. With hypercalciuria
    1. Resorptive
      a. Hyperparathyroidism
      b. Idiopathic hypercalciuria (normocalcemic primary hyperparathyroidism)
      c. Hyperthyroidism
      d. Immobilization
      e. Senile osteoporosis
      f. Metastatic cancer
      g. Multiple myeloma
      h. Vitamin D intoxication
    2. Absorptive
      a. Idiopathic hypercalciuria (primary hyperabsorptive type)
      b. Vitamin D intoxication
      c. Milk alkali syndrome
      d. Sarcoidosis
      e. Beryllium poisoning
    3. Reabsorptive (defective renal tubular ion excretion)
      a. Idiopathic hypercalciuria
        i. Defective renal calcium reabsorption
        ii. Defective renal phosphate reabsorption
      b. Metabolic acidosis
      c. Corticosteroids (exogenous or endogenous)
  B. With normocalciuria
    1. Impaired excretion of inhibitor substance
      a. Magnesium
      b. Pyrophosphate
      c. Citric acid
      d. pH
    2. Transient excess urinary supersaturation for calcium oxalate or calcium phosphate
    3. Association with uric acid
II. Oxalate-containing stones
  A. Inflammatory bowel disease
    1. Crohn's disease
    2. Ulcerative colitis
  B. Intestinal bypass
  C. Primary hyperoxaluria
    1. Type I (glycolic aciduria)
    2. Type II (L-glyceric aciduria)
  D. Methoxyflurane anesthesia
  E. Excess ingestion of oxalate (rhubarb poisoning)
    or of oxalate precursors (ethylene glycol poisoning)
  F. Pyridoxine deficiency
III. Urate-containing stones
  A. Hyperuricosuria
    1. Gout
    2. Secondary hyperuricemia
      a. Lymphoproliferative diseases
      b. Psoriasis
      c. Glycogen storage disease type I
      d. Myxedema
      e. Hyperparathyroidism
      f. Drugs, e.g. diuretics
    3. Hypersecretors (hyperuricosuria with normouricemia)
  B. Persistent acid pH of urine
    1. Inflammatory bowel disease with diarrhea
    2. Ileostomy

Table 5-2—continued

3. Acidifying medications
4. Loss of normal alkaline tide
IV. Magnesium ammonium calcium phosphate (triple phosphate stones)
A. Urine infection with urea splitters
V. Cystinuria
VI. Xanthinuria

Excessive levels of circulating parathyroid hormone (PTH) exert their action on three organs: bone, intestine, and kidney. In bone, PTH stimulates both osteoclastic and osteoblastic activity but with the balance strongly in favor of bone resorption. The consequent release of calcium into the circulation is a major factor in producing hypercalcemia, which is the hallmark of the disease. At the renal level, PTH stimulates the conversion of 25-hydroxycholecalciferol to 1,25-dihydroxycholecalciferol (1,25 OH-Vit D_3), which plays an important role at the level of both the bone cells and the intestine. The interaction between PTH and 1,25 OH-Vit D_3 at the level of bone is not understood completely, but 1,25 OH-Vit D_3 is required for full biologic activity of PTH. In the intestine, 1,25 OH-Vit D_3 increases calcium absorption, thereby contributing to the hypercalcemia of hyperparathyroidism. Despite an increase in intestinal calcium absorption, calcium balance studies reveal negative balances of approximately 50–100 mg of calcium per day. Most of the negative calcium balance is due to hypercalciuria.

The renal effects of PTH as they relate to the pathogenesis of stone formation are many and complicated. Hypercalciuria results from a high filtered load of calcium, despite a direct action of PTH increasing distal tubular calcium reabsorption. The small capacity of distal tubular calcium transport (normally responsible for reabsorption of 5% to 10% of the filtered calcium load) is easily overwhelmed by the increased calcium delivery to this reabsorptive site. PTH also depresses renal tubular phosphate transport, resulting in increased renal phosphate clearance and hypophosphatemia. Fractional excretion of phosphate is determined by expressing the clearance of phosphate

$$\left(\frac{U_P V}{P_P}\right)$$

as a percent of the creatinine clearance

$$\left(\frac{U_{Cr} V}{P_{Cr}}\right),$$

that is,

$$\frac{C_P}{C_{Cr}} \text{ x } 100.$$

It is customary to convert this to fractional tubular reabsorption of phosphate (% TRP), which is

$$\left(1 - \frac{C_P}{C_{Cr}}\right) \text{ x } 100.$$

The volume term (V) of the clearance equations can be cancelled, yielding

$$1 - \frac{U_{PO_4} \text{ x } P_{Cr}}{U_{Cr} \text{ x } P_{PO_4}} \text{ x } 100 =$$

fractional tubular resorption of phosphorus (TRP), in which U_{PO4} and P_{PO4} represent urinary and plasma phosphorus concentrations and U_{cr} and P_{cr}, urinary and plasma creatinine concentrations. The TRP in normal fasting subjects varies from 80% to 95%. Hyperparathyroid subjects have low TRP values in relationship to their plasma phosphorus. Prior to the development of radioimmunoassays for PTH, great reliance was placed on TRP values in diagnosing primary hyperparathyroidism. Its current importance is in assessing the renal transport rate for phosphorus in many disease states, including hypercalciuria.

The high urinary calcium and phosphate concentrations in patients with primary hyperparathyroidism frequently exceed the capacity of urine to keep these substances in solution. This is especially so when the effect of PTH on renal bicarbonate handling is considered. PTH depresses proximal tubular reabsorptive rates of sodium, phosphorus, and bicarbonate. Thus the pH of the urine tends to be higher than normal in hyperparathyroid subjects, and some even develop a proximal form of renal tubular acidosis. The solubility of apatite (a complexed calcium phosphate) decreases markedly in urine pH's above 6. The tendency of hyperparathyroid subjects with high urine calcium and phosphorus concentrations to exhibit higher urine pH's is important in the development of calcium phosphate precipitation. Once the initial crystal nidus forms, further calcium precipitation may occur as calcium oxalate. Thus, renal stones in hyperparathyroid subjects almost always have at least a core of calcium phosphate, either apatite [Ca_{10} $(PO_4)_6$ OH_2] or brushite ($CaHPO_4 \bullet 2H_2O$), and the major factor producing renal calculi in hyperparathyroidism is the tendency for urinary calcium phosphate concentrations to exceed the urine's capacity to maintain these salts in solution.

Diseases associated with secondary hyperparathyroidism, such as intestinal malabsorption and renal tubular acidosis, are also frequently associated with calcium stones. These patients are generally mildly hypocalcemic and have low filtered loads of calcium. The increased bone resorption due to PTH is not sufficient to offset the calcium malabsorption of certain intestinal diseases, and the pathogenesis of stones is not dependent on PTH-induced hypercalciuria. In renal tubular acidosis, hypercalciuria may be present, probably as a consequence of the acidosis itself. These disorders will be discussed later in this chapter in relation to the pathogenesis of stone formation associated with them.

Not infrequently, hypercalciuric patients forming calcium stones will have normal total serum calcium and high PTH levels. This is especially remarkable, since not all hypercalcemic primary hyperparathyroid patients are hypercalciuric. These patients usually manifest mild elevations of plasma ionized calcium, and when their renal calcium reabsorption is stimulated by thiazide administration, they become frankly hypercalcemic. These patients respond to partial parathyroidectomy with normocalciuria and disappearance of their stone-forming diathesis. This group of patients can be alternatively considered as having "normocalcemic primary hyperparathyroidism" or, as they present, hypercalciuria of resorptive origin. The pathogenesis of stone formation in this disorder, which is also applicable to primary hyperparathyroidism with hypercalcemia, is shown in Figure 5-1.

This chain of events may be difficult to differentiate from defective renal calcium reabsorption, since both disease states result in high PTH levels in plasma. However, thia-

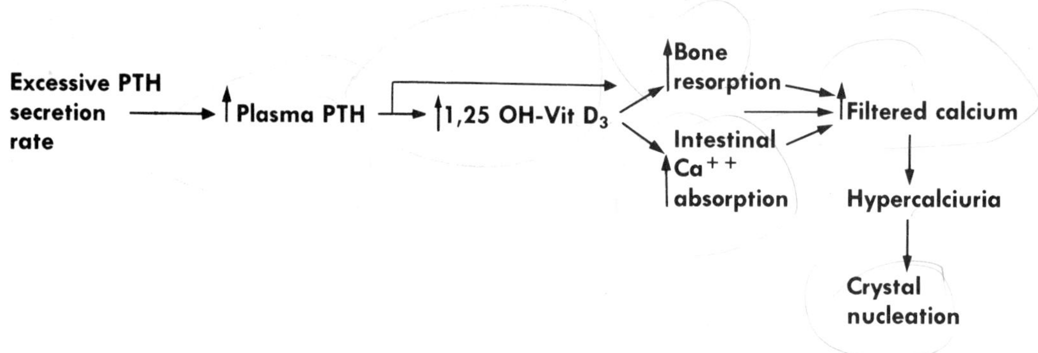

Fig. 5-1.

Pathogenesis of resorptive hypercalciuria.

zide administration in the latter condition results in normocalcemia, normocalciuria, and normalization of plasma PTH in contradistinction to the effects of thiazides in patients with resorptive hypercalciuria.

The differential diagnosis of resorptive hypercalciuria includes several entities that cause renal stones much less frequently than they do hypercalciuria. They include *hyperthyroidism, immobilization, osteoporosis,* and *malignancies.* They will not be discussed here in depth. *Multiple myeloma* not only causes hypercalciuria but also hyperuricosuria. This combination is especially prone to permit crystallization of calcium salts, because uric acid decreases the capacity of urine to maintain them in metastable supersaturation. However, calcium or uric acid stones in multiple myeloma are less common than acute renal failure due to uric acid deposition or Bence-Jones protein precipitation.

Vitamin D intoxication is very uncommon, although its occurrence may be seen with greater frequency with the increased clinical use of potent hydroxylated metabolites of cholecalciferol. It carries a high occurrence rate of nephrocalcinosis and renal stones. The hypercalcemia and hypercalciuria result from both increased bone resorption and intestinal calcium absorption.

2. Absorptive Hypercalciuria

Primary absorptive hypercalciuria, presenting as calcium stones in patients with hypercalciuria and normocalcemia, is the single most frequent diagnosis made in the author's series of patients with nephrolithiasis. The pathogenesis of this disease is shown in Figure 5-2.

The basis for intestinal hyperabsorption of calcium is incompletely understood, but high levels of 1,25 OH-Vit D_3 have been found in preliminary investigations by Haussler. The finding of hypercalciuria without hypercalcemia in this setting may be due in part to decreased levels of PTH to stimulate renal calcium reabsorption. This category of patients is similar to patients with a renal phosphate leak (discussed below), except that these patients have normal plasma phosphate and normal values for TRP. An adequate treatment regimen remains to be defined for this patient population, but inhibitors of calcium absorption may constitute logical choices. Thiazides or neutral phosphate therapy would be expected to be less effective, although definitive data on this point do not exist.

Other Causes of Absorptive Hypercalciuria. Other forms of absorptive hypercalciuria are less common. *Vitamin D intoxication* is an obvious cause of hyperabsorption. Patients with *sarcoid* demonstrate hypersensitivity to normal levels of vitamin D metabolites, hyperabsorb calcium, develop hypercalcemia, and exhibit low PTH levels. Treatment with adrenal steroids, which impair the action of vitamin D on calcium absorption, represents effective therapy. The *milk alkali syndrome* is an uncommon entity characterized by ingestion of calcium and alkali in combination and sufficient quantity to result in hyperabsorption, hypercalcemia, and hypercalciuria in the presence of alkaline urines. The result is

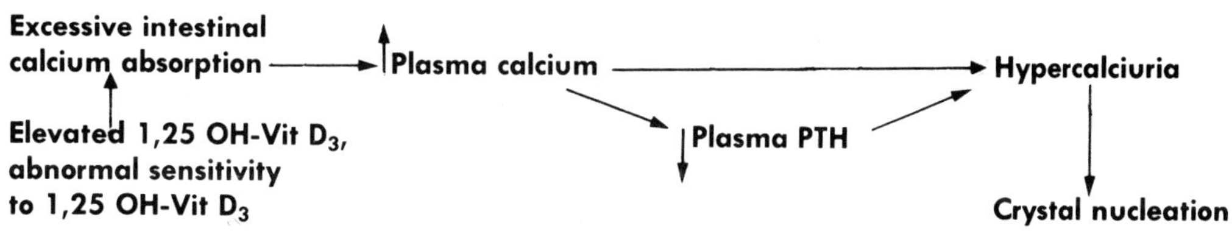

Fig. 5-2.

Pathogenesis of primary absorptive ("idiopathic") hypercalciuria.

the development of nephrocalcinosis and calcium phosphate stones. *Beryllium poisoning* is rare but also stimulates intestinal calcium absorption through an unknown mechanism.

3. Reabsorptive (Defective Renal Tubular Excretion)

The final mechanism of hypercalciuria is defective renal reabsorption. There are two disease categories listed here that were previously categorized as idiopathic hypercalciuria: *defective calcium reabsorption* and *defective phosphate reabsorption.* The pathogenesis of hypercalciuria and the diagnostic tests of defective renal calcium reabsorption are shown in Figure 5-3.

This disease mimics resorptive hypercalciuria or normocalcemic hyperparathyroidism very closely, except that treatment with thiazides results in maintained normocalcemia, normal PTH levels, and normocalciuria. It is less common than the other forms of hypercalciuria in the author's experience.

The pathogenesis of hypercalciuria associated with defective renal phosphate handling is portrayed in Figure 5-4. Low phosphate concentrations are a potent stimulus to the production of 1,25 OH-Vit D_3, thus explaining the tendency of patients with severe phosphate depletion to exhibit hypercalcemia. In patients with renal stones, low plasma phosphorus, and low values of TRP, the high levels of 1,25 OH-Vit D_3 and low PTH levels mimic the findings of the primary intestinal hyperabsorption syndrome discussed above. However, the hypophosphatemia and low TRP are differentially diagnostic. Treatment with neutral phosphates in these patients has been shown to correct the hypercalciuria.

Hypercalciuria is often seen in disease states associated with either *acute or chronic metabolic acidosis.* Although the pathogenesis is not completely certain, the most likely cause is that acidosis directly depresses renal calcium reabsorption. Experimentally induced acute metabolic acidosis was found to be associated with hyperphosphatemia and mild elevations of parathyroid hormone. The former depressed ionized calcium slightly despite the effect of acidosis to decrease albumin binding of calcium and thereby increase ionized calcium. Thus, increased bone resorption from the effects of acid or PTH was not the basis for the observed hypercalciuria, since the filtered calcium load decreased. Chronic metabolic acidosis is also associated with high PTH levels and slight hypocalcemia, making a resorptive basis for hypercalciuria unlikely.

In *renal tubular acidosis (RTA),* hypercalciuria, nephrocalcinosis, and calcium phosphate renal stones are seen frequently. PTH levels may be elevated or normal. Bone histology demonstrates osteomalacia rather than the osteitis fibrosa and increased osteoclastic activity that would be expected from excess PTH. In addition, patients with RTA tend to be hypocalcemic, although ionized calcium levels are closer to normal than total plasma calcium. Thus the cause of the hypercalciuria is more likely a result of a direct effect of chronic acidosis on renal calcium reabsorption. However, patients with incomplete forms

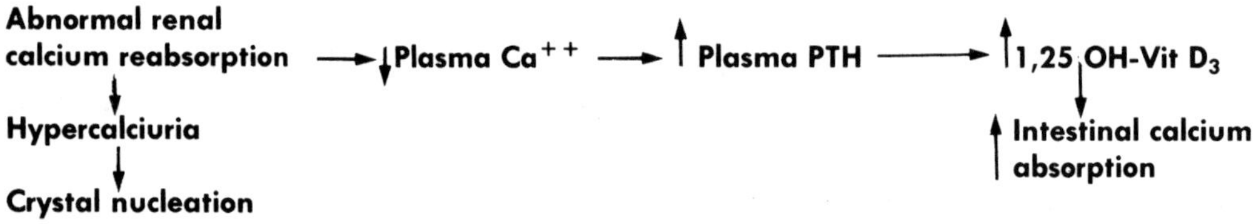

Fig. 5-3.

Pathogenesis of reabsorptive hypercalciuria—renal calcium leak.

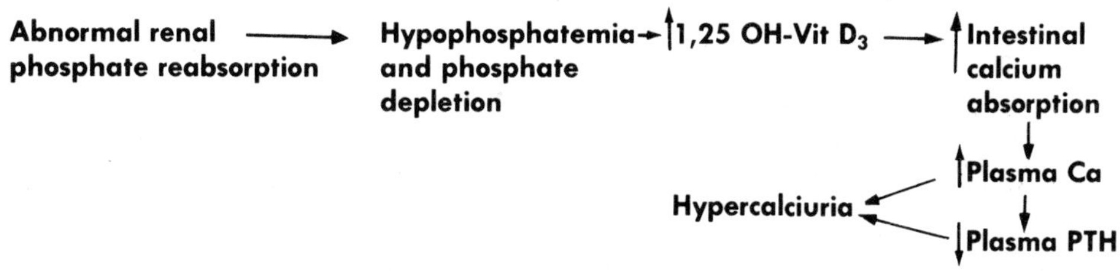

Fig. 5-4.

Pathogenesis of reabsorptive hypercalciuria—renal phosphate leak.

of RTA also manifest hypercalciuria approximately 20% of the time, while a discernible abnormality of plasma pH is not detectable. This may represent an inherited tendency, since family members of patients with RTA also manifest a high incidence of hypercalciuria without associated acidification defects. The nephrocalcinosis and calcium phosphate stone-forming tendency of patients with RTA are also contributed to importantly by decreased urine solubility for brushite or apatite as compared to normal urine. This is due to low excretion rates of citrate, which chelates calcium, and the tendency for high urine pH's, which decreases apatite solubility. These latter factors may produce renal stone disease and nephrocalcinosis in the absence of hypercalciuria.

Chronic acetazolamide (Diamox) therapy is another cause of metabolic acidosis, mild hypercalciuria, mild hyperphosphaturia, and high urine pH's that routinely results in nephrocalcinosis and renal stone formation. Diamox is most commonly employed to decrease intraocular pressure in glaucoma patients. Calcium phosphate stone formation results from the now familiar triad of increased urinary calcium and phosphate concentrations and high urine pH's.

The *chronic administration of corticosteroids and Cushing's disease* are both associated with the development of osteoporosis, a tendency to hypercalciuria, and a definite increased incidence, though not great, of renal stone formation. The hypercalciuria is thought to result from both the mineralocorticoid and glucocorticoid activity of the agents. The former causes expansion of extracellular fluid volume and decreases proximal tubular sodium and calcium reabsorption. The rejected sodium is reabsorbed distally under the influence of aldosterone, but the calcium tends to be excreted. Glucocorticoids also increase bone resorption, and increases in filtered calcium may be demonstrated on occasion. However, the tendency toward hypercalcemia is, in part, compensated by steroidal inhibition of vitamin D activity, which decreases intestinal calcium absorption. The exact nature of the pathogenesis of hypercalciuria and renal stones in states of steroid excess remains to be fully elucidated.

B. With Normocalciuria

Patients with calcium-containing stones who do not exhibit hypercalciuria constitute a group of stone-forming patients difficult to define and to treat; the condition is here referred to generically as normocalciuric calcium lithiasis. Many theories for the basis of stone formation in this group of patients have been suggested. Currently, three general concepts regarding normocalciuric calcium stone formation merit consideration: impaired excretion of inhibitor substances, transient periods of excess urinary supersaturation with calcium oxalate or calcium phosphate, and finally, the role of uric acid in promoting calcium salt precipitation.

Urine normally contains substances that give it the capability of maintaining in solution concentrations of calcium phosphate or oxalate that would precipitate out of an aqueous mixture. These precipitation inhibitory substances are chiefly magnesium, pyrophosphates, citric acid, and urine pH.

Some investigators have reported low magnesium to calcium excretion ratios in patients with calcium stone-forming processes. Other investigators, including this author, have been unable to document this finding. However, magnesium is known to inhibit calcium oxalate precipitation by binding with oxalate, rendering it unavailable for calcium binding. Magnesium supplements may thus be beneficial if magnesium-to-calcium excretion ratios are less than 0.3.

Pyrophosphates are potent inhibitors of calcium phosphate precipitation. Normal excretion of pyrophosphate is 1–4 mg/day. Because of this small amount in normal urine and difficulty with accurate determinations, an adequate test of the role of pyrophosphate in preventing crystal nucleation has yet to be developed. Also, controversy exists as to whether excretion of pyrophosphates is normal or low in calcium stone-forming states.

Citric acid is a strong chelator of calcium, thus removing it from association with oxalate and phosphate ions. It is the one inhibitory substance known to play a role in stone formation. In RTA patients, both deficient citrate excretion and high urine pH are critical to the development of nephrocalcinosis and renal stones. The role of urine pH in the solubility of other substances is also critical for uric acid and cysteine, which are discussed below.

With the development of the capability to measure urinary ion activity products, several investigators have found that normocalciuric calcium oxalate stone formers are more prone to oversaturate their urine with calcium oxalate at some time during the day than normals. Patients with mixed calcium phosphate and calcium oxalate stones tend to oversaturate with calcium phosphate. Yet, when 24-hour urinary saturation levels are examined, these patients may not differ significantly from normal subjects. The factors producing this tendency to exceed the formation production for crystal nucleation have not been clarified. But attention must be directed toward the measurement of urinary activity and formation products as the best means of assessing the patient's urine in terms of its current ionic strength and its propensity to crystal nucleation, the first step in stone formation.

The determination of activity products has demonstrated the important role of oxalate in the pathogenesis of normocalciuric calcium oxalate nephrolithiasis. Studies by Robertson et al. (1968, 1969) have demonstrated that addition of calcium to normal urine does not produce oversaturation of calcium oxalate because much of the calcium is complexed to citrate, sulfate, and phosphate. However, the addition of oxalate in the presence of normal amounts of calcium results in oversaturation for calcium oxalate and precipitation of the salt. Thus, transient changes in urinary oxalate concentrations seem to play an important role in normocalciuric nephrolithiasis.

The final factor for consideration in the pathogenesis of normocalciuric calcium lithiasis is the association, made with increasing frequency, of hyperuricosuria and small amounts of uric acid in calcium oxalate or mixed calcium oxalate-calcium phosphate stones. Coe et al. (1975) found hyperuricosuria in 55 of 146 calcium stone formers, 58 of whom were hypercalciuric. The overlap between hyperuricosuria and hypercalciuria was not given. The basis for the hyperuricosuria was thought to be dietary in origin with a shift in the patient's dietary patterns to high purine foods, which is a common occurrence when avoiding calcium-containing dairy products. Also, some patients demonstrated hyperuricosuria at relatively low plasma urate concentrations, suggesting a defective renal tubular urate handling. Hyperuricosuria is important in terms of calcium oxalate crystal growth through promotion of epitaxial growth due to shared interatomic dimensions of sodium urate and calcium oxalate.

II. Oxalate-containing Stones

After calcium, oxalate is the most frequent constituent in urinary stones and is found in about two thirds of all stones. These may be pure calcium oxalate stones or, frequently, calcium oxalate with other constituents (calcium phosphate, uric acid, and magnesium ammonium phosphate). In the vast majority of cases, patients with calcium oxalate stones have no detectable abnormality in oxalate excretion or oxalate metabolism. They either have disordered calcium metabolism leading to hypercalciuria, or they fit into the group of normocalciuric calcium stone formers. Both of these disorders were discussed above. The normal excretion of oxalic acid is 20–55 mg/24 hours. Most of urinary oxalate excretion is derived from endogenous production and very little from dietary sources. Average oxalate ingestion is 100 mg/day, but only 3% to 5% is absorbed normally. Oxalic acid is a nonmetabolizable end product of glycine metabolism, and all that is synthesized is excreted. The six known conditions that result in excess oxalate excretion are listed in Table 5-2. Those that are involved through excess synthesis are shown in Figure 5-5 by the letter corresponding to the condition as listed in Table 5-2.

A. Inflammatory Bowel Disease and Intestinal Bypass

The hyperoxaluria seen in patients with inflammatory bowel disease and in patients with intestinal bypasses for obesity is related to hyperabsorption of dietary oxalate, now the most common cause of hyperoxaluria. The mechanism for hyperabsorption is not understood but appears to be related to the degree of steatorrhea, the extent of bowel resection in operated patients (greater than 30 cm of ileum), and the delivery of bile salts to the large intestine where they stimulate oxalate absorption. Treatment with cholestyramine in these patients decreases the diarrhea and reverses the hyperoxaluria. Also, decreased dietary oxalate ingestion is effective.

B. Primary Hyperoxaluria

Primary hyperoxaluria represents an autosomal recessive inborn error of metabolism. Type I is caused by deficient concentration of the enzyme alpha-ketoglutarate: glyoxalate carboligase in the liver, kidney, and spleen. Type II is caused by a defective enzyme in serine metabolism that also converts glyoxalate to glycolate, accounting for the increased excretion of both oxalate and L-glyceric acid.

C. Other Causes of Hyperoxaluria

Methoxyflurane anesthesia causes several metabolic abnormalities related to the kidney, including a nephrogenic diabetes insipidus and an acute renal failure associated with varying degrees of intratubular and interstitial calcium oxalate deposition. The mechanism of calcium oxalate precipitation has not been elucidated.

Ethylene glycol intoxication results in acute renal failure characterized by increased excretion of oxalate and deposition of oxalate crystals in the tubules.

Pyridoxine deficiency leads to increased endogenous production of oxalate through decreased transamination of glyoxalate to glycine, but only rarely has this led to stone production.

III. Urate-containing Stones

Uric acid stone formers can be divided into two general groups as shown in Table 5-2. Uric acid is the major constituent of 5% to 10% of kidney stones. From 10% to 25% of patients with gout have uric acid stones, and 30% to 40% of patients with lymphoprolifer-

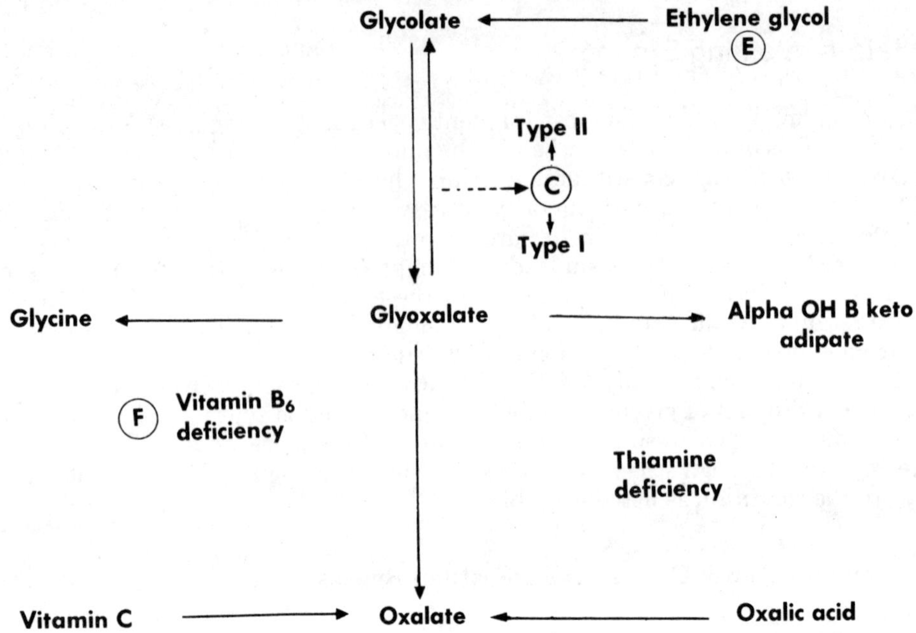

Fig. 5-5.

Pathways of oxalate synthesis.

ative disorders and hyperuricemia manifest uric acid precipitation. However, most patients with hyperuricosuria do not have clinical gout or a lymphoproliferative disease. They manifest disordered renal uric acid handling or display increased urine acidity.

Normal uric acid synthesis is approximately 1 gm/day. About 25% to 30% is excreted into the gut and destroyed by uricase from intestinal bacteria. About 500–700 mg/day is excreted in the urine. Plasma urate is completely filterable and net reabsorption is usually 90% to 95%. Urinary urate represents the balance between that filtered and reabsorbed and that secreted. A few patients with uric acid stones exhibit hyperuricosuria without hyperuricemia, and most of these have enhanced tubular secretion of uric acid.

The solubility of uric acid is much less than its sodium or potassium salts. The result is that stones are uric acid rather than urates. Thus, urine pH is a major determinant of uric acid solubility. The pK of the N-9 position of uric acid is 5.75, and at urine pH's of 5, 85% of the urate is undissociated uric acid. At this pH, only 6–8 mg% of urate is soluble, so that supersaturation occurs easily. At urine pH of 7, 158 mg% of urate is soluble. Any condition that results in decreased urinary water and/or persistently acid urine has a significant chance of precipitating uric acid. One postulate of uric acid stone formation supports a defect in renal tubular ammonia production as the primary defect. This requires excretion of a more acid urine to balance the normal metabolic acid load. This postulate has been both supported and disproven. Another possibility is the loss of the normal "alkaline tide" that occurs after meals, and since urine is often supersaturated with urate, patients have impaired ability to maintain a metastable state of uric acid supersaturation despite normal mechanism of ammonia and titratable acid production.

IV. Stones with Magnesium Ammonium Phosphate

Patients with chronic infection of the urinary tract manifest renal stones composed of magnesium ammonium phosphate (struvite) and variable amounts of calcium phosphate—thus the term "triple phosphate stones." The urine of these patients has high levels of ammonia produced from urea by bacteria containing urease. Ammonia production results in alkalinization of the urine and consequent oversaturation of the urine for triple phosphates that are less soluble at alkaline pH. These stones grow rapidly and are the type most prone to fill the pelvicalyceal system (staghorn calculi). They require surgical extirpation before successful treatment of the urinary tract infection can be accomplished, since urea-splitting organisms, especially *Proteus* species, have been cultured from and are harbored in the stone itself. These stones also recur after removal unless extirpation is complete and the infection is eradicated.

Triple phosphate precipitation is often superimposed on another stone-forming process when the original stone causes urinary tract infection. An important tool in establishing the primacy or the secondary nature of infection-related stone formation is topographical stone analysis. A central core of crystalloid other than triple phosphate suggests that the infection was a secondary process.

V. Cystine Stones

The appearance of hexagonal crystals of cystine in the urine is never a normal finding and identifies the disease state of congenital cystinuria. This autosomal-recessive trait results in defective renal tubular reabsorption of cystine, lysine, arginine, and ornithine (dibasic amino acids). When the resulting cystinuria reaches cystine to creatinine concentration ratios of .25 or greater or when total cystine excretion exceeds 400 mg/24 hours, then stone formation occurs.

Cystinuria accounts for 1% to 3% of all renal stones, but since 10% of the stones passed by cystinurics do not contain measurable cystine, the urine of all stone formers should be tested for cystine. The microscopic analysis of urine for cystine crystals is only adequate for a concentrated urine. Therefore, the cyanide-nitroprusside reaction should be performed. The nitroprusside test for the detection of urinary cystine is easily performed by the method of Brand et al. (1930). The reagents necessary to perform the test are (1) concentrated ammonium hydroxide, (2) 5% sodium cyanide, and (3) 5% sodium nitroprusside (this solution should be recently prepared). To 5 ml of urine, add one drop of ammonium hydroxide and 2 ml of sodium cyanide. Mix and allow to stand for 10 minutes. Add sodium nitroprusside drop by drop and shake. A permanent purplish-red color indicates the presence of cysteine or cystine. Confirmation of positive nitroprusside tests is obtained by quantitative estimation of cystine by paper chromatography.

VI. Xanthine Stones

Xanthine stones are very uncommon. Elevated urinary xanthine is seen as an autosomal recessive trait associated with deficiency of xanthine oxidase. The effect of this enzyme deficiency is reproduced by the administration of the drug allopurinol, which has the potential of increasing urinary xanthine excretion, although this has not been reported in the absence of increased purine synthesis. Normal urinary xanthine excretion is 5–9 mg/day, and its solubility is 5 mg/100 ml of urine at pH 5 and 13 mg/100 ml at pH 7. Stone formation results from oversaturation of xanthine due to higher than normal excretion rates.

Diagnostic Protocol

The stone-forming disorders described above can be diagnosed either on an outpatient or an inpatient basis with an appropriate metabolic protocol that involves several 24-hour urine collections. The number of 24-hour urines required is greater than expected because precipitation of calcium salts must be prevented by addition of a strong acid to the collection receptacle. Therefore, urinary uric acid cannot be determined on the same specimen as calcium. The tests involved in the evaluation of stone formers are listed in Table 5-3

Table 5-3

Diagnostic Protocol for Nephrolithiasis

Test	Day 1	2	3	4	5
Bloods					
Electrolytes*	+				
Calcium	+	+	+	+	
Phosphorus	+	+	+	+	
Parathyroid hormone level	+				
1,25 Dehydroxycholecalciferol level†	o				
Magnesium	o				
Uric acid	+		+	+	
Arterial blood gases††					o
Ionized calcium	+				
Creatinine	+	+	+	+	
Urines					
24-Hour calcium excretion	+	+			
24-Hour phosphorus excretion	+	+			
24-Hour uric acid excretion			+	+	
24-Hour oxalate excretion					o
24-Hour creatinine excretion	+	+	+	+	
24-Hour citrate excretion					o
24-Hour magnesium excretion	o				
Cystine screening	+				
Urinalysis	+				
Urine culture	+				
Urinary acidification test					o
Urine pH	+	+	+	+	
Urinary activity/formation product for calcium oxalate and calcium phosphate†					o

* Sodium, potassium, chloride, carbon dioxide combining power.
† Limited availability, primarily of research use.
†† pH, pCO_2 and (HCO_3^-).
\+ Should be done when indicated.
o Optional test.

with the appropriate days for obtaining them. Crosses indicate required tests and circles represent optional tests to be ordered if indicated. Certain of the tests are currently of limited availability and are of major research use. These are indicated as such but are listed because their use will eventually become more widespread. Performance of these tests and an adequate history and physical examination will result in categorization of more than 95% of all stone formers and detection of 70% of patients with a remediable disease.

The blood and urine calcium and phosphorus should be measured on multiple occasions because of day-to-day variations in their levels. The urine pH is an important determination and should be performed on fresh urine collected under mineral oil by a pH electrode and not by reliance on dipstick analysis alone. If on repeated determinations, preferably of first voided morning urines, the urine pH is not spontaneously less than 6, then an acid-loading test should be performed. The short ammonium chloride loading test of Wrong and Davies (1965) is adequate for this purpose. Capsules of ammonium chloride are administered as a single dose of 0.1 gm/kg body weight over a 1-hour period to avoid gastric irritation and vomiting. After ingestion, hourly urine samples are collected under oil for pH, and a venous blood sample is drawn 2 to 4 hours after ingestion. The normal response is a drop in venous CO_2 combining power of 3 to 6 millimol/liter and a fall in urine pH into the range of 4.5–5.2 within 2 to 4 hours. Failure to decrease urine pH below 5.3 is an indication of an acidification defect and renal acid excretion may be further examined with a standard 3-day ammonium chloride loading test of Elkington et al. (1960).

The results of the above-described protocol require careful interpretation of each result and application to each situation. However, this process is direct and has been placed on a computer program (Coe, 1974).

Clinical Problem

W. S., a 35-year-old white male, was admitted to the hospital for right costovertebral angle pain with a presumptive diagnosis of renal colic. His first episode of renal colic occurred 8 years prior to the present diagnostic evaluation. In the intervening 8 years, he had had bimonthly episodes of renal colic, with numerous episodes of stone passage. There had been three associated urinary tract infections, all of which were treated successfully. Of the numerous stones that had been passed, two had been sent for analysis, which revealed calcium oxalate mixed with calcium apatite. The patient was on no prescribed medication and followed no set diet.

Physical examination was unremarkable, revealing a normal well-developed young male, appearing his stated age with normal vital signs. Moderate right costovertebral angle tenderness was noted. Genital and rectal exams were normal.

Intravenous pyelography revealed a nonobstructing radiopaque stone 1 x 2 mm in size in the right renal pelvis. There was no evidence of nephrocalcinosis on laminograms. The patient's pain resolved spontaneously without stone passage, and after a pain-free day in the hospital, a diagnostic evaluation was begun.

Laboratory evaluation revealed a normal complete blood cell count; the SMA-6 revealed a sodium concentration of 140 mEq/liter; serum potassium, 4.0 mEq/liter; serum chloride, 102 mEq/liter; and a CO_2 combining power of 26 mEq/liter. The serum creatinine was 0.9 mg%; serum calcium concentration was 10 mg%; serum phosphorus, 4.2 mg%; total protein was 7 gm% with albumin of 4.5 gm%. The alkaline phosphatase level was 75 IU (normal: 50–100). Parathyroid hormone level was 5 μlEq/ml (normal: 2–10), and the ionized calcium level was 5.0 mg%. The 24-hour urine collections revealed urinary calcium excretion of 350–500 mg/24 hours on three determinations and phosphate excretion from 900–1200 mg/24 hours. The tubular reabsorption of phosphorus was 85% to 90% on three determinations. Twenty-four-hour urinary uric acid excretion was 700 mg/day. The urine pH on four determinations was never lower than 6.3 An ammonium chloride loading test was performed by the administration of 2 gm of ammonium chloride q.i.d. for eight doses. The lowest urine pH was 5.4, which is distinctly abnormal maximal urinary acidification. Urinary citrate excretion was 200 mg/24 hours, normal being 275–400 mg/24 hours. The patient was treated with chlorthalidone (100 mg/day), low calcium diet (600 mg/day), and high fluid intake. Follow-up at three 6-month intervals showed no recurrence of stones.

Questions

1. What is the pathophysiologic basis for the hypercalciuria in this patient, and what were the critical tests performed in establishing the diagnostic category?
2. What is the relationship between hypercalciuria and renal acidification defects?
3. What is the significance of the 24-hour urinary citrate excretion?

Discussion

The evaluation here clearly revealed hypercalciuria in the presence of normocalcemia. Thus, this patient fits the diagnostic term "idiopathic hypercalciuria" previously used to describe these patients. The presence in this patient's serum of normal levels of parathyroid hormone indicated that the mechanisms of resorptive hypercalciuria or of renal reabsorptive (calcium leak) hypercalciuria were not the basis of the hypercalciuria. In addition, the evidence of normal phosphate metabolism, evidenced by repeatedly normal serum phosphorus concentrations and normal tubular reabsorption of phosphorus, indicated that the renal reabsorptive (phosphate leak) mechanism was not the basis of the hypercalciuria in this patient. Rather, the most likely diagnosis was an absorptive hypercalciuria. The finding of the impaired urinary acidification in this patient established the diagnosis of an incomplete renal tubular acidosis. Whether the impaired acidification manifested by the patient was the result of nephrocalcinosis or whether the patient had two associated defects, renal tubular acidosis and hypercalciuria, could not be determined. The use of thiazides in cases of demonstrated absorptive hypercalciuria has not clearly been shown to be of therapeutic benefit. Their use in patients with acidification defects, especially of the proximal tubule variety, is helpful in decreasing associated hypercalciuria. Until selective calcium binders such as cellulose phosphate become available, thiazides will remain the mainstay of therapy for hypercalciurics.

References

Brand, E., Harris, M. M., and Biloon, S. "Cystinuria: The excretion of a cystine complex which decomposes in the urine with the liberation of free cystine." J. Biol. Chem. *86:* 315–331, 1930.

Coe, F. L. "The performance of a computer system for metabolic assessment of patients with nephrolithiasis." Comput. Biomed. Res. *7:* 40, 1974.

Coe, F. L., and Kavalach, A. G. "Hypercalciuria and hyperuricosuria in patients with calcium nephrolithiasis." N. Engl. J. Med. *291:* 1344–1350, 1974.

Coe, F. L., Firpo, J. J., Hollandsworth, D. L., Segil, L., Canterbury, J., and Reiss, E. "Effect of acute and chronic metabolic acidosis on serum immunoreactive parathyroid hormone in man." Kidney Int. *8:* 262–273, 1975.

Elkington, J. R., Huth, E. J., Webster, G. D., and McCance, R. A. "The renal excretion of hydrogen ion in renal tubular acidosis. I. Quantitative assessment of the response to ammonium chloride as an acid load." Am. J. Med. *29:* 554–560, 1960.

Hodgkinson, A., and Pyrah, L. N. "The urinary excretion of calcium and inorganic phosphate in 344 patients with calcium stones of renal origin." Br. J. Surg. *46:* 10–18, 1958.

Lonsdale, K. "Human stones: Limited studies give some details of composition, rates of growth, distribution, and possible causes." Science *159:* 1199–1207, 1968.

Morris, R. C., Jr., Sebastian, A., and McSherry, E. "Renal acidosis." Kidney Int. *1:* 322, 1972.

Nordin, B. E. C. Metabolic Bone and Stone Disease. Churchill Livingstone, London, 1973.

Pak, C. Y. C. "Disorders of stone formation." *In:* The Kidney, B. M. Brenner and F. C. Rector, Jr. (eds.). W. B. Saunders, Philadelphia, pp. 1326–1354, 1976.

Pak, C. Y. C., Ohata, M., Lawrence, E. C., and Snyder, W. "The hypercalciurias: Causes, parathyroid functions, and diagnostic criteria." J. Clin. Invest. *54:* 387–400, 1974.

Robertson, W. G., Peacock, M., and Nordin, B. E. C. "Activity products in stone-forming and non-stone-forming urine." Clin. Sci. *34:* 579–594, 1968.

Robertson, W. G., Peacock, M., and Nordin, B. E. C. "Calcium crystalluria in recurrent renal stone formers." Lancet *II:* 21–24, 1969.

Williams, H. E. "Nephrolithiasis." N. Engl. J. Med. *290:* 33–38, 1974.

Wrong, O., and Davies, H. E. F. "The excretion of acid in renal disease." Q. J. Med. *28:* 259–313, 1965.

Chapter 6

Hypertension

General Considerations

At the present time in the United States, 23 million people are known to be affected by hypertension, although the actual number of persons with this condition may approach 40 million. Of the total with known hypertension, only 50% are treated, and of these, only 20% are adequately treated. Thus, hypertension is a major diagnostic and therapeutic consideration for the practicing physician and requires intense evaluation and thorough, complete medical follow-up.

Maintenance of Normal Blood Pressure

Blood pressure may be considered as the product of the cardiac output and the total peripheral vascular resistance. Under most circumstances, adequate blood pressure is maintained by changes in total peripheral vascular resistance. Although cardiac output may acutely affect blood pressure, chronic deviations in blood pressure are difficult to attribute to changes in cardiac output alone. Several conditions, such as renal failure, toxemia of pregnancy, and acute glomerulonephritis, may have markedly increased cardiac outputs associated with a hypertensive state.

Maintenance of peripheral resistance and thus blood pressure is dependent upon many factors. One parameter that plays a critical role in the maintenance of adequate pressures is the circulating blood volume. Under normal circumstances, intake of adequate salt and water is necessary to maintain circulating volume. The kidney will respond to changes in salt intake with an appropriate salt output. Homeostasis of sodium is dependent upon an adequate cardiac output and thus an appropriate filtered load of sodium. Physical factors such as the peritubular hydrostatic or oncotic pressure will also affect the rate of proximal tubular sodium reabsorption. The intrarenal distribution of blood flow, the presence of natriuretic substances ("natriuretic hormone"), and the like may also be important in sodium homeostasis. Hormonal factors, such as aldosterone, regulate distal sodium reabsorption and are responsive to volume changes via the renin-angiotensin system. Blood volume and thus blood pressure is integrally related with the renin-angiotensin-aldosterone system. Figure 6-1 outlines the proposed interrelationships. Renin is produced by specialized cells located in the afferent arteriole, referred to as the juxtaglomerular cells. The release of renin is dependent upon several factors that primarily affect the stretch receptors in the afferent arteriole. Juxtaposed to the afferent arteriolar cells is a specialized area of the distal tubule called the macula densa. This area is sodium-responsive, and thus release of renin by the afferent arteriole can be affected by the amount of sodium being delivered to the distal nephron. The juxtaglomerular cells and the macula densa constitute the juxtaglomerular apparatus. Other factors affecting the release of renin include renal sympathetic innervation, catecholamines, and adrenergic stimula-

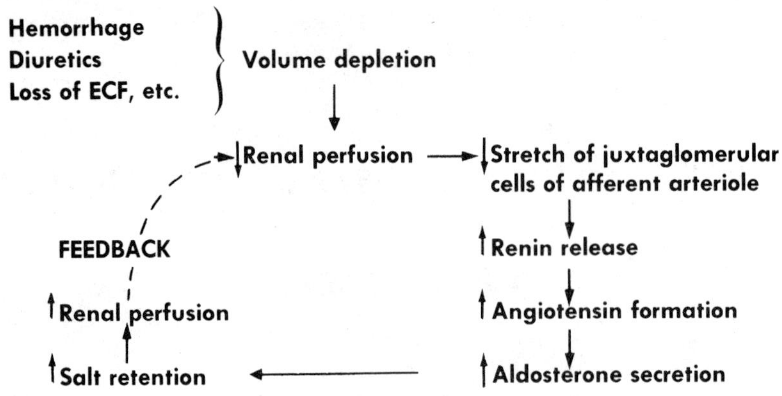

Fig. 6-1.

Renin-angiotensin-aldosterone interrelationships.

tion. As shown in Figure 6-1, aldosterone and the renin-angiotensin system are closely associated with renal regulation of renin release and thus maintenance of blood volume and blood pressure.

While volume is a critical factor in the maintenance of normal blood pressure, other factors may directly affect peripheral vascular resistance. There are, of course, many factors, and only the most important will be discussed here. The most potent vasoactive peptide produced in the body is angiotensin II. The generation of angiotensin II is outlined in Figure 6-2. Angiotensinogen, or renin substrate, is a circulating α_2 globulin, which, in the presence of renin, is cleaved in plasma to angiotensin I, a decapeptide. This decapeptide, on circulation through the pulmonary vascular bed, is converted to angiotensin II, a vasoactive octapeptide. There is recent evidence that angiotensin II may be converted to angiotensin III, but clear documentation is still lacking. Therefore, any factor directly increasing renin release will affect angiotensin II, producing an increase in total peripheral resistance.

Other conditions affecting peripheral resistance include the sympathetic innervation of the vascular bed, the amount of catecholamine release, the response of the baroreceptors to changes in plasma volume and cardiac output, and possibly release of vasodepressor substances from the kidney. While the exact role of each of the above factors may be difficult to document, maintenance of normal blood pressure requires the interaction of these as well as that of yet undefined factors. Hypertension, therefore, may be considered in the context of a perturbation of this normal control system.

Definition

Hypertension is defined as a blood pressure of greater than 140 mm Hg systolic or 90 mm Hg diastolic, obtained on two or three successive measurements on at least two separate days, in patients below the age of 40. For patients older than 40, the pertinent levels are higher: 160 mm Hg systolic and/or 90 mm Hg diastolic. For the elderly, predominantly elevated systolic pressures may occur, presumably reflecting rigidity of the vasculature. Of course, for children the blood pressure levels that indicate the presence of hypertension are somewhat lower. Eighty-five percent of all hypertensive patients presenting to the physician have essential hypertension. Thus, evaluation of the patient will primarily depend

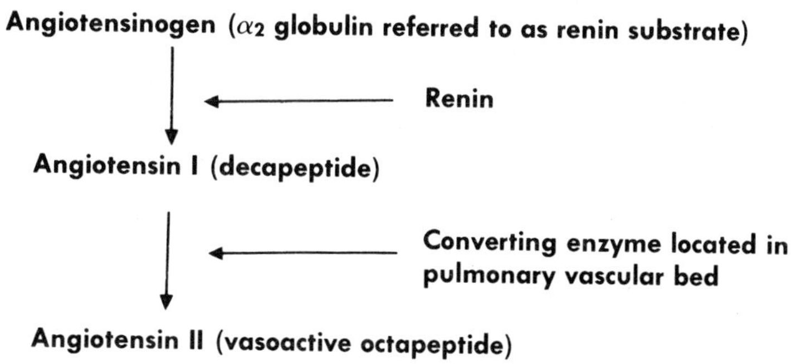

Fig. 6-2.

Generation of angiotensin II.

upon history, physical examination, and response to therapy. Table 6-1 outlines the differential diagnosis of hypertension. While the list is quite extensive, the majority of diagnoses will be excluded by a careful history and physical examination. The approach to the patient's diagnosis, therefore, will be oriented toward the sequential evaluation of the patient, realizing the most likely diagnosis to be essential hypertension.

Differential Diagnosis of Hypertension

I. Essential Hypertension

Clinical Features and Systemic Effects of Hypertension

Most patients with essential hypertension have a family history of hypertension, premature death, renal disease, cardiovascular disease, or cerebrovascular accidents. It is important when initially evaluating the patient to determine these facts and to establish the duration of hypertension. A prolonged labile hypertension with gradually increasing levels of blood pressure is characteristic of essential hypertension. Dietary habits, specifically the amount of sodium intake, have in many studies been directly related to the severity of hypertension. For those individuals with excessive salt intake (greater than 15 gm/day), the incidence of hypertension is considerably higher than for those with low salt intakes. The association with cigarette smoking must also be elicited, since the cardiovascular effects of cigarette smoking are directly proportional to the number of cigarettes smoked. Although the potentially reversible causes of hypertension must be evaluated, the majority of patients will not present with histories or physical examinations that would clue the physician toward their possible presence. Pertinent historical and physical examination data will be outlined later, directing the physician to pursue reversible causes of hypertension.

Other important points to evaluate in the patient's history are the effects of hypertension on target organs, including the brain, the cardiovascular system, and the kidneys. The association with headache, intermittent cerebrovascular attacks, dizziness, lightheadedness, vertigo, intermittent loss of memory, or frank cerebrovascular accidents is very

Table 6-1

Differential Diagnosis of Hypertension

- I. Essential hypertension
- II. Other forms of hypertension
  - A. Nonrenal causes
    - 1. Adrenal cortical overactivity
      - a. Cushing's syndrome
      - b. Primary hyperaldosteronism
        - i. adrenal adenoma
        - ii. Adrenal hyperplasia
        - iii. Dexamethasone suppressible hyperldosteronism
        - iv. Glucocorticoid suppressible hyperaldosteronism
      - c. Hypertension associated with congenital hyperplasia of the adrenal cortex
        - i. 11-β-hydroxylase deficiency
        - ii. 17-α-hydroxylase deficiency
    - 2. Adrenal medullary overactivity
      - a. Pheochromocytoma
    - 3. Acromegaly
    - 4. Preeclampsia
    - 5. Use of estrogen-containing oral contraceptives
    - 6. Coarctation of the aorta
    - 7. Syndrome of hyperdynamic circulation
    - 8. Miscellaneous causes
      - a. Porphyria
      - b. Lead poisoning
      - c. Increased intracranial pressure
      - d. Administration of monoanine oxidase inhibitors
      - e. Licorice
  - B. Renal causes
    - 1. Renal artery stenosis
    - 2. Hypertension associated with chronic renal failure
    - 3. Renoprival hypertension

important. On the other hand, the patient may present with evidence of coronary insufficiency or congestive heart failure associated with such symptoms as exertional dyspnea, orthopnea, paroxysmal nocturnal dyspnea, and pedal edema. Despite the fact that the kidney is a frequent target organ of hypertension, few symptoms may be associated with its involvement, and evidence of renal involvement will usually require laboratory evaluation. On the other hand, if severe renal failure is present, symptoms associated with uremia may be the presenting complaints in patients with severe hypertension. Typically the patient will present with recent weight loss, nausea and vomiting, confusion, tremor, pallor, uremic frost, nocturia, or decreased urine output.

Physical Examination

A complete and thorough physical examination is indicated in any patient with documented hypertension.

General Appearance. Certain forms of hypertension can be partially excluded by the presence of general physical findings, and these will be outlined subsequently.

Evaluation of Blood Pressure. Blood pressure should be obtained in both arms after the patient has been lying quietly for at least 5 minutes. For purposes of standardization, the fifth Korotkoff phase (disappearance of all sounds) should be used as the diastolic pressure. If there is a marked disparity between the fourth (muffling of sounds) and fifth phases, both should be recorded. Blood pressure should also be determined with the patient standing for at least 60 seconds to determine any orthostatic changes. If a disparity between both arms is present (<10 mm Hg), this should be confirmed by repeated measurements. If coarctation is excluded by x-ray examination, then the arm with the highest blood pressure should be used for follow-up. Blood pressures in the legs are extremely difficult to evaluate and require a large cuff; thus they are only helpful for evaluation of coarctation.

The Optic Fundi. Evaluation of the optic fundus may help in determining both the severity and the duration of hypertension. To visualize the peripheral arterioles and veins, pupils should be dilated. The degree of arteriolar constriction correlates well with the level of the diastolic blood pressure. Furthermore, the presence of arteriolar sclerosis, indicated by silver or copper wire changes and arteriovenous (A-V) nicking, indicates the chronicity of the disease. Severe retinal hemorrhages, cotton-wool exudates, and papilledema signify an accelerated or malignant phase of hypertension, requiring immediate therapy. Associated with these retinal changes is the presence of severe necrotizing arteriolitis in the kidneys and elsewhere. The patient presenting for initial evaluation without evidence of sclerosis of the vessels but with severe constriction and spasm most likely has had recent onset of hypertension. In the absence of constriction of the vessels, but with high-grade sclerosis, the hypertension is usually mild and chronic. The initial evaluation should include a classification of the funduscopic examination according to the Kirkendall-Armstrong classification, as outlined below. This classification is comparable to the Keith-Wagener-Barker classification but includes sclerosis, making determination of chronicity easier.

Grade I: Narrowing in terminal branches of vessels
Grade II: General narrowing of vessels with severe local constriction and moderate local sclerosis
Grade III: Severe local sclerosis and segmentation associated with striate hemorrhages and soft exudates
Grade IV: Papilledema added to the preceding signs

Cardiac Examination. Patients with sustained hypertension typically develop left ventricular hypertrophy, which may progress to dilatation and failure. The association with arteriosclerotic heart disease is high, and the patient may have angina pectoris with coronary insufficiency and myocardial infarction. Since hypertension is associated with decreased left ventricular compliance, one of the first signs of cardiac involvement is the presence of a fourth heart sound (atrial gallop). This abnormality may be detectable before any cardiac enlargement or dilatation is present. Left ventricular hypertrophy is often associated with an increased cardiac impulse and evidence of a hyperdynamic precordium. As the hypertension progresses, evidence of left ventricular failure becomes more evident. The patient may present with evidence of either left ventricular or biventricular failure. Frequently the patient with severe prolonged hypertension will have a third heart sound (ventricular diastolic gallop) that is a manifestation of severe left heart failure. With severe hypertension (diastolic blood pressure over 130 mm Hg), aortic incompetence may be a prominent finding, causing a decrescendo diastolic murmur along the left sternal border and in the second right intercostal space. This murmur will usually disappear as the hypertension is treated.

Examination of Peripheral Pulses. Since hypertension is associated with an accelerated vascular disease, abnormalities in flow along peripheral vessels are a frequent physical finding. The carotid, subclavian, and vertebral-basilar systems are frequently involved, as are the aortic and femoral vessels. Bruits along the carotid, subclavian, or femoral arteries are an indication of prolonged significant hypertension. With sustained hypertension, aneurysms are also formed, typically in the abdominal aorta. The presence of an expanding abdominal aortic aneurysm, found on examination typified by a mass pulsating laterally, is an ominous physical finding. With severe peripheral vascular disease, a to-and-fro bruit may be present, which is indicative of a significant gradient. A systolic bruit alone suggests only intimal disease of the vessel without stenosis. Carotid artery bruits are a significant physical finding and must be differentiated from a cardiac murmur propagated into the carotid arteries. These bruits are frequently associated with evidence of cerebrovascular disease, such as intermittent ischemic attacks or frank cerebrovascular accidents. Patients presenting with evidence of renal vascular hypertension on occasion have bruits audible over the abdomen due to stenotic renal arteries. The bruit is usually heard in the mid-epigastrium or over the upper quadrant or flank of the side involved. It must be remembered, however, that bruits in the abdomen need not be renal in origin and may relate to stenotic involvement of either celiac or superior mesenteric arteries.

Neurological Examination. Initial neurological examination is required to exclude the possibility of a silent neurological deficit. Specific references must be made as to the presence of symmetrical reflexes; presence of unilateral weakness; long track signs, such as Babinski's reflex; and sensorineural deficits in the lower or upper extremities. Cranial nerves should also be evaluated.

Abdominal Examination. Abdominal examination of the patient with hypertension rarely reveals significant abnormalities in the absence of severe right heart failure, where marked liver enlargement may occur. In this instance the liver may be tender, enlarged, and, on occasion, pulsatile. Of course, the presence of renal enlargement must be excluded, since hypertension is a frequent presenting sign in patients with polycystic renal disease. Abdominal bruits have been discussed in the section on examination of the peripheral vessels.

Laboratory Findings

Since the average hypertensive patient will have essential hypertension, it is not necessary to evaluate the patient for all forms of potentially curable disease. A patient initially presenting with hypertension should have a complete blood cell count, including a white blood cell count with differential, hemoglobin level, and hematocrit. A routine urinalysis is indicated to determine the presence of formed elements in the urine and the ablity to concentrate the urine as depicted by specific gravity. The urine pH, protein excretion, and the presence of glucose should all be recorded. A routine set of electrolytes is indicated. The presence of alkalosis or a depressed serum potassium concentration may be helpful in differentiating the patient with primary hyperaldosteronism. Serum cholesterol and triglyceride analyses are indicated in any hypertensive patient below the age of 60. Since hypertension is frequently associated with diabetes mellitus, a fasting and a 2-hour postprandial blood glucose are necessary. Since hypertension may affect the kidney, both a blood urea nitrogen (BUN) and a serum creatinine level are required as part of an initial evaluation. Finally, a chest roentgenogram and an electrocardiogram are necessary to exclude significant cardiac involvement. The above should be an adequate evaluation for the patient who initially presents to the physician with hypertension. Evaluation of the peripheral plasma renin activity is not indicated initially, since it requires hospitalization, a stable sodium intake, and certain provocative tests. Random determinations of plasma renin activities are of little value.

Further Diagnostic Considerations

If the patient initially evaluated responds to conservative management, that is, administration of a diuretic and antihypertensive therapy, with stabilized blood pressure and no evidence of progressive vascular disease, further diagnostic tests are not indicated. However, if the blood pressure is labile or relentlessly progressive, despite therapy, or if evidence of renal impairment exists, then a more thorough evaluation is necessary.

II. Other Forms of Hypertension

The reversible or curable forms of hypertension and hypertensive states associated with other systemic diseases, and their diagnostic considerations, are discussed below (see also Table 6-1):

A. Nonrenal Causes

1. Adrenal Cortical Overactivity

Cushing's syndrome is produced by the excessive secretion of cortisol from the adrenal gland or excessive, nonsuppressible ACTH secretion from the pituitary. Adrenocortical tumors may secrete cortisol, and other neoplasms themselves may secrete cortisol or ACTH. Cushing's syndrome is extremely rare, but the patient will present with classical physical findings that should alert the physician to its presence. They include central obesity, moon facies, oligomenorrhea, purpura and striae, muscle atrophy, hirsutism, and edema. The patients will usually be hypertensive with impaired glucose tolerance and occasional hypokalemia. Since hypertension is rarely a manifestation of Cushing's syndrome without at least one or two of the above findings, the diagnosis can most often be suspected from history and physical findings. The definitive tests require hospitalization. Most patients with Cushing's syndrome will have elevated urinary 17-hydroxycorticosteroid levels. Elevated plasma cortisol levels cannot be suppressed by dexamethasone (1 mg by mouth the night before the test). Further diagnostic studies required to confirm ectopic ACTH production or carcinoma are beyond the scope of this text but should be performed prior to initiation of therapy.

Primary hyperaldosteronism results from the overproduction of aldosterone or one of its precursors. Hypertension is associated with at least four specific disease entities related to the overproduction of aldosterone or one of its analogs by the adrenal cortex. The most frequent entity causing primary hyperaldosteronism is adrenal adenoma associated with hypokalemic alkalosis and hypertension. Plasma aldosterone levels are significantly elevated in this disease state, and plasma renin levels are low. Surgery is usually curative. Idiopathic hyperaldosteronism associated with hyperplasia of the zona glomerulosa is not remediable by surgery, although the hypertension may be more easily controllable after adrenalectomy. A small group of patients will have the classic signs of hyperaldosteronism, which are suppressible by the administration of deoxycorticosterone acetate. The exact mechanism for this observation is unclear. The final type of hyperaldosteronism is observed most frequently in children and is suppressible by the administration of glucocorticosteroids.

While the true incidence of hyperaldosteronism is not known, it may account for up to 5% of all cases of hypertension. The patients will typically present with modest to severe hypertension and hypokalemic alkalosis. For a further discussion of this metabolic condition the reader is referred to the chapters on hypokalemia and metabolic alkalosis. No overt historical findings will alert the physician to this disease state with the exception of mild to moderate weakness related to the hypokalemia. Edema is usually not present. The excessive ingestion of licorice must be excluded, since it produces a clinical syndrome similar to hyperaldosteronism. Primary hyperaldosteronism should be suspected if the serum potassium concentration is less than 3.5 mEq/liter and is associated with a urinary potassium level greater than 40 mEq/24 hours. It must be remembered that diuretic therapy must be discontinued for at least 72 hours prior to the determination. Usually the patient with hypokalemia will also be mildly alkalotic on initial screening. The diagnosis of primary hyperaldosteronism can be ruled out if the serum concentration of potassium is greater than 4 mEq/liter when the patient is ingesting at least 100 mEq of sodium daily. Many patients on initial evaluation may have mild hypokalemia and low urinary potassium levels or may have borderline hypokalemia and increased urinary potassium levels. Repeated observation of these patients is indicated before further diagnostic considerations are made.

If the patient is suspected of having primary hyperaldosteronism, hospitalization is indicated. The patient should be fed a normal sodium chloride diet and peripheral plasma renin activity determined. The patient should then be placed on a .5 gm sodium diet and furosemide or thiazides administered each morning for 2 to 4 days. Patients with primary hyperaldosteronism will have low levels of renin that will not increase substantially on a low salt diet and diuretics. The second major diagnostic criterion is evidence of an increased urinary aldosterone level, which cannot be suppressed by greater than 100 mEq sodium chloride per day or the administration of deoxycorticosterone acetate. The hypokalemia of primary hyperaldosteronism can be corrected by the administration of potassium supplements and spironolactone (200–400 mg/day). Although this therapy may correct the metabolic consequences of hyperaldosteronism, definitive surgical exploration to document adrenal adenoma or hyperplasia is the treatment of choice if the hyperaldosteronism is not suppressible by deoxycorticosterone acetate or glucocorticoids.

Hypertension associated with congenital hyperplasia of the adrenal cortex may occur with either 11-β-hydroxylase or 17-α-hydroxylase deficiency. 11-β-Hydroxylation deficiency presents in childhood and is associated with virilization and hypertension. Secretion of 11-deoxycortisol and deoxycorticosterone are increased. Plasma aldosterone levels are either normal or decreased. The disease state is responsive to dexamethasone (.25–1.0 mg/day). The 17-α-hydroxylation deficiency syndrome manifests itself during puberty. The patients present with hypertension, hyperkalemia, and amenorrhea or male pseudohermaphroditism. Because the 17-α-hydroxylase enzyme is necessary for the production of both androgens and estrogens, both are reduced or absent. Cortisol production is also reduced, leading to increased production of ACTH. The nonsuppressed production of ACTH causes increased progesterone, deoxycorticosterone, and 18-hydroxycorticosterone production. Plasma aldosterone levels are reduced or absent. Plasma renin levels are also decreased as a result of increased deoxycorticosterone production leading to sodium retention, volume expansion, and hypertension. The disease state is also responsive to dexamethasone (.25–1.0 mg/day).

2. Adrenal Medullary Overactivity

Pheochromocytoma is a rare chromaffin tumor that often produces a typical symptom complex. The patient may present with paroxysms of hypertension associated with headache, excessive perspiration, palpitations, tachycardia, tremor, anxiety, episodic facial pallor, and recent weight loss. Another clue to the diagnosis of pheochromocytoma is a paradoxical response to antihypertensive agents or severe hypertension associated with the use of generalized anesthesia. Patients with pheochromocytoma have an increased incidence of diabetes mellitus. Hypertensive retinopathy, Kirkendall-Armstrong classification group II or III, is a usual finding. The blood pressure is usually labile, but there is often associated weight loss, hypermetabolism, and an abnormal carbohydrate tolerance test. Because of the severity of the hypertension, the patient usually has a short history, less than 2 years. The most reliable screening procedure for pheochromocytoma is a urinary metanephrine or vanillylmandelic acid (VMA) obtained over a 24-hour urinary collection. Abnormally elevated excretion rates of VMA may be seen with the ingestion of vanilla, alpha-methyldopa, bananas, certain nuts, and monoamine oxidase (MAO) inhibitors, and these must be excluded for 3 to 5 days before measuring VMA excretion. Sometimes VMA excretion is intermittent, and the test will be abnormal only when the tumor is stimulated. If the results are normal on original screening, then a histamine (24–50 mg of histamine base given intravenously) or a glucagon (1 mg I.V.) stimulation test is indicated. Careful monitoring of the blood pressure is required during the procedures.

3. Acromegaly

Acromegaly is a rare disease produced by the oversecretion of growth hormone from the acidophilic cells of the pituitary. It affects both men and women equally, usually in the third and fourth decades. Growth hormone stimulates the growth of almost all tissues leading to chondrogenesis, osteogenesis, and soft tissue increase, resulting in thickened and enlarged hands, feet, lips, tongue, and skin folds. There is also diffuse organomegaly including the heart, lungs, liver, spleen, intestines, and kidneys. Glands such as the adrenal cortex, thyroid, and parathyroids may also increase in size.

The patients are often mildly diabetic and will frequently have hypercalciuria as well as occasional hypercalcemia. Pituitary insufficiency may occur late in the course of the disease. From 20% to 50% of the patients will be hypertensive, possibly as a result of the increased cardiac output.

The diagnosis most frequently is made by physical examination. Measurements of growth hormone by radioimmunoassay will confirm the diagnosis. The disease is usually treated by irradiation of the sella, although the results are variable.

4. Preeclampsia

Pregnancy is associated with expanded blood volume, increased renin substrate, and, on occasion, hypertension in the last trimester, sometimes accompanied by proteinuria and edema (preeclampsia). While the hypertension usually subsides after delivery, occasional sustained hypertensive states occur and must be documented by careful history.

5. Estrogen-containing Oral Contraceptives

The use of oral contraceptive agents containing estrogen is associated with increased renin substrate and renin activity. Ten percent of all women using these medications will develop some degree of hypertension, and this is probably the most frequent curable cause of hypertension in young females. The use of the drugs may be elicited by history, and their cessation is usually associated with a return of the blood pressure to normal.

6. Coarctation of the Aorta

Coarctation of the aorta is a disease of young adults frequently causing death by age 30 to 35. The coarctation usually occurs in a location just distal to the origin of the left subclavian artery. The major associated abnormalities include bicuspid aortic valve and aneurysms of the circle of Willis. The major symptoms associated with the disease include congestive heart failure, infective endocarditis, aortic rupture, and cerebral hemorrhage. Congestive heart failure occurs in infancy, while aortic rupture is most common in individuals over the age of 20. Typically the patient will have a large upper torso with thin legs. Pulses in the upper extremities are disparate, with marked variation in blood pressure between both arms or the arms versus the legs. The femoral pulse will reveal a significantly reduced amplitude compared to the upper extremities. The major increase in blood pressure is systolic and is thus associated with a wide pulse pressure. Cardiomegaly is frequent, often with associated aortic regurgitation and an aortic ejection sound. Chest x-ray reveals posterior notching of the ribs, which may be unilateral depending upon the location of the coarctation. Poststenotic dilatation of the aorta will help localize the area of coarctation. Under most circumstances, angiographic delineation is not necessary. Definitive surgical correction is required.

7. Syndrome of Hyperdynamic Circulation

The syndrome of hyperdynamic circulation is seen in adolescents and young adults and is characterized by labile, predominantly systolic hypertension; resting tachycardia; a hyperactive precordium; prominent pulsations in the carotid arteries; and a systolic flow murmur along the left sternal border. Careful follow-up of these cases is indicated, but no definitive therapy is necessary, although propranolol has been beneficial.

8. Miscellaneous Causes

Other miscellaneous causes of hypertension include acute intermittent porphyria, lead poisoning, and increased intracranial pressure.

Acute intermittent porphyria is a disease primarily affecting young women in the third and fourth decades. It is inherited as a dominant trait. During acute attacks the patient may present with severe colicky abdominal pain associated with protracted vomiting. Diffuse neurological deficits are frequently present, including isolated peripheral neuropathy, cranial nerve deficits, occasional respiratory paralysis, and wasting and contracture of affected muscles. Occasional psychiatric disturbances have been documented. Sinus tachycardia and nonspecific electrocardiographic changes are seen during acute attacks. During these attacks, the blood pressure may rise significantly requiring medical intervention. The cause for the hypertension is unclear. The diagnosis is confirmed by documenting elevated urinary levels of δ-aminolevulinic acid (ALA) and porphobilinogen (PBG).

Acute lead intoxication produces a symptom complex indistinguishable from acute intermittent porphyria. Lead inhibits ALA synthetase and dehydrase, causing an increased urinary excretion of ALA and coproporphyrin III. The disease is differentiated from acute intermittent porphyria by the absence of PBG in the urine. The hypertension associated with lead intoxication presumably relates to the altered porphyrin metabolism, but the exact mechanism is not defined.

Hypertension is also associated with *increased intracranial pressure.* Usually the increase in blood pressure is rapid and severe. Progressive bradycardia due to vagal stimulation is a frequent associated finding. The hypertension occurs as the intracranial pressure approaches arterial diastolic pressure, inducing medullary ischemia and compensatory systemic vasoconstriction. Adequate ventilation to reduce CO_2 retention (which may acutely elevate intracerebral pressure) and decompression is required.

Ingestion of monoamine oxidase inhibitors will induce severe hypertension in patients ingesting tyramine-containing foods such as unpasteurized cheese and imported Chianti wines. The syndrome is caused by excessive catecholamine release.

Licorice, on the other hand, produces a syndrome indistinguishable from hyperaldosteronism, due to its content of glycyrrhizic acid, which has aldosterone-like properties.

B. Renal Causes

1. Renal Vascular Hypertension

Renal vascular hypertension is probably the most frequent cause of curable hypertension in males. It accounts for approximately 3% to 5% of all cases of hypertension. It is typically of acute onset and short duration, most often affecting individuals in their mid-20s or younger or individuals older than 55. The diagnosis is most frequently suspected by rapid sequence intravenous pyelography as an initial screening procedure. Although abdominal bruits may alert the physician to its presence, the bruit is frequently absent and cannot be relied upon as a screening procedure. The hypertension is most often accelerated, with grade III or IV hypertensive retinopathy being observed. Often the patient will have hematuria and may have had a past history of renal trauma or flank pain. The hypertension is occasionally resistant to medical therapy.

Rapid sequence intravenous pyelograms (IVP) should be performed on any patient under the age of 30 with a diastolic blood pressure greater than 110 mm Hg or, regardless of age, if the diastolic blood pressure is greater than 130 mm Hg. If the patient has significant renal vascular hypertension, the IVP will demonstrate reduction in renal size on the involved side. If the right side is involved, it will be at least 1.5 cm smaller than the left, and if the left side is involved, it will be 0.5 cm smaller than the right, because the left kidney is usually 1 cm larger than the right. There will also be delayed appearance of the contrast material on the involved side followed by delayed excretion and increased concentration of the contrast material on that side. If the IVP is suggestive of renovascular hypertension, then differential renal venous renins should be obtained. In about 20% of patients with renovascular hypertension, the IVP may be negative.

The kidney involved by renal artery stenosis is ischemic, there is increased renin release, production of angiotensin II, and subsequent systemic hypertension. Differential renal venous renins will demonstrate a renin release 1.5 times greater from the involved side when compared to the uninvolved side. Renal venous renins should be obtained only after the patient has been maintained on a .5 gm sodium diet and has received an oral diuretic for at least 48 hours prior to the tests. Care should be taken to discontinue any drugs that may interfere with renin release prior to the above measures. In conditions in which bilateral artery stenosis is present, renal venous renins may be difficult to interpret. The role of split renal function studies has not been clearly defined at this point. If the renal venous renins demonstrate a significant increase in release from the involved side, arteriography should then be performed to document the location of the lesion.

Under many circumstances, medical management will suffice. If sustained hypertension is present despite vigorous medical management, surgical correction of the stenotic lesion is indicated.

2. Hypertension Associated with Chronic Renal Failure

Many patients will have hypertension secondary to renal disease or will have secondary renal involvement from hypertension. During the original screening procedure, a carefully performed urinalysis can alert the physician to the presence of renal disease. A low specific gravity, variable degrees of proteinuria, red or white blood cells in the urine, or the presence of casts may suggest renal compromise. The BUN and serum creatinine levels will determine the degree of renal impairment. Any patient presenting with hematuria, proteinuria, formed casts in the urine, a BUN level greater than 20 mg/dl, or a creatinine level over 1.2–1.4 mg/dl should be carefully evaluated for renal impairment. Twenty-four-hour urine collections for protein, sodium, and creatinine are indicated, as are appropriate urine cultures. Documentation of the creatinine clearance is essential as a baseline value. Intravenous pyelography should also be performed to evaluate renal size, the collecting system, bladder, and the presence of postvoiding residual. Under most circumstances with creatinine clearances greater than 20 ml/min, adequate visualization will occur. If the patient presents with severe azotemia, intravenous pyelography may not be adequate to visualize renal silhouettes or collecting systems. The IVP should, however, be attempted with tomography, and often this will suffice. If the IVP is inadequate, then renal scanning procedures with hippurate and pertechnitate will at least demonstrate the presence of blood supply to both kidneys. Recently described techniques using computerized axial tomography have been extremely helpful in documenting the presence of two kidneys and in excluding obstruction in individuals with severe azotemia. Retrograde pyelography should be reserved for those patients in whom obstruction is suspected but cannot be proven by the above techniques.

Hypertension is a frequent complication of chronic renal failure, but the mechanisms causing it have not been fully delineated. Most patients will develop hypertension only after the glomerular filtration rate has been significantly reduced. However, those patients with severe vasculitis, such as polyarteritis nodosa or systemic lupus erythematosus, may present with significant hypertension before renal function is compromised. The hypertension is thought to be related to ischemic changes within the kidney, leading to accelerated renin release and angiotensin II production.

Many patients, however, will present with acute or chronic renal failure and hypertension with no prior history of vasculitis. Most of these patients have increased total body sodium and water with plasma renin levels that are normal or only slightly increased. This relationship between plasma volume and plasma renin is inappropriate. In other words, for the degree of volume expansion, the plasma renin levels are too high, thus leading to a hypertensive state. While cardiac output may be increased in these patients, the increase is usually appropriate for the degree of anemia and is probably not a contributing factor. These patients usually respond to antihypertensive medications and to volume control by hemodialysis.

A smaller population of patients with chronic renal failure have more severe hypertension with significantly elevated plasma renin levels and respond poorly to antihypertensive agents. Furthermore, these patients are poorly responsive to volume control by dialysis and, in fact, may accelerate their hypertension during the procedure. The disease state is felt to result from an accelerated renin release associated with an altered renin-sodium interrelationship. Since the renin is not suppressible by the expanded plasma volume, release may actually increase as volume is reduced. Despite the newer forms of antihypertensive agents, nephrectomy may be necessary for blood pressure control in a small number of these patients.

3. Renoprival Hypertension

A rare cause of hypertension that must be considered of renal origin is renoprival hypertension. Under certain circumstances, bilateral nephrectomy may be indicated (infection, carcinoma, trauma, etc.). Previously normotensive patients then become hypertensive. With the inability to control salt and water excretion, hypertension may occur solely on a volume basis. It is also possible that the hypertension may occur secondary to loss of a vasodepressor substance normally liberated by the kidney. The presumed substance is a prostaglandin, probably of the E series. The hypertension may be severe but is usually responsive to antihypertensive medications or to adequate control of the blood volume by hemodialysis.

Clinical Problem

M. B. is a 33-year-old black woman who presents with a chief complaint of mild headache. The patient was in generally good health until the last trimester of her second pregnancy, when she developed mild hypertension. She was treated by her obstetrician with diuretics alone for control of blood pressure. She delivered a normal child and subsequently was lost to follow-up. She stated she was in good health for the past 2 years, but noted the onset of mild headaches for the 2 months prior to this visit. Headaches are predominantly occipital, pounding in nature, and usually progress throughout the day. They are occasionally relieved by aspirin but are most frequently relieved by rest. She has noted no diplopia, blurred vision, or other neurological signs. She denies urinary frequency or urgency, dysuria, or nocturia. She admits to intermittent shortness of breath, usually induced by exertion, and has had occasional swelling of the feet, for which she had taken diuretic medications prescribed for her during her pregnancy. She has continued to have the prescription renewed despite not visiting her physician for the past 2 years. She denies, however, palpitation, chest pain, cough, hemoptysis, or the like.

Her past medical history is essentially negative. She is gravida II, para II. The only medications she uses are diuretics for "swelling of the feet" and occasionally aspirin for headache. She denies the use of estrogen-containing medications. She eats an "average" diet and does not heavily salt her food.

Social History. She is married, lives with her husband, and does not abuse drugs, cigarettes, or alcohol.

Family History. Her mother is 54, alive and well, but has a history of adult onset diabetes mellitus. Her father is 57 and has had hypertension for 10 years but is adequately treated. She has two siblings, a brother 34, alive and well, and a sister 27, who is also said to have hypertension.

Review of systems is negative with the exception of that noted in the present illness. She denied the use of laxatives or enemas and has had no gastrointestinal disturbances.

Physical Examination. The patient presented as a healthy-appearing 33-year-old woman. She was thin, relaxed, and alert. Blood pressure in the right arm, supine, was 180/110 mm Hg, and in the left arm, supine, 180/108 mm Hg. Standing blood pressure, right arm, was 180/114 mm Hg. Blood pressure in the right leg was 190/114 mm Hg. Repeat blood pressures at the end of the examination were the same. The pulse was 86 beats per minute and regular, and the respirations, 18 per minute. The temperature was 37° C orally.

The funduscopic examination revealed grade II hypertensive retinopathy, Kirkendall-Armstrong classification. Cardiac examination demonstrated the point of maximal impulse (PMI) to be in the sixth intercostal space, midclavicular line. There was a forceful left ventricular heave with mild cardiomegaly to percussion. Auscultatory examination demonstrated a normal S1 and an S2 with a slightly increased aortic component. An atrial diastolic gallop was present, but no ventricular diastolic gallop or murmurs were heard. Peripheral pulses revealed carotid, radial, femoral, popliteal, and dorsalis pedis pulses to be normal. There was no organomegaly on abdominal examination and no bruits were heard. Examination of the extremities was completely normal, without evidence of pedal edema. The skin was clear. The neurological examination was normal.

Questions

1. What is the most likely cause of hypertension in a young black female not taking oral contraceptive medications?
2. Is there a need for obtaining intravenous pyelography in this patient?
3. Could the diagnosis of hyperaldosteronism be suspected from laboratory data at this time in this patient?
4. What end organ involvement caused by the hypertension might be suspected in this patient?

Discussion

Because of the fact that this is a young black female who had developed hypertension at the latter part of her last pregnancy and because of the family history of diabetes mellitus and hypertension, the most likely diagnosis is essential hypertension. It becomes necessary, however, to obtain screening tests as outlined above and, based upon these tests, to either treat the patient or to continue evaluation. As part of the initial evaluation, chest x-ray, electrocardiogram, serum electrolytes, BUN and creatinine levels, as well as a 2-hour postprandial blood glucose and a urinalysis were obtained. The results were as follows: Chest roentgenogram revealed no evidence of notching, clear lung fields, normal aortic arch but mild left ventricular prominence. The electrocardiogram was within normal limits. The plasma chemistries revealed: sodium, 139 mEq/liter; potassium, 3.1 mEq/liter; chloride, 98 mEq/liter; CO_2, 31 mEq/liter; BUN, 21 mg%; creatinine, 1.2 mg%; and 2-hour PC glucose of 140 mg%. The urine was clear with a specific gravity of 1.014. The urine was negative for glucose but there was 1+ proteinuria. There were two to four white cells per high-power field and no formed elements on microscopic examination.

Based upon the preliminary evaluation of this patient, it was obvious that several abnormalities existed, including mild hypokalemia with alkalosis and very mild elevations in both the BUN and creatinine levels. For complete evaluation of this patient with borderline changes, further diagnostic tests were indicated. To evaluate the hypokalemia, it was necessary to document the intake and to discontinue all diuretic usage. After the patient had discontinued all diuretic therapy and was on an adequate potassium intake of approximately 100 mEq/day for at least 1 week, 24-hour urines for potassium, protein, and creatinine levels were obtained. Serum creatinine and potassium concentrations were also obtained at the termination of the collection to determine creatinine clearance and plasma potassium levels. Results were as follows: 24-hour urinary protein, 700 mg/day; 24-hour urinary potassium, 80 mEq/day, with a plasma potassium of 4.1 mEq/liter; creatinine clearance 85 ml/min, and when corrected for 1.73 square meters, 95 ml/min. The plasma bicarbonate level was 26 mEq/liter at that time. Follow-up urinary and plasma potassium determinations as well as plasma bicarbonate levels were obtained to fully exclude the possibility of hyperaldosteronism. Because of a mildly reduced creatinine clearance in the presence of proteinuria with a negative sediment, evaluation of the urinary tract was necessary. Rapid sequence urography demonstrated bilaterally symmetrical concentration of the dye, with normal renal size and silhouettes, normal pelves, ureters and bladder, no evidence of reflux, and no evidence of intrinsic disease.

Based upon the fact that she became mildly hypertensive with the second pregnancy and had a normal IVP with a creatinine clearance that was only modestly reduced, the most likely diagnosis was essential hypertension with mild hypertensive nephrosclerosis. No further workup was indicated at this time. Since there were no physical findings or history to suggest potentially reversible causes of hypertension, such as pheochromocytoma or Cushing's syndrome, appropriate medications were started, and the blood pressure was found to be easily controlled. Monthly follow-ups for the following year demonstrated persistently normal plasma potassium and bicarbonate levels as well as controlled blood pressures and a serum creatinine level that has remained in the range of 1.1–1.2 mg%.

References

Beeson, P. B., and McDermott, W. Text Book of Medicine. W. B. Saunders, Philadelphia, pp. 981–991, 1975.

Biglieri, E. G., Stockigt, J. R., and Schombelon, M. "Adrenal mineralocorticoids causing hypertension." Am. J. Med. *52:* 623–632, 1972.

Brenner, B. M., and Rector, F. C. The Kidney. W. B. Saunders, Philadelphia, pp. 477–483, 1976.

Laragh, J. H. (ed.). "Symposium on hypertension." Am. J. Med. *60:* 733, 1976.

Maxwell, M. H., and Kleeman, C. R. Clinical Disorders of Fluid and Electrolyte Metabolism. McGraw-Hill, New York, pp. 855–872, 1972.

Papper, S. Clinical Nephrology. Little, Brown, Boston, pp. 293–306, 1971.

Schalehamp, M. A. et al. "Hypertension in chronic renal failure." Am. J. Med. *55:* 379–390, 1973.

Chapter 7

Azotemia

General Considerations

Azotemia is the accumulation in the blood of endogenously produced nitrogenous substances that are normally cleared by the kidneys. The term is used synonymously with renal failure. Renal failure is detected and its severity estimated by the extent to which the serum creatinine and/or the blood urea nitrogens concentrations are elevated above normal. The evaluation of changes in the concentrations of serum creatinine or BUN requires an understanding of some basic principles of physiology and metabolism.

Blood Urea Nitrogen

Urea is the final product of protein catabolism. It is distributed throughout the total body water and is in equal concentration in the intracellular and extracellular fluid. The concentration of urea in the blood serves as a convenient index of the kidney's ability to excrete metabolic waste, and an increase in BUN often signals a deterioration in the excretory functions of the kidney. In health, the rate of excretion of urea is equal to its rate of production in the body. Urea is excreted by filtration at the glomerulus, although about half of the amount filtered diffuses back into the blood during passage of the filtrate down the tubule. The relationship between BUN and glomerular filtration rate is such that at any given rate of urea production their product remains constant. This relation is shown graphically in Figure 7-1. When GFR falls, the BUN rises until constancy of their product is restored. In this way, the rate of urea excretion is kept equal to its rate of production. It is apparent from this relationship that the most important factor determining the concentration of urea in blood is the GFR, although it will also be influenced by the rate of urea production. The rate of urea production depends on protein catabolism and protein intake. At any given level of GFR, the greater the protein catabolism, the greater the urea concentration would be.

In Figure 7-1, note that the BUN begins to rise after small reductions in the GFR; but the increase is gradual and may lie within the arbitrarily defined "normal range" until GFR is reduced to about 50% of normal. Further reduction in the GFR below this level then results in a rapid increase in the BUN. Although the BUN is determined by the GFR even within the normal range, interpretation of normal variations is not warranted without precise knowledge of the rate of protein catabolism. For this reason, the upper limit of normal is set at 20 mg/dl. Values above this level usually signify depression of glomerular filtration rate.

From the above considerations, it can be inferred that the BUN is not a precise measure of renal function. Considerable deterioration of renal function must usually be present before the BUN rises above the normal range. The degree of depression of renal function at which the BUN rises may be markedly affected by the rate of protein catabo-

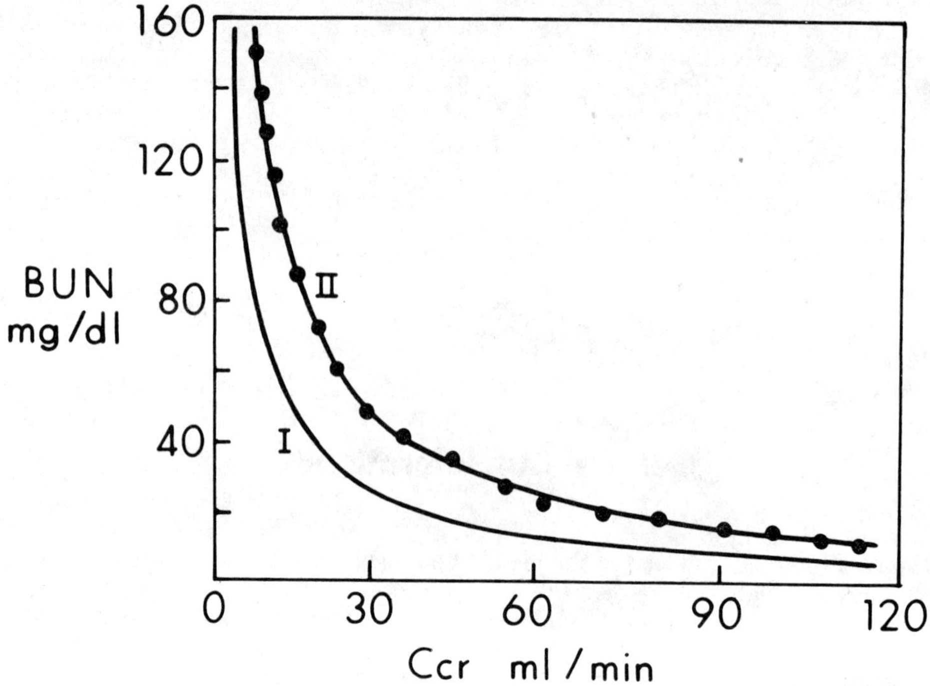

Fig. 7-1.

Relationship of BUN level to creatinine clearance at two different levels of protein intake. High protein intake is depicted by II and normal protein intake by I.

lism. If protein catabolism is rapid, as it is during acute febrile illnesses, following trauma, surgery, or after administration of cytolytic drugs, the BUN may rise above normal limits even when the GFR is diminished by less than 50%. Conversely, when protein catabolism is slow, as it is during protein starvation or with chronic debilitating diseases, the rise of BUN into the abnormal range may be delayed until the GFR is reduced to as little as 20% of normal. In practice, factors influencing the rate of protein catabolism must always be considered in interpreting BUN levels. The high BUN that is often seen following acute gastrointestinal hemorrhage, for example, represents the combined effect of a fall in GFR due to blood loss and increased urea production secondary to absorption of blood from the gastrointestinal tract.

Since urea production depends primarily on the intake of protein, blood urea will exhibit diurnal variations related to ingestion of food. The increase is usually maximal 3 to 4 hours after meals. However, these diurnal variations are small (0–3 mg/dl), and for clinical purposes, it is usually not necessary to obtain blood in the fasting state.

Serum Creatinine (S_{Cr})

Creatinine is produced from creatine and phosphocreatine in muscle. The quantity produced and excreted depends on skeletal muscle mass and is relatively constant in any individual from day to day. It is virtually unaffected by variations in the rate of protein catabolism and is affected only slightly by variations in the protein content of the diet. Creatinine excretion is almost exclusively dependent on the rate of filtration, since tubular reabsorption does not occur and only small quantities are secreted. Therefore, the S_{Cr} concentration rises when the filtration rate falls. The relation between S_{Cr} concentrations and GFR is similar to that depicted for BUN in Figure 7-1, except that significant alterations in the rate of creatinine production do not commonly occur. For this reason an abnormally elevated S_{Cr} concentration is a more reliable indication of decreased renal function than the BUN. A normal level of S_{Cr} at the time when the BUN is elevated usually means that a great portion of the BUN elevation may be due to increased urea production rather than to depression of renal function. This may occur following acute gastrointestinal hemorrhage or in other conditions where protein catabolism is increased. Again, it should be mentioned that S_{Cr} does not become elevated into the arbitrarily defined abnormal range until the GFR is depressed to some 50% of normal. A normal S_{Cr} concentration, therefore, cannot be interpreted as an indication of unimpaired renal function. The average values for S_{Cr} concentrations vary somewhat with the method of analysis. In general, normal values range from 0.7–1.3 mg/dl, with the upper limit of normal being 1.5 mg/dl in adults.

Blood Urea Nitrogen to Serum Creatinine Ratio

As mentioned above, BUN is disproportionately elevated above S_{Cr} in conditions where there is increased catabolism of protein leading to greater urea production. In addition, conditions that would decrease the clearance of urea to a greater extent than GFR is decreased may result in a greater elevation of BUN than S_{Cr}. The clearance of urea varies from 40% to 60% of GFR values, depending on the state of urine flow. For example, with decreased renal perfusion or acute urinary tract obstruction the clearance of urea falls more than GFR. Under these conditions, BUN increases to a greater extent than S_{Cr}. Therefore, additional information may be obtained from examining the ratio of BUN to S_{Cr}. This ratio is about 10 to 15 under normal conditions and in patients with stable chronic renal disease. However, under conditions of avid sodium and water reabsorption and low urine flow rates, as in hypovolemia, relatively less urea will be cleared compared to creatinine and the BUN to S_{Cr} ratio may be greater than 15.

Differential Diagnosis of Azotemia

When evaluating azotemia one should first consider whether the azotemia has developed acutely or chronically and second whether the azotemia is due to intrinsic renal disease or to extrarenal causes. If previous values for BUN or S_{Cr} are available, it is easy to evaluate the acuteness or chronicity of the azotemia. If this information is not available, it may be difficult, except under certain circumstances, to judge the acuteness or chronicity of the process. The acuteness of onset may be judged by clinical features such as nausea, vomiting, central nervous system (CNS) symptoms, absence of pallor, and decreased urine output or laboratory findings of severe hyperkalemia, acidosis, and hypocalcemia. On the other hand, the differentiation between prerenal azotemia and azotemia due to intrinsic parenchymal renal disease is based on laboratory considerations.

Differentiation of Prerenal Azotemia from Azotemia Caused by Intrinsic Renal Disease

Renal handling of salt and water in patients with intrinsic kidney disease differs from that in patients with hemodynamic alterations (prerenal azotemia). If salt and water intake remain constant as the nephron population decreases, homeostasis is maintained by a progressive increase in the fractional excretion of salt and water; that is, a greater percentage of the filtered salt and water is excreted in the final urine. This leads to a urine characterized by a low urine to plasma (U/P) creatinine ratio, decreased osmolality, and a relatively high sodium concentration (U_{Na}). If the concentration of sodium (U_{Na}) divided by the U/P creatinine ratio (referred to as the renal failure index, RFI) exceeds unity, this favors the presence of intrinsic renal disease (see Table 7-1). If the blood flow to a normal

Table 7-1

Laboratory Tests Useful in the Differential Diagnosis of Causes of Azotemia

Type of Renal Failure	U/P Creatinine	RFI	U/P Osmolality	Urinary Sodium Concentration (mEq/liter)	BUN/S_{Cr}	GFR (ml/min)	Urine Volume per 24 hours (ml)
Oliguric ARF	< 20	> 1	< 1.2	> 20	10	< 1	< 500
Nonoliguric ARF	< 20	> 1	< 1.2	> 20	10	2–10	> 500
Prerenal azotemia	> 20	< 1	> 1.2	< 20	> 10	20–50	Inversely related to U/P creatinine
Obstructive uropathy							
Acute	> 20	< 1	> 1.2	< 20	10	Variable	Anuria to polyuria
Chronic	< 20	> 1	< 1.2	> 20	10	Variable	

Note: ARF, acute renal failure; U, urine; P, plasma.

kidney is impaired as in congestive heart failure, severe dehydration, hypotension, and the like, a large fraction of the filtered salt and water will be reabsorbed, resulting in a concentrated urine with a low sodium concentration (U_{Na}). The U/P creatinine ratio and U/P osmolality ratio will be elevated, the BUN to S_{Cr} ratio will exceed 15, and the RFI will be less than 1 (see Table 7-1). These relatively simple laboratory tests will, under most conditions, distinguish between prerenal azotemia and azotemia resulting from intrinsic renal disease. When prerenal failure is superimposed on intrinsic renal disease, one must rely on other clinical parameters, because differentiation using U/P creatinine ratios and urinary sodium concentrations becomes invalid, since intrinsic renal disease will alter the hemodynamic response of the kidney to a decrease in renal perfusion.

Temporal Considerations

If the rate of change of S_{Cr} or BUN is known, it is possible to determine whether the renal disease (azotemia) is acute, subacute, or chronic based on the following criteria. Acute renal failure implies a sudden (hours to a few days) decrease in GFR. If GFR falls acutely from normal to zero in a 70 kg person, in whom total body water remains constant, the S_{Cr} concentration would rise by 2–3 mg/dl/day. This is based on the fact that creatinine is distributed in total body water (50 liters), normal serum creatinine concentration is 1 mg/dl, and thus the total body creatinine is about 500 mg. Assuming a daily creatinine production of 1000 mg with no excretion at the end of 24 hours, the total body creatinine would be 1500 mg, giving a S_{Cr} of 3 mg/dl. Subsequent daily increments are based on similar calculations. Thus, a daily rise in S_{Cr} of 1–3 mg/dl is evidence of acute renal failure. Subacute renal failure, in this discussion, refers to a rate of disease progression (from inception to termination) in months to a year. Chronic renal failure has a course greater than a year. Although these are arbitrary criteria, they do have considerable utility.

If an azotemic patient presents with no previous laboratory studies, one must rely on historical data, other laboratory tests, and subsequent examination to distinguish between acute and chronic renal disease. When functional renal impairment occurs slowly, a number of adaptations occur such that a patient with far-advanced renal disease (as little as 10% of normal renal function) may be asymptomatic. On the other hand, patients with acute renal disease are subjectively quite ill. A useful test under these circumstances is evaluation of kidney size by a roentgenogram of the abdomen. Small kidneys (less than 10 cm or the length of 2.5 vertebral bodies) imply chronic disease; if renal size is normal, no conclusion may be drawn because end-stage chronic renal disease may be present with normal-sized kidneys (diabetes mellitus, amyloidosis, renal vein thrombosis, and other entities). Very large kidneys suggest polycystic renal disease.

Causes of Prerenal Azotemia

The syndromes producing azotemia secondary to decreased renal perfusion in the absence of intrinsic renal damage are referred to as prerenal. They include *congestive heart failure, dehydration, blood loss, and severe decompensated liver disease.* The common denominator for each of these syndromes is maximal renal conservation of salt and water. The U/P creatinine and osmolality ratios are greater than 20, the urinary sodium concentration (U_{Na}) is low ($<$ 20 mEq/liter), and the RFI is low (Table 7-1). While these diagnostic indices almost always indicate prerenal failure, important exceptions include acute incomplete urinary tract obstruction and acute diffuse glomerular damage. These entities may be differentiated from prerenal states by intravenous or retrograde pyelography or by the changing pattern of urine chemistries (increased U_{Na}, decreased U/P creatinines) 48 to 72 hours after the onset of azotemia. The urine analysis is generally normal in prerenal azotemia but may contain hyaline casts. On the other hand, examination of the urine of patients with acute diffuse glomerulonephritis or the vasculitides may reveal numerous red blood cells, granular casts, and red blood cell casts.

The prerenal syndromes are usually distinguishable from each other by the presence or absence of signs, symptoms, or history of congestive heart failure, blood loss (usually from the gastrointestinal tract), or dehydration (judged by skin turgor and/or a history of vomiting, diarrhea, perspiration, or excessive diuretic therapy). If there is decreased intravascular volume, hypotension is frequently present and may be exaggerated by the assumption of the upright position and accompanied by an increase in heart rate. In dehydration, the hematocrit reading and the concentration of plasma proteins may be increased.

The hepatorenal syndrome is a specific condition, not synonymous with intrinsic renal failure occurring in a patient with liver disease. It is only seen in patients with severe decompensated hepatic failure with ascites, jaundice, and markedly abnormal liver function tests. After the onset of liver failure the patients develop oliguria with a very low urine sodium (<5 mEq/liter) and a high U/P creatinine ratio. The BUN/S_{Cr} ratio may not be as elevated as seen in the other causes of prerenal azotemia because hepatic synthesis of urea is diminished. Death usually results from hepatic failure and rarely from alterations imposed by diminished renal function (Table 7-2).

Causes of Postrenal Azotemia

One must always consider obstruction in the differential diagnosis of azotemia. Demonstration of obstruction to the normal outflow of urine provides the basis for the diagnosis of postrenal azotemia. During the first 24 to 48 hours of incomplete obstruction, there may be a decrease in fractional salt and water excretion, thus suggesting prerenal azotemia. However, the pattern rapidly changes, and the characteristic diagnostic indices of postrenal azotemia are a decrease in U/P creatinine ratio, an increase in U_{Na}, and an increase in RFI. If anuria is present, complete obstruction must be ruled out; a history of anuria followed by polyuria and recurrent anuria is pathognomonic of intermittent complete obstruction. Slowly progressive obstruction is usually not associated with a decrease in urine output; rather polyuria is frequently a feature of incomplete obstruction.

Nephrolithiasis may cause obstruction without overt symptoms, although renal colic and hematuria are expected. Since obstruction of the urinary tract is frequently associated with infection, fever and pyuria require a thorough examination to exclude obstruction. Intravenous pyelography may be diagnostic, although complete obstruction of one ureter may be associated with nonvisualization of the affected kidney. Repeated injections of contrast material with reexamination several hours later may visualize collecting systems that are not seen by routine pyelography. Computerized axial tomography or retrograde studies may be indicated if obstruction cannot be excluded by intravenous pyelography. Bladder outlet obstruction may be rapidly diagnosed by palpation and rapidly corrected by the insertion of a bladder catheter.

Causes of Intrinsic Renal Disease with an Acute Course

The common features of diseases in this category are rapid deterioration of renal function, an elevated U_{Na}, a decreased U/P creatinine ratio, an RFI of 1.0 or greater, and normal-sized kidneys. The diagnostic considerations in Table 7-2 are discussed below.

Acute Tubular Necrosis (ATN)

This is the most common cause of acute intrinsic renal failure. Oliguria is present in 50% of cases, while anuria is rare, and the remainder are nonoliguric. The urine output is most diminished in those patients with the greatest degree of renal functional impairment; that is, patients with nonoliguric ATN usually have GFRs in excess of 3 ml/min. Those with oliguric ATN have clearances of less than 1 ml/min. Urinary microscopic findings in-

Table 7-2

Acute Renal Failure

Prerenal	Intrinsic Disease	Postrenal
1. Congestive heart failure 2. Decreased intravascular volume a. Blood loss b. Dehydration (1) Excessive diuretic therapy (2) Vomiting (3) Diarrhea (4) Excessive perspiration 3. Liver failure a. Cirrhosis with ascites b. Hepatorenal syndrome	1. Acute tubular necrosis (ATN) a. Hypovolemia b. Septic shock c. Drug-induced d. Hemolytic anemia e. Rhabdomyolysis 2. Pregnancy related a. Eclampsia b. Bilateral cortical necrosis c. Irreversible postpartum renal failure 3. Malignant hypertension 4. Acute diffuse pyelonephritis 5. Atheroembolic disease 6. Acute glomerulonephritis a. Poststreptococcal b. Other infections (1) Endocarditis (2) Infected shunts 7. Hypersensitivity angiitis 8. Uric acid nephropathy 9. Associated with multiple myeloma	1. Incomplete and complete obstruction a. Bladder outlet obstruction (1) Prostatic hypertrophy (2) Neurogenic b. Nephrolithiasis

clude dark granular casts and renal epithelial cells; red blood cell casts are rare but do occur. Heme-pigmented casts are rare except in patients with rhabdomyolysis and/or hemolytic anemia.

Severe dehydration increases the likelihood of developing ATN regardless of the etiologic agent or precipitating event. Shock secondary to trauma, blood loss, sepsis, burns, cardiovascular collapse, tamponade, and the like is the most common precipitating event. Nephrotoxic drugs, particularly the aminoglycosides, cephalosporins, and penicillins (those drugs that most avidly bind in the renal cortex) are a major cause of ATN. Oliguria and azotemia may not appear for as long as a week following cessation of therapy with nephrotoxic drugs. Myoglobinuria from traumatic or non-traumatic rhabdomyolysis or hemoglobinuria from hemolytic anemia are important precipitating events in the development of ATN, particularly in the dehydrated patient. No precipitating event may be found in 30% of patients with ATN.

Pregnancy-related Acute Renal Failure

Acute renal failure early in pregnancy usually results from ATN; it is usually seen following unskilled abortions, which result in sepsis, intravascular hemolysis, or severe blood loss. Acute renal failure in the third trimester is usually secondary to eclampsia, a syndrome characterized by hypertension, proteinuria, edema, and convulsions. Acute renal failure at parturition may be related to abruptio placentae or intrauterine hemorrhage, which result in diffuse or patchy bilateral cortical necrosis. Anuria and permanent renal functional impairment are common in this syndrome. Patients with patchy cortical necrosis may regain some renal function after weeks to months.

Acute renal failure occurring in the early postpartum period (1 day to several months) with microangiopathic hemolytic anemia, thrombocytopenia, hypertension, and unexplained fever often leads to irreversible renal failure. The renal lesions in these patients are similar to those seen in the experimental generalized Schwartzman reaction, and the entity is considered to be a form of the adult hemolytic-uremic syndrome.

Hypertension

Although hypertension is frequently associated with nephrosclerosis and chronic progressive renal disease, it may result in acute renal failure when a sudden and marked increase in blood pressure (malignant hypertension) occurs. Furthermore, acute renal failure may also occur after vigorous therapy for severe hypertension.

Acute Diffuse Pyelonephritis

It is a rare cause of acute renal failure unless bilateral papillary necrosis occurs. The patients are critically ill with sepsis, fever, and flank pain. Obstruction is a frequent underlying condition.

Atheroembolic Disease

Atheroembolic disease with occlusion of both renal arteries or the arterial supply to a solitary kidney may cause azotemia, especially in the elderly. The diagnosis is established by arteriography.

Acute Glomerulonephritis

Acute poststreptococcal glomerulonephritis is the prototype of acute diffuse glomerulonephritis. This clinical syndrome is characterized by hematuria with red blood cell casts, proteinuria, edema, and hypertension. The edema typically involves the face, eyelids, and hands, being most noticeable in the morning. Hypertension is usually mild and not accompanied by retinal alterations. Pulmonary edema, circulatory overload, and congestive heart failure are common. Oliguria is present in severe cases, and anuria has been reported.

Acute syndromes clinically resembling the poststreptococcal syndrome may occur with other infections: viral—varicella, hepatitis, mumps, infectious mononucleosis, ECHO and coxsackie; parasitic—malaria and toxoplasma; bacterial—infected shunts or fistulas and bacterial endocarditis. Appropriate cultures or serological studies or both are required for differentiation.

The majority of causes of acute renal failure of parenchymal origin are associated with a high U_{Na}, a low U/P creatinine ratio, and a high RFI. Diseases producing an acute diffuse glomerulonephritis or severe protein loss or both may be important exceptions and are mentioned again for emphasis. Urinary diagnostic indices in this latter entity will be like those seen with prerenal failure. This should not be a source of diagnostic confusion, since the urinalysis will reveal red blood cells, frequently with casts or massive proteinuria. These latter findings are not seen in uncomplicated prerenal azotemia.

Causes of Intrinsic Renal Disease with a Subacute Course

Diagnostic considerations under this heading include diseases that result in complete functional renal impairment within a month to a year. A common denominator is damage to the glomerulus or renal vasculature. Syndromes in this category are listed in Table 7-3. The differential diagnosis of these causes of azotemia is described in detail in the chapters on hematuria and proteinuria. Most of the entities in this group are associated with systemic disease; idiopathic rapidly progressive glomerulonephritis, malignant hypertension, and obstruction are exceptions (Table 7-3).

Causes of Intrinsic Renal Disease with a Chronic Course

Diagnostic indices in chronic progressive renal disease are uniform and include a decreased U/P creatinine ratio, a high U_{Na}, and an RFI greater than unity; consequently, the assignment of patients to this group rarely presents a problem. The finding of small kidneys on a roentgenogram of the abdomen or intravenous pyelogram strongly suggests chronic renal disease. However, it must be remembered that patients with chronic renal disease may have normal-sized kidneys (diabetic nephropathy, amyloidosis, etc.) or large kidneys (polycystic disease). Chronic obstruction of the urinary tract must always be considered, and appropriate studies must be conducted to exclude this possibility.

The differential diagnosis of chronic renal disease is facilitated by determining whether the disease involves the kidneys exclusively or is associated with disease in other organs and whether the disease primarily affects the glomerulus or the interstitium. Glomerulopathy may be distinguished from interstitial nephritis by the presence of the nephrotic syndrome, which is usually not a feature of interstitial disease (see chapter on proteinuria). The urinary sediment of patients with glomerular disease is usually more "active" than that of patients with interstitial disease. The number of red blood cells and granular casts is an index of activity. A renal biopsy is usually necessary for a conclusive diagnosis. The various diseases responsible for chronic renal disease are listed in Table 7-4. The reader is referred to the chapters on hematuria and proteinuria for specific details.

Marked azotemia, anemia, hypocalcemia, hyperphosphatemia, metabolic acidosis, and clinical manifestations of uremia point to the diagnosis of advanced chronic renal disease. However, patients with chronic renal disease with a moderate decrease in renal function may present as patients with far advanced disease if there is an intercurrent problem. Infection, dehydration, or obstruction should always be sought as potentially reversible causes for increased azotemia in patients with chronic renal disease.

Table 7-3

Subacute Renal Failure

Without Systemic Symptoms	With Systemic Symptoms
1. Idiopathic rapidly progressive glomerulonephritis	1. Goodpasture's syndrome
2. Malignant hypertension	2. Polyarteritis a. Periarteritis nodosa b. Hypersensitivity angiitis c. Allergic granulomatosis
3. Obstruction a. Prostatic hypertrophy b. Neurogenic bladder c. Tumor d. Retroperitoneal fibrosis	3. Adult hemolytic-uremic syndrome
	4. Thrombotic thrombocytopenic purpura
	5. Henoch-Schonlein purpura
	6. Wegener's granulomatosis
	7. Progressive systemic sclerosis

Table 7-4

Chronic Renal Disease

Glomerular Involvement without Systemic Symptoms	Glomerular Involvement with Systemic Symptoms	Tubulo-interstitial Disease
1. Focal glomerular sclerosis	1. Polyarteritis	1. Pyelonephritis
2. Membranous glomerulopathy	2. Progressive systemic sclerosis	2. Papillary necrosis
3. Mesangio-capillary glomerulonephritis	3. Henoch-Schonlein purpura	3. Hereditary a. Polycystic renal disease b. Medullary cystic disease c. Fanconi syndrome
4. Proliferative glomerulonephritis	4. Systemic lupus erythematosus	4. Metabolic a. Urate nephropathy b. Oxalate nephropathy c. Nephrocalcinosis
5. Heroin-associated nephropathy	5. Amyloidosis a. Primary b. Secondary	5. Toxic a. Analgesic nephropathy (papillary necrosis) b. Antibiotics c. Heavy metals
6. Hereditary nephritis	6. Diabetic nephropathy	6. Radiation nephritis
	7. Neoplastic disease a. Lungs b. GI tract c. Hodgkin's and other lymphomas	7. Obstruction (see Table 7-3)
		8. Infarction

Clinical Problem

A 51-year-old white female was admitted to the hospital with a 24-hour history of shortness of breath, difficulty swallowing, and dizziness. She had a 1-year history of migratory symmetric polyarthralgias associated with alopecia and pruritus. Her past history was unremarkable except for primary hypothyroidism with current thyroid replacement. On admission to the hospital, she was alert and afebrile with a blood pressure of 140/86 mm Hg, pulse rate of 84 beats per minute, and a respiratory rate of 16 per minute. The remainder of the physical examination was normal. Laboratory data included a normal urinalysis, a T_4 of 5.6 μg/ml, a normal liver profile, BUN, creatinine, and electrolytes. The hemoglobin level was 11.6 gm/dl; hematocrit, 34.4%; white blood cell count (WBC), 5.800. Radiographic studies included normal chest x-ray, IVP, barium enema, and upper GI series. Oral cholecystogram demonstrated numerous opaque gallstones in a functioning gallbladder. Cholecystectomy was performed on the eighth hospital day without complication. Postoperatively, the patient was treated with sodium cephalothin because of daily temperature elevations to 37.8° to 38°C. On the seventh hospital day, cefazolin sodium was started. She then noted arthralgias and pruritus, although physical examination was unremarkable. Antibiotics were changed to gentamicin and tetracycline on the ninth hospital day. Bibasilar rales, left basilar dullness, minimal periungual erythema, and minimal metacarpal and proximal interphalangeal (PIP) joint thickening were noted. Laboratory data included a white count of 8700; hematocrit, 31%; and arterial blood with a pH of 7.54, a pCO_2 of 30.3 mm Hg, and a pO_2 of 88 mm Hg. Sputum and urine cultures were negative. Liver function tests were normal except for an alkaline phosphatase value of 306 mU/ml. Antinuclear antibodies (ANA), rheumatoid arthritis (RA) factor latex, heterophil, HB_sAg and Ab tests, and the intermediate purified protein derivative (PPD) were negative. Urinalysis revealed 1+ blood and 1+ protein. Chest x-ray revealed left lower lobe atelectasis and a left pleural effusion. Lung scan was nondiagnostic. Bronchoscopy and sinus x-rays were negative. Pleural fluid cultures were negative; pleural fluid amylase was 60 units /dl.

Over the next several days, fever spikes continued; multiple blood cultures were negative. The white blood cell count rose to 13,400 with a left shift. On the 25th hospital day, oxacillin, 2 gm I.V. q. 6 hr and gentamicin, 80 mg I.V. q. 8 hr were started. The BUN level at that time was 17. A repeat urinalysis revealed many red blood cells and 4+ proteinuria. On the 27th hospital day the temperature rose to 41°C and a pericardial friction rub was noted. Chest x-ray was unchanged. The WBC rose to 19,500 with a left shift. The BUN level increased to 42. Repeat cultures of blood, sputum, and urine were negative. Pleural fluid from the left chest now revealed 30,800 white cells, with 93% polymorphonuclear leukocytes. On the 31st hospital day, an erythematous rash was noted over the abdomen. The BUN level increased to 54, and the creatinine level rose to 6.8 mg/dl. An IVP revealed the kidneys to be slightly enlarged but with no evidence of obstruction. On the 33rd hospital day, she was alert, oriented, and in mild respiratory distress with chest pain. Her blood pressure was 155/75, with 5 mm Hg pulsus paradoxus; respiratory rate, 30 per minute; pulse rate, 130 beats per minute; and temperature, 39° C. There was an erythematous maculopapular rash over the face and upper back. Examination of the head, neck, eyes, ears, nose, and throat was unremarkable. Physical findings were consistent with bilateral pleural effusions. A 2/6 systolic ejection murmur was heard at the lower left sternal border, and there was a two-component pericardial friction rub but no gallop. Abdominal examination revealed only a healing surgical scar. Neurological examination was unremarkable. The patient's hemoglobin level was 8.6 gm/dl; hematocrit, 26.7%; WBC, 26,200 with a left shift. Serum sodium level was 129 mEq/liter; potassium, 5.2 mEq/liter; carbon dioxide, 17 mEq/liter; chloride, 93 mEq/liter; creatinine, 8.7 mg/dl; glucose, 82 mg/dl; and amylase, 84 units/dl. Arterial blood gases revealed a pH of 7.36; pCO_2, 26 mm Hg; and pO_2, 75 mm Hg. An electrocardiogram showed sinus tachycardia. The serum bilirubin level was 0.8 mg/dl, alkaline phosphatase, 158 mU/ml; SGOT, 22 mU/ml; LDH, 403 mU/ml; CPK, 64 mU/ml. The urine specific gravity was 1.014, pH 5.0, 2+ blood, 2+ protein, and the sediment showed 5–6 WBC/hpf, 3–4 RBC/hpf, and a few granular casts. Urinary creatinine level was 62 mg/dl; sodium, 50 mEq/liter. Chest x-rays revealed a left pleural effusion and bibasilar air bronchograms.

Because of progressive azotemia, hemodialysis was begun on the 37th hospital day. The patient's fever continued. Pleural fluid, blood, sputum, cerebrospinal fluid, and urine cultures were all negative. The erythrocyte sedimentation rate was 125 mm/hr, the platelet count was 935,000, and serum complement levels were normal. An LE prep was negative; direct Coomb's test and ANA and DNA antibody tests were negative. Febrile and fungal serologies were negative. During the patient's hospitalization, the WBC rose to as high as 42,000, with a differential showing 1 blast, 8 myelocytes, 6 metamyelocytes, 34 bands, 45 segs, 2 lymphocytes, 2 eosinophils, and 1 monocyte. A bone marrow examination revealed increased cellularity, an increased myeloid:erythroid (M:E) ratio, and a pronounced left shift with megaloblastoid changes. Abdominal sonograms and computerized axial tomography (CAT) scans were normal; pulmonary angiography failed to reveal pulmonary emboli. Liver spleen scans revealed markedly diminished splenic uptake and mild hepatocellular dysfunction. Gallium scan revealed a constant increase in activity in the region of the hepatic flexure and portions of the transverse colon. Spleen scans showed a significant decrease in uptake of the radiocolloid interpreted as evidence of splenic infarction. The patient continued to spike temperatures to 39.5° C and complained of dizziness and on occasion left pleuritic chest pain. Repeated physical examinations showed a persistent pleural effusion, varying degress of congestive heart failure, a persistent pericardial friction rub, and vague right and left upper quadrant discomfort. On the 42nd hospital day, an exploratory laparotomy was performed.

Questions

1. Is the course compatible with acute, subacute, or chronic renal failure?
2. Is the azotemia due to prerenal, postrenal, or intrinsic renal disease?
3. Is the azotemia associated with systemic disease?
4. Are drugs or infection responsible for the renal failure?

Discussion

The intravenous pyelogram ruled out obstruction as a cause of azotemia and revealed normal-sized kidneys. There was a high U_{Na} (50 mEq/liter), a U/P creatinine ratio of 7, and a renal failure index of 7. The rate of progression of disease from inception to renal failure occurred over a period of almost 1 month. The renal failure was not antedated by shock, hypovolemia, trauma, or massive hemolysis. Malignant hypertension was excluded as was infection of the kidney.

Acute tubular necrosis must be considered because it sometimes occurs in the absence of overt clinical precipitating events and because various nephrotoxic antibiotics were prescribed. The large number of red blood cells and protein in the urine argue against drug induced ATN and favor a glomerular lesion of the type listed in Table 7-3 under subacute renal failure associated with systemic disease. Goodpasture's syndrome should be considered because of the pulmonary involvement. However, hemoptysis was not present, and more importantly, the other systemic manifestations that this patient had are not part of this syndrome. The adult hemolytic-uremic syndrome has been described in patients with various infections including typhoid fever, *Escherichia coli,* and suspected viral infections. Infection was not demonstrated in this patient; however, this is difficult to evaluate because cultures were obtained while she was on antibiotics. Burr and helmet cells were not seen, although anemia was present. Again the other symptoms are not a part of this syndrome. Wegener's granulomatosis is unlikely, based on the absence of rhinorrhea and sinusitis. The lack of CNS symptoms and thrombocytopenia rules out thrombotic thrombocytopenia purpura. The skin rash that the patient had was not purpuric. The most likely diagnosis is polyarteritis, which includes periarteritis nodosa, hypersensitivity angiitis, and allergic granulomatous angiitis. This diagnosis is compatible with the past history of arthralgias, the pulmonary and pericardial involvement, and the suspicion of splenic infarction. The time course and skin rash are compatible with hypersensitivity angiitis.

An exploratory laparotomy was performed with splenectomy and renal biopsy. The pathological diagnosis was necrotizing small vessel vasculitis.

References

Berns, A. S., Llinas, S. L., Miller, R. R., Heinrich, W. L., Anderson, R. J., and Schrier, R. W. "Urinary diagnostic indices in acute renal failure." Proc. Am. Soc. Nephrol., Washington, November 1976, p. 495.

Bleiler, R. E., and Schedl, H. P. "Creatinine excretion; variability and relationship to diet and body size." J. Lab. Clin. Med. *59:* 945, 1962.

Coe, F. L. "The clinical and laboratory assessment of the patient with renal disease." *In:* The Kidney, B. M. Brenner and F. C. Rector (eds.). W. B. Saunders, Philadelphia, p. 765, 1976.

Enger, E., and Bligen, E. M. "The relationship between endogenous creatinine clearance and serum creatinine in renal failure." Scand. J. Clin. Lab. Invest. *16:* 273, 1964.

Glassock, R. J., and Bennett, C. M. "The glomerulopathies." *In:* The Kidney, B. M. Brenner and F. C. Rector (eds.). W. B. Saunders, Philadelphia, p. 941, 1976.

Levinsky, N. G., and Alexander, E. A. "Acute renal failure." *In:* The Kidney, B. M. Brenner and F. C. Rector (eds.). W. B. Saunders, Philadelphia, p. 806, 1976.

Suki, W. N., and Eknoyan, G. "Tubulo-interstitial disease." *In:* The Kidney, B. M. Brenner and F. C. Rector (eds.). W. B. Saunders, Philadelphia, p. 1113, 1976.

Walser, M., and Bodenlos, L. J. "Urea metabolism in man." J. Clin. Invest. *38:* 1617, 1959.

Chapter 8

Oligurìa and Anuria

General Considerations

Oliguria and anuria usually signify decreasing renal function and may or may not mean intrinsic renal failure. Oliguria is defined as the excretion of less than 400–500 ml of urine per 24 hours. Anuria is literally no urine output. Many clinicians, however, have defined anuria as the excretion of less than 50 ml of urine in 24 hours. In the present discussion, the literal definition will be used.

The organism's requirement for osmolar balance is the physiological basis for the definition of oliguria. The average diet and metabolic processes result in the daily production of about 600 milliosmoles (mOsm) of solute which must be excreted by the kidney to maintain homeostasis. A large portion of osmolar content of foodstuffs is oxidized to carbon dioxide and water. Thus the osmolar content of foodstuffs that must be excreted by the kidney for homeostasis, that is, the 600 mOsms, involves such compounds as phosphorus, sodium, sulfur, nitrogen, chloride, and the like. The human can maximally concentrate urine to 1200 mOsm/kg H_2O. Therefore, the minimum volume for the excretion of the normal osmolar load is 500 ml of maximally concentrated urine. Urine volumes less than this and less than maximally concentrated are distinctly abnormal.

Oliguria and anuria signify one of the following events: decreased renal perfusion or decreased glomerular filtration rate per nephron; intrinsic renal disease; or obstruction to the efflux of urine from the tubules, ureters, bladder, or urethra. Thus, in the evaluation of decreased urine flow (oliguria), prerenal, renal, or postrenal causes must be differentiated.

Clinical Evaluation and Differential Diagnosis of Oliguria

Prerenal Causes of Oliguria

Prerenal causes of oliguria (see Table 8-1) are related to a decrease in "effective" or absolute blood volume. A decrease in "effective" blood volume is illustrated by congestive heart failure, where the intravascular volume is actually increased, but renal perfusion is decreased. Absolute reduction in the intravascular volume, however, is the most common cause of oliguria.

The kidney responds in either instance by attempting to preserve intravascular volume, that is, by increasing fractional salt and water reabsorption. The urine is concentrated maximally; urine sodium concentration is less than 20 mEq/liter and the U/P creatinine ratio is greater than 20 (See Table 7-1, Chapter 7). Urea clearance decreases to a greater extent than GFR (urea clearance varies with urine flow); consequently the BUN to S_{cr} ratio will be greater than 10 to 15 except when the production of urea is impaired as in

Table 8-1

Differential Diagnosis of Anuria and Oliguria

	Anuria	Oliguria

Prerenal:	Bilateral renal artery occlusion
	  Bilateral emboli
	  Dissecting aneurysm
	Cardiogenic shock
		Decreased intravenous volume
		  Dehydration
		  Blood loss
		  Hypoalbuminuria
		Osmotic diuresis
		Left ventricular failure
		Shock, vasodilatation

Renal:	Acute diffuse renal disease
	  Bilateral cortical necrosis
	  Vasculitis
	  Glomerulonephritis
		Patchy cortical necrosis
		Acute tubular necrosis
		Glomerulonephritis
		Nephrotoxins
		Hemolysis
		Myoglobinuria
		Multiple myeloma
		Interstitial nephritis
		Postpartum renal failure
		Sepsis
		Abruptio placentae
		Bacterial endocarditis

Postrenal:	Bilateral ureteral obstruction
	  (or ureteral obstruction when
	  only one kidney)
	Neurogenic bladder
	Urethral obstruction
	Bladder neck obstruction
	Plugged urinary catheter
		Neurogenic bladder
		Partial ureteral or bladder obstruction

liver failure or malnutrition. In general plasma constituents will be more concentrated when there is decreased intravascular volume, for example, increased hematocrit and albumin concentrations.

Prerenal causes of oliguria include *decreased intravascular volume, heart failure,* and *shock* or *profound vasodilatation.* Diuretics are probably one of the most common causes of decreased intravascular volume. This can proceed to oliguria when the reduction is severe and persistent. Dehydration is also quite common and is usually secondary to gastrointestinal fluid losses, heat exhaustion, osmotic diuresis, water deprivation, or, rarely, failure of thirst mechanisms, inadequate fluid replacement, or blood loss. Hypercalcemia induces a renal concentrating defect such that patients with severe hypercalcemia may become dehydrated, lethargic, oliguric, and ultimately develop renal failure unless the intravascular volume is corrected.

Left ventricular failure leads to lower renal perfusion and can produce oliguria. This occurs in arteriosclerotic heart disease, myocardial infarction, some valvular insufficiencies, cardiomyopathies, and arrhythmias. These patients are usually fluid-overloaded and may even have pulmonary edema, but the effective renal plasma flow is depressed. Improvement of myocardial contractility or arrhythmias or both help to resolve the oliguric state. Shock and profound vasodilatation from bacteremia and the like also produce oliguria. Oliguria is common in the evolution of the hepatorenal syndrome where the effective renal blood flow is decreased.

Intrarenal Causes of Oliguria

Oliguria commonly occurs in acute, severe, diffuse intrarenal disease whether of tubular or glomerular origin. Diffuse intrarenal disease usually leads to the inability to concentrate the urine. Therefore, the biochemical indices and characteristics of the urinary sediment are crucial in assessment. Patients often have systemic acidosis and are hypertensive. Serum urea nitrogen and creatinine levels are increased in the normal proportion, that is, a ratio of 10–15 to 1. The exception to this is when the patient is extremely catabolic, an instance when the BUN may be considerably increased. The serum calcium concentration is low and frequently less than 8 mg/dl. The serum phosphorus concentration is increased. Urine sodium concentration is high, that is, greater than 20 mEq/liter. The urine osmolality is not markedly different from serum osmolality, since the kidney loses its ability to concentrate in diffuse intrarenal disease. The U/P creatinine ratio is less than 20. In acute tubular disease the urine often contains granular casts that may be pigmented by hemoglobin or myoglobin but will rarely contain red cells. White cells are few. There may be many renal tubular cells seen. The urine may have a characteristic brown, muddy color. In glomerular diseases the urinary sediment contains red blood cell casts, protein, granular casts, and free red cells. Early in glomerulitis the urine sodium may be low, resembling prerenal failure. After 48 to 72 hours, however, the urine sodium concentration is characteristically high.

By far the most common intrarenal cause of oliguria is acute tubular necrosis. In many instances the cause of ATN is idiopathic. There are, however, several known etiologies. Often the onset of ATN is preceded by periods of dehydration and marked decrease in renal perfusion. Superimposed, however, is a specific inciting event or entity. ATN is frequently seen secondary to various nephrotoxins such as the heavy metals mercury, bismuth, arsenic, cadmium; organic compounds including such pesticides as chlordane, creosol, carbon tetrachloride, methanol, toluene, ethylene glycol, oxalic acid, aniline; anesthetics such as methoxyflurane; antibiotics such as the aminoglycosides, cephalosporins, colistin, amphotericin; and roentgenographic contrast media. Intravascular hemolysis and rhabdomyolysis are also recognized causes of ATN. Rhabdomyolysis may be traumatic or secondary to myositis, heat stroke, vigorous muscle contraction as in seizures and strenuous exercise, crush injury, electric shock, burns, and severe potassium depletion. Rarely does the oliguria of ATN persist beyond 1 month. Anuria is very rarely seen in ATN. Nonoliguric ATN differs from oliguric ATN only in the degree of functional renal impairment; that is, the GFR is usually greater than 3 ml/min in nonoliguric ATN.

Acute glomerulonephritides and arteritides may present with oliguria. These entities often accompany a systemic disorder with characteristic manifestations that help to define the underlying disease. Acute glomerulonephritis, such as poststreptococcal or rapidly progressive glomerulonephritis, Goodpasture's syndrome or periarteritis nodosa, may have an abrupt onset with oliguria, hematuria, proteinuria, and hypertension. The urinary sediment in glomerular disease is distinctive in that proteinuria is heavy and red cells and red cell casts are plentiful in contrast to the tubular diseases.

Oliguria may also be associated with small vessel occlusion as in scleroderma, malignant hypertension, and polyarteritis. Patchy cortical necrosis may present as oliguria. An abrupt decrease in blood pressure or the treatment of severe hypertension may lead to oliguria. Oliguric renal failure may also occur in patients with multiple myeloma and diabetes mellitus who are particularly sensitive to radiographic contrast media, especially if dehydrated or with moderately advanced renal failure, that is, serum creatinine level greater than 5 mg/dl.

Uric acid nephropathy may present with oliguria or anuria. The urinalysis reveals many urate crystals and usually an acid pH. The spun sediment may be heavy sludge with a pinkish tinge to the crystals. Uric acid nephropathy most often occurs in the myeloproliferative disorders as chronic lymphocytic leukemia and may develop suddenly, coincident with chemotherapy of the underlying disease. Interstitial nephritis secondary to drug sensitivity, such as methicillin, may present with oliguria. Hematuria and eosinophilia are characteristically associated with this disorder.

Obstetrical causes of oliguria include abruptio placentae, sepsis, abortafacients, septic abortions, and postpartum renal failure.

Postrenal Causes of Oliguria

Postrenal failure is always caused by obstruction. In anuric or oliguric states, obstruction must be a primary consideration. Alternating episodes of oliguria or anuria and polyuria are pathognomonic of obstruction. Ureteral obstruction must be bilateral to produce sudden anuria or oliguria. It may be unilateral if only one kidney is present. Bladder outlet obstruction or a neurogenic bladder, as in acute urinary retention, may be a cause of anuria or oliguria. Bilateral papillary necrosis with obstruction of ureters, though rare, may be seen in diabetics or patients with phenacetin abuse or sickle cell disease.

The urinary sediment in obstruction may be relatively benign, unless infection plays an important part; then white blood cells, WBC casts, and bacteria may be seen in the sediment. Diagnosis of outlet obstruction is aided by quick, temporary catheterization under sterile conditions with a French catheter. Intravenous pyelography, nephrotomography, and computerized axial tomography may also be of diagnostic help.

Anuria

Anuria results from bilateral obstruction to renal arterial perfusion, complete obstruction of the efflux of urine via the collecting system, cortical necrosis, and sometimes acute glomerulitis. Bilateral renal artery occlusion may be produced by emboli or rarely thrombosis. Over 75% of renal artery occlusions are associated with cardiac events. Large emboli may be flipped from the left ventricle in patients with atrial fibrillation, myocardial infarction, cardiomyopathy, mitral stenosis, and bacterial endocarditis. Rarely, large cholesterol plaques from the aorta may be occlusive. Patients with dissecting aneurysms or cardiogenic shock may be anuric. Renal venous obstruction is a remote cause of oliguria in adults. However, it is a cause of oliguria or anuria in infants. Renal venous obstruction has been associated with sepsis and septic thrombophlebitis in adults. Cortical necrosis associated with obstetrical causes or diethylene glycol poisoning produces anuria.

Clinical Problem

A 42-year-old man was admitted to the hospital with a history of 7 days of shaking chills and fever. The patient had been seen 3 months earlier, at which time he was diagnosed as having chronic myelocytic leukemia. He had a course of hydroxyurea at which time his WBC had fallen to 20,000. The patient had been followed by hematologists at weekly intervals on a treatment consisting of Myleran, 6 mg q.i.d., allopurinol, 300 mg q.i.d., and Valium, 5 mg P.O. t.i.d. On physical examination, the patient appeared chronically ill in moderate respiratory distress. His vital signs were blood pressure, 130/80; temperature, 40°C; pulse, 130 beats per minute and regular; and respiratory rate, 32 per minute. Skin was moist. Noted to have tonsillar inflammation. Chest was clear to auscultation and palpation. He had a grade 2/6 systolic ejection murmur at the base of the heart. He had massive hepatosplenomegaly. There was no pretibial or sacral edema. Twenty-four hours after admission, his total urinary output had been 450 ml. Serum electrolytes were sodium, 144 mEq/liter; chloride, 83 mEq/liter; bicarbonate, 36 mEq/liter; potassium, 5.0 mEq/liter; and BUN, 132 mg/dl. Serum creatinine level was 2 mg/dl and uric acid, 12.5 mg%. Total serum protein was 6.4 gm%; with serum albumin, 2.2 gm%; WBC, 360,000/mm^3. Urine examination revealed pH 6, 2+ protein, and granular casts. No bacteria were seen on an unspun specimen. However, there were large amounts of amorphous urate crystals. Urine chemistries were sodium, 4 mEq/liter; and creatinine, 120 mg%.

Questions

1. What is the cause of this man's acute renal failure?
2. What is the significance of the serum bicarbonate concentration?
3. What is the urgency for rapid evaluation of this man's status and treatment?

Discussion

This is a young man who was acutely worse from his underlying hematological disease. His oliguria resulted from a marked decrease in renal perfusion, that is, dehydration from a week's febrile illness and probable anorexia in addition to a marked decrease in intravascular volume as evidenced by severe hypoalbuminemia. This was deduced from the diagnostic indices, that is, a urine sodium concentration less than 20 mEq/liter and a U/P creatinine level greater than 20. The BUN level was disproportionately greater than the serum creatinine level. Further evidence of volume contraction is a serum bicarbonate concentration of 36 mEq/liter and tachycardia. No edema with a serum albumin level of 2.2 mg% indicates a marked decrease in total body water. The diagnosis of a prerenal cause for oliguria in this patient is certain when the urine sodium level is found to be very low and U/P creatinine ratio is high. The urgency for evaluation and treatment in this man with an elevated serum uric acid and amorphous urates in the urine is to prevent renal obstruction by uric acid crystals, that is, superimposing uric acid nephropathy on dehydration. With a central venous line, hydration with 3 liters normal saline and the administration of 75 gm of human serum albumin in the next 24 hours resulted in a decline of the BUN level to 35 mg% and the bicarbonate concentration to 25 mEq/liter. The urine output increased to 1100 ml/24 hours. With establishment of urine flow, exogenous sodium bicarbonate and acetazolamide were started to alkalinize his urine to a pH of 7 or above in order to increase the solubility of filtered uric acid.

References

Bricker, N. S., and Klahr, S. "Obstructive nephropathy." *In:* Diseases of the Kidney, 2nd ed., M. B. Strauss and L. G. Welt (eds.). Little, Brown, Boston, pp. 997–1037, 1971.

Harrington, J. T., and Cohen, J. J. "Current concepts: Acute oliguria." N. Engl. J. Med. *292:* 89, 1975.

Kerr, D. N. S. "Acute renal failure." *In:* Renal Disease, 3rd ed., D. Black (ed.). Blackwell Scientific Publications, Oxford, pp. 417–461, 1972.

Schoolwerth, A. C., Sandler, R. S., Klahr, S., and Kissane, J. "Nephrosclerosis post-partum and in women taking oral contraceptives." Arch. Int. Med. *136:* 178, 1976.

Chapter 9

Edema

General Considerations

Edema is the clinical manifestation of expansion of the interstitial fluid space, or extravascular component of the extracellular fluid volume. Edema may occur in only a localized area or may be generalized, in which case it is termed anasarca.

Regulation of Extracellular Fluid Volume

About one third of total body water is confined to the extracellular fluid (ECF) space. This compartment, in turn, is composed of the plasma volume and the interstitial space. The sodium ion is the principal cation of the extracellular fluid, and with its two major anions, chloride and bicarbonate, comprises 90% or more of the total solute contained in the extracellular fluid. On the other hand, the sodium content of the intracellular fluid is extremely low by virtue of mechanisms capable of extruding sodium ions from cell water back into the extracellular fluid. Water molecules, in contrast to sodium ions, move freely across most cell membranes in the direction of an osmotic gradient. Thus, if there is retention of sodium ions in the extracellular fluid, there will be an attendant increase in the osmotic pressure of this fluid compartment and a concomitant decrease in the chemical activity of water. The chemical activity of water in the cells will exceed that of the extracellular fluid, and water will move out of the cell across the cell membrane into the extracellular space. Moreover, the rise in osmolality of the extracellular fluid imposed by the sodium retention will result in an increase in the rate of release of antidiuretic hormone (ADH), and positive water balance will ensue. The thirst mechanism may also be activated, and water intake will increase. Thus the overall effect of a primary increase in sodium mass will be an increase in extracellular fluid volume. Conversely, a decrease in sodium mass will initiate a corresponding decrease in extracellular fluid volume. Therefore, the control system regulating sodium balance is, in effect, an integral part of the volume control system.

Distribution of Fluid Between the Vascular and the Interstitial Spaces

The ECF is divided between the vascular and interstitial spaces and the movement of fluid between these two spaces is governed largely by Starling's forces. First, however, the blood vessels and the lymphatics running through the interstitial compartment must both be intact. Alteration in the integrity of either will lead to the local accumulation of edema fluid. This is exemplified in burns where blood vessel injury allows leakage of fluid into the area, and lymphatic injury inhibits removal of that excess fluid from the interstitial space.

In general terms, two forces tend to promote the movement of fluid from the vascular to the interstitial space; these forces are the hydrostatic pressure within the vascular system and the colloid osmotic pressure in the interstitial fluid. In contrast, the factors that promote a movement of fluid into the vascular compartment are the colloid oncotic pressure contributed by the plasma proteins and the hydrostatic pressure within the interstitial fluid, referred to as the tissue tension. These forces are balanced in the microcirculation such that water and diffusible solutes move from the vascular space at the arteriolar end and into the vascular compartment at the venous end. In addition, fluid is returned from the interstitial space into the vascular system by way of the lymphatics, and unless these channels are obstructed, lymph flow tends to increase if there is a tendency toward a net movement of fluid from the vascular compartment to the interstitium.

The Starling's forces normally favoring movement of fluid from the arteriolar end of capillaries are the relatively high intracapillary arteriolar pressure and the relatively low interstitial osmotic pressure. At the venule end of the capillary, the relatively high intracapillary oncotic pressure and the elastic tension of the tissues promote return of fluid to the vascular space. Edema develops when the imbalance of these forces results in the accumulation of interstitial fluid. When the forces again are balanced, no more fluid accumulates.

It would appear, then, that as edema fluid accumulates in the interstitial compartment, the volume of the intravascular compartment would decrease, tissue tension would soon make intracapillary and interstitial forces equal, and expansion of the interstitial compartment would cease. However, the change in volume of the intravascular compartment will be a stimulus for the renal retention of salt and water. Such stimulus will cease only when "effective" volume is restored.

Renal Regulation of Extracellular Fluid Volume

In normal subjects, ECF volume and sodium balance vary through only a narrow range, even in the phase of substantial changes in intake or extrarenal losses of water or salt or both. Although some degree of regulation of extrarenal losses of salt seems to exist in humans, by far the major role in achieving sodium homeostasis is attributable to the kidney.

The regulation of sodium excretion in reality depends on controlling the difference between the amount of sodium filtered and the amount of sodium reabsorbed. Theoretically, excretion of sodium could be regulated through changes in the GFR or sodium reabsorption. However, marked changes in the GFR may result in very slight changes in sodium excretion in the final urine. This suggests that most of the alterations in sodium excretion are the result of changes in net reabsorption of sodium along the nephron. The control system for sodium probably operates by changing either the active reabsorption of sodium or by increasing the backleak of sodium from the peritubular capillaries back into the lumen. There are, at present, several known factors that play a role in the regulation of sodium excretion. The relative importance of these factors in the day-to-day regulation of sodium excretion has not been completely defined. These factors include (1) the intrarenal distribution of glomerular filtrate, (2) hormonal effects, (3) peritubular physical factors, and (4) the possible existence of a natriuretic material.

Generalized Edema

Edema-forming states are thus characterized by the renal retention of salt and water as a result of alterations in the above factors regulating sodium excretion. It would appear that one of the strongest stimuli resulting in sodium and water retention is a decrease in "effective" intravascular volume. This decrease may, in turn, lower "effective" renal blood flow resulting in a reduced GFR and, hence, a fall in the filtered load of sodium and sodium excretion. Sodium retention resulting from a reduced GFR is clinically significant only when the reduction is acute. A slow reduction of the GFR (as seen in chronic progressive renal disease) is associated with appropriate compensatory tubular changes that prevent the retention of sodium and water until the GFR is very low.

Moreover, decreased "effective" intravascular volume often results in a decrease in renal plasma flow (RPF) proportionately greater than the decrease in the GFR, thus increasing the filtration fraction (GFR/RPF). This increase in filtration fraction results in an increased peritubular capillary oncotic pressure, thereby enhancing sodium and water reabsorption in the proximal tubule.

Decreased "effective" renal blood flow may result in a redistribution of blood flow with a greater proportion of the renal blood flow perfusing the juxtamedullary nephrons. These nephrons comprise only 15% of the total nephron population but, because of the long loops of Henle, are particularly adapted to afford greater sodium and water reabsorption.

Hormones are also involved in effecting the increased salt and water retention responsible for edema. Again, decreased effective plasma volume is important because it stimulates renin release, which ultimately results in increased adrenal release of aldosterone. Aldosterone then enhances distal tubular sodium reabsorption.

Antidiuretic hormone, found in increased concentrations in the plasma of some patients with cirrhosis, congestive heart failure, and nephrotic syndrome, may contribute to increased water retention. There may be additional factors involved in the handling of sodium and water by the kidney that are as yet unelucidated. A hormone, "natriuretic hormone," that may depress sodium reabsorption and is released in response to volume expansion has been implicated in the regulation of sodium excretion. The relevance of this postulated hormone in edema-forming states is unknown.

A combination of the above-mentioned factors appears to be involved in the formation of edema.

Localized Edema

Localized edema can be explained by the change in one of several or sometimes a combination of Starling's forces. One such factor is *increased capillary hydrostatic pressure.* In thrombophlebitis, for example, the occlusion of a large vessel and the consequent impairment of blood flow results in increased hydrostatic pressure distal to the obstruction that exceeds the intracapillary oncotic pressure and tissue tension that would promote return of fluid to the capillary. Localized edema of the extremity is the result. Other examples of this clinical situation include the edema of varicose veins, dependent stasis, and local venous obstruction, such as that produced by tumor.

Increased capillary membrane permeability may also result in localized edema. Inflammation occurring with infections or burns is associated with edema formation at the site. This mechanism may also produce local edema in vitamin E deficiency and angioneurotic edema.

Burns, especially in the healing phase, may also lead to *lymphatic obstruction,* hindering the return of fluid to the venous system. Other examples of lymphatic obstruction are seen in the cases of tumors that obstruct major lymphatic vessels (e.g. lymphoma), in elephantiasis, in congenital lymphatic obstruction (Milroy's disease), and in gonadal dysgenesis.

An increase in oncotic pressure of tissue fluid may occur, especially when there is either increased capillary permeability leading to the accumulation of large amounts of albumin in the interstitial space or when lymphatic obstruction inhibits its return. Quickly the oncotic pressure of the tissue fluid may equal that of the intravascular fluid, cancelling any effective method of returning excess fluid to the vascular space.

It would also be possible that a *decrease in tissue pressure* might lead to edema accumulation. This happens in the case of administration of hyaluronidase locally, a practice that at one time allowed the administration of fluids subcutaneously but which, in the era of intravenous fluid administration, is no longer necessary nor advisable.

Differential Diagnosis of Edema

A list of edema-associated conditions is presented in Table 9-1 and the clinical features of each will be briefly reviewed.

I. Localized Edema

A. Local Increase in Venous Pressure

1. Varicose Veins

Varicose veins are dilated and tortuous superficial veins, usually of the lower extremities, which may result from constitutionally defective valves in the veins or as compensa-

Table 9-1

Clinical Causes of Edema

- I. Localized edema
  - A. Local increase in venous pressure
    1. Varicose veins
    2. Dependent stasis
    3. Venous obstruction (thrombophlebitis, tumor)
  - B. Lymphatic obstruction
    1. Lymphoma and other neoplasms
    2. Filariasis
    3. Gonadal dysgenesis
    4. Milroy's disease
    5. Burns
    6. Resection of regional lymph nodes
- II. Local or generalized edema
  - A. Altered capillary integrity
    1. Vitamin E deficiency
    2. Idiopathic edema
    3. Angioneurotic edema
    4. Inflammation, burns
- III. Generalized edema
  - A. Decrease in vascular colloid osmotic pressure
    1. Nephrotic syndrome
    2. Protein-losing enteropathy
    3. Malabsorption
    4. Starvation
    5. Catabolic states
    6. Cirrhosis (late)
  - B. Decreased cardiac output
    1. Heart failure
    2. Cirrhosis
  - C. Absolute decrease in glomerular filtration rate
    1. Acute renal failure
    2. Preeclampsia, eclampsia
    3. Chronic renal failure (advanced)
  - D. Idiopathic edema
    1. Cyclic edema
    2. Oral contraceptives
  - E. Administration of drugs (mineralocorticoids, glucocorticoids)

tion for obstructed deep veins. When the valves are incompetent the venous return of blood to the heart is impeded and an increase in local hydrostatic pressure may result in increased transudation of fluid. Physical examination easily demonstrates the tortuous vessels. It is important to distinguish venous dilatation due to defective valves from that secondary to deep venous obstruction. A family history for varicosities is often obtainable in the constitutionally defective type.

2. Dependent Stasis

Dependent stasis may occur in individuals without defective venous valves but whose activities require that they stand without moving for long periods. Surgeons are often prone to the edema of dependent stasis, particularly in long, involved operations.

3. Venous Obstruction

The most common causes of venous obstruction are thrombophlebitis and tumor. Signs of thrombophlebitis include tenderness over the area, particularly when the muscles surrounding the vein are contracted (pain on dorsiflexion of the foot is a sign of deep thrombophlebitis in the calf). There may be a measurable difference in the circumference of the two extremities, slight cyanosis of the affected limb, slight prominence of the superficial veins, and increased warmth, as well as edema.

Venous obstruction from tumor invasion or compression is suggested not only by edema distal to the obstruction but also by a deepening in color. For example, when tumor-invaded lymph nodes compress the superior vena cava the face and neck become edematous and bluish red, signs of venous congestion. Diagnosis is often suggested by enlarged lymph nodes of the region demonstrable by radiograph. Definitive diagnosis often rests with biopsy of lymph nodes.

B. Lymphatic Obstruction

1. Lymphoma and Other Neoplasms

Neoplasms that invade lymph nodes may result in obstruction to the flow of lymph. Thus, lymph accumulates proximal to that point. In addition to the local accumulation of edema in that area, the obstruction of lymph flow may be so great as to prevent the return of adequate amounts of intravascular fluid, so that "effective" plasma volume decreases. In that case, mild generalized edema may result. The association of painless, enlarged, hard, fixed lymph nodes in the area of fluid accumulation should lead one to consider neoplasm. Other features may include splenomegaly and, in advanced stages, pallor and pain. Lymphangiography may be necessary to diagnose lymphatic obstruction. Tumors may also produce localized edema by extrinsic compression or invasion of blood vessels.

2. Filariasis

This is a disorder produced by infection with nematodes of the family Filarioidea. The worms invade the subcutaneous tissues and lymphatics of humans, producing disorders of acute inflammation to chronic scarring. The greatest edema results from scarred, obstructed lymphatics. History reveals travel to India, Ceylon, Vietnam, China, New Guinea, and other surrounding areas. The inflammatory filariasis is associated with brief febrile attacks over a period of weeks, beginning after a long incubation period of 3 to 12 months. Lymphangitis may be very common, usually associated with lymphadenitis. As the disease becomes chronic the primary findings are the effusions and edema distal to the lymphatic obstruction associated with continued lymphadenopathy, which occasionally produces draining sinuses. The disease is diagnosed definitively by demonstration of the parasite in blood or effusion fluid.

3. Gonadal Dysgenesis (Turner's Syndrome)

This is a chromosomal disorder comprised of a 45-X chromosome constitution. One third of patients, however, are 45-X–46-XX mosaics. The clinical features include short stature, webbing of the neck, short metacarpals, and sometimes coarctation of the aorta. The clinical findings and the absence of any other cause for edema may suggest that the edema arises from the occasional lymphatic obstruction of Turner's syndrome.

4. Milroy's Disease

This is a familial disease in which there is widespread obstruction of lymphatics. Usually there is a family history, and the signs of lymphedema develop in childhood. In time the lymphedema produces fibrosis of the tissues, and they become hard and brawny. Fortunately, the abnormality is usually restricted to a particular area of the body such as an extremity.

5. Burns

The inflammation of burns and other disorders, in addition to its effect on capillary permeability, results in lymphatic obstruction and promotes further accumulation of edema fluid. Once again, physical examination and history provide the cause and diagnosis of the edema.

II. Local or Generalized Edema

A. Altered Capillary Integrity

Localized or generalized edema may occur depending on whether or not the altered capillary integrity is localized or general.

1. Vitamin E Deficiency

This condition is associated with malabsorption syndromes, such as seen in cystic fibrosis and acanthocytosis, and is also seen in premature neonates. In addition to the capillary leakage leading to edema, this condition involves anemia produced by exaggerated hemolysis.

2. Idiopathic Edema

This syndrome is characterized by episodes of edema without obvious cause. A detailed description of this condition(s) is provided later in this chapter.

3. Angioneurotic Edema

Angioneurotic edema results, as the name suggests, from allergies, usually to food, physical allergens, or drugs. It is often seen on the face or extremities in which large wheals may become confluent. It may be associated with other signs of allergy such as itching, sneezing, and increase in tearing and mucous membrane secretions. The history often reveals a prior history or family history of allergies.

4. Inflammation

Inflammation due to many causes, including infection and burns, results in altered capillary integrity, so that the area becomes edematous. Physical examination reveals the redness, heat, and localized pain of inflammation in addition to the swelling. Extensive burns or infections may result in the loss of so much albumin-containing plasma that generalized edema may result.

III. Generalized Edema

As noted above, alterations in Starling's forces may be the sole mechanisms in the production of localized edema. However, to develop generalized edema, which may indeed be massive, sodium and water must be excessively retained. Many clinical conditions result when a primary disease process results in the secondary retention of fluid. Several will be briefly discussed.

A. Decrease in Vascular Colloid Osmotic Pressure

Generalized edema may be the result of a decrease in vascular oncotic pressure. In the initial evaluation of generalized edema, serum albumin should be measured. When it is decreased (edema usually develops when the serum albumin is below 2 gm/dl), evaluation must be directed toward the cause of the lowered albumin.

1. Nephrotic Syndrome

Nephrotic syndrome (a symptom complex characterized by proteinuria, hypoproteinemia, edema, and hypercholesterolemia) may be seen as a disease entity with no outstanding histopathological characteristics (minimal change or lipoid nephrosis) or as a secondary manifestation (e.g. in chronic glomerulonephritis, diabetes mellitus, systemic lupus erythematosus, etc.). See Chapter 2 on proteinuria for a more detailed differential. Although the inciting factors for development of the nephrotic syndrome may be different, many of the pathophysiological features are similar.

Because of an alteration in glomerular permeability, the kidneys lose massive amounts of protein daily. Many grams of protein, with albumin as a primary constituent, may appear in the urine. This amount is in excess of the ability of the liver to manufacture albumin, and this, plus increased catabolism of albumin, leads to a reduction in the concentration of serum albumin. Edema begins to form at albumin concentrations less than 2 gm/dl. This can be initially explained by changes in Starling's forces. No longer is there adequate oncotic pressure to promote the return of fluid from the interstitial space at the venular end of the capillary. Lymphatic flow is increased markedly in an attempt to remove the excess interstitial fluid, but the fluid accumulates despite that. With less fluid returning to the vascular space, there is concentration of the vascular volume. The appropriate response would be to retain salt and water at the level of the nephron. Thus the renal retention of salt and water will serve the physiologic purpose of trying to preserve the volume of the intravascular compartment. However, the decrease in oncotic pressure within the capillaries as a consequence of the decreased plasma albumin content would result in the constant translocation of fluid from the intravascular compartment into the interstitial space. As a consequence, the volume of the intravascular compartment will not be expanded despite salt and water retention, and stimuli for the need for further expansion will continue to be signaled to the nephron.

The mechanisms by which salt and water retention occur at the level of the nephron in the nephrotic syndrome are not completely understood. Patients with the nephrotic syndrome and hypoalbuminemia present an interesting theoretical inconsistency with respect to salt and water retention. On the basis of experimental observations, it would be expected that hypoalbuminemia and decreased plasma protein oncotic pressure would lead to decreased proximal tubular reabsorption and natriuresis, yet patients with the nephrotic syndrome avidly retain sodium, If proximal tubular reabsorption is indeed decreased in these patients as a result of hypoalbuminemia, then the retention of sodium must relate to augmented distal tubular reabsorption. Recent evidence by Grausz et al. in five patients with the nephrotic syndrome suggests that, indeed, proximal sodium reabsorption may not be increased in this entity and that the retention of salt and water results from increased reabsorption beyond the proximal tubule.

Aldosterone levels are usually elevated in the nephrotic syndrome, and this, as already mentioned, will increase the reabsorption of sodium. Edema formation in the nephrotic syndrome certainly can occur in the absence of any decrease in the GFR. The role of a possible redistribution of filtrate from superficial nephrons toward juxtamedullary units has not been explored in the nephrotic syndrome. The inability of nephrotic patients to expand intravascular volume despite retention of salt and water, due to the constant translocation of fluid toward the interstitial space, may prevent the release of a natriuretic substance. Suggestive evidence regarding this mechanism has been obtained in uremic patients with the nephrotic syndrome. While most uremic patients exhibit in their blood the presence of a material that is natriuretic in the rat, blood obtained from nephrotic patients with far-advanced uremia failed to demonstrate the presence of this material. These observations suggest the absence of a natriuretic material in the blood of patients with the nephrotic syndrome. Whether this material is a natriuretic hormone remains to be established.

In summary, there may be initial contraction of the intravascular volume in the nephrotic syndrome, with renal retention of salt and water as a compensatory mechanism for preservation of plasma volume. While this scheme in general applies to most nephrotic patients, edema can be seen in the absence of marked hypoalbuminemia, and the chain of events here would not resemble the simpler approach that we have presented regarding the pathogenesis of salt retention in this syndrome.

2. Protein-losing Enteropathy

Patients with this entity may describe frequent, loose stools, often with weight loss, prior to the onset of edema. Causes of such enteropathy include regional ileitis, ulcerative colitis, nontropical sprue, intestinal tuberculosis, and neoplasms. A definitive diagnosis is based on quantitation of protein loss which can be made by the intravenous administration of a substance like ^{51}Cr-albumin and measurement of the amount recovered in the stool.

3. Malabsorption

Malabsorption syndromes, of which protein-losing enteropathy is one, are associated with many symptoms, the most frequent of which are malnutrition, weight loss, and diarrhea. In childhood, growth failure may be prominent. Other symptoms and signs reflect the malabsorption of substances such as iron, vitamin K, and vitamin B_{12}. Symptoms include anemia, weakness, paresthesias, and glossitis. The edema that develops is probably a consequence of impaired absorption of amino acids, protein depletion, and hypoproteinemia. The diagnosis can be confirmed by measuring stool fat as well as by noting decreased serum levels of iron, carotene, and folic acid.

4. Protein-calorie Malnutrition

The edema of malnutrition is the result of decreased intake of calories and protein. There is a diminished presentation of amino acids and peptides to the intestinal mucosa for absorption. Like malabsorption, many other substances are also lacking, and so anemia, weakness, paresthesias, and bone pain are associated symptoms and signs. The history of deficient intake makes the diagnosis. Serum cholesterol level is markedly depressed.

5. Chronic Diseases Accompanied by Malnutrition

Patients who have suffered *severe injuries* and those with *widespread carcinoma* are examples of catabolic states that may result in hypoproteinemia and edema. Often, decreased intake accompanies these situations and compounds the hypoproteinemia. History and physical examination are most important in delineating these causes.

6. Cirrhosis (Late)

Late in the course of cirrhosis, when the liver can no longer manufacture adequate amounts of albumin, hypoproteinemia develops. The diagnosis of cirrhosis is suggested by the history, which may include excessive alcohol ingestion, acute bouts of jaundice, and occasionally right upper quadrant pain. Demonstrable signs may include ascites, jaundice, splenomegaly, spider nevi, palmar erythema, caput medusus, hemorrhoids, and esophageal varices demonstrable on radiograph. In men, loss of body hair, gynecomastia, and testicular atrophy may also be noted. Abnormal liver function tests confirm the diagnosis, although a liver biopsy may be required to determine the cause of the "cirrhosis."

B. Decreased Cardiac Output

1. Congestive Heart Failure

Failure of the myocardium to deliver adequate amounts of blood to the arterial tree results in a decrease of blood flow to the kidneys. The juxtaglomerular cells of the kidney respond to this decreased "effective" renal blood flow, no matter how small, by increasing renin production, leading to the eventual formation of angiotensin II. Increased angiotensin II levels stimulate the release of aldosterone, which then enhances distal tubular sodium reabsorption. With retention of sodium, water is also retained, resulting in hypervolemia and increased venous and capillary hydrostatic pressure. The increased hydrostatic pressure leads to transudation of fluid and edema. This mechanism is termed the "forward failure" theory.

The "backward failure" theory suggests that with the failure of the myocardium to empty the heart sufficiently, an increase in venous and capillary pressure results, leading to transudation of fluid. This, in turn, decreases the "effective" plasma volume and promotes the retention of sodium and water by the kidney. It is likely that the mechanisms of both these theories play a part in the formation of the generalized edema of congestive heart failure; the exact time sequence is still in dispute.

Besides aldosterone, many other sodium excretion regulatory factors, as discussed earlier in the chapter, participate in the sodium and water retention. In congestive heart failure, RPF falls to a greater extent than the GFR, raising the filtration fraction and increasing the oncotic pressure in the peritubular capillary blood. This may, as in experimental situations, lead to an increase in the reabsorption of fluid from the proximal tubule. In addition, it has been demonstrated in experimental congestive failure that renal blood flow is redistributed so that the juxtamedullary nephrons, with their long, sodium-retaining loops of Henle, receive a greater proportion of the blood flow. It is probable that all these mechanisms act together to produce generalized edema.

The edema of congestive heart failure is associated with signs and symptoms of increased hydrostatic pressure of the venous system. The first signs may be cough, dyspnea on exertion, orthopnea, and paroxysmal nocturnal dyspnea to be followed by dyspnea even at rest. Hepatomegaly, basal pulmonary rales, and jugular venous distention with the patient at a 45° angle are common findings. Hepatojugular reflux may occur, demonstrated by an increase in jugular venous distention when pressure is applied over the liver.

Cardiac enlargement, diastolic murmurs, and gallop rhythm, in addition to evidence of cardiac failure, usually provide abundant evidence that the edema is the result of heart failure. Once the cause of the edema is ascribed to heart failure, the cause of the cardiac failure should be investigated. The differential diagnosis of heart failure is beyond the scope of this book.

2. Cirrhosis

In cirrhosis, portal hypertension develops. The increase in hydrostatic pressure results in transudation of fluid across the capillaries and leak into the peritoneal cavity. When the lymphatics can no longer keep up with the transudation, ascites develops. Removal of this fluid from the circulating volume then leads to a decreased "effective" renal blood flow and renal retention of sodium and water follows.

Late in the course of cirrhotic liver disease, significant hypoproteinemia may lead to a decrease in oncotic pressure that increases the loss of vascular volume. Generalized edema then occurs.

In addition to the usual mechanisms for salt and water retention by the kidney, other factors may be at play in cirrhotics. Such patients may retain water in excess of salt; the explanation for this has been postulated to be sustained production of antidiuretic hormone. Definitive proof of this occurrence is not yet available. Ascites plus evidence of hepatic disease (see above) characterize edema of hepatic origin.

C. Absolute Decrease in Glomerular Filtration Rate

1. Acute Renal Failure

Edema may result from the fluid retention that occurs when normal intake of salt and water continues in the face of a sudden decrease in the GFR. Such may be the case in *acute glomerulonephritis* when inflammation of the glomeruli is present. The diagnosis is suggested by hematuria, oliguria, hypertension, and azotemia. *Acute tubular necrosis* with its concomitant decrease in filtration may also result in edema formation. This diagnosis is suggested by a history of hypotension resulting from surgery, trauma, or dehydration, and associated with oliguria and inability to concentrate the urine (see Chapter 7 on azotemia). Other causes of acute renal failure (cortical necrosis, obstruction, etc.) may also lead to the development of edema if salt and water intake is not markedly curtailed.

2. Preeclampsia

Preeclampsia is the occurrence of hypertension, edema, and proteinuria during the third trimester of pregnancy. With increasing severity, convulsions and coma may supervene *(eclampsia)*. The edema has been attributed to hypoalbuminemia, although levels are usually not below 2 gm/dl. Since the histological findings in the kidney in eclampsia are swelling of endothelial and epithelial cells with glomerular fibrin deposition, this inflammation of the kidney may be responsible for the major part of the fluid accumulation. Observation for preeclampsia should be most careful in primiparas, women over age 35, and in twin births. A rise in blood pressure in the third trimester of pregnancy, when blood pressure usually declines, should alert the physician to the possibility of preeclampsia. Proteinuria, the presence of granular casts in the urine, and a mild increase in blood urea nitrogen levels add credence to this diagnosis.

3. Chronic Renal Failure

If the GFR falls slowly (chronic renal failure), the level must be very low before edema develops. Until filtration is lower than 10% of normal (and sometimes as low as 1%), tubular rejection of filtered fluid will maintain fluid balance. At low levels of GFR, however, the great decrease in reabsorption of filtered fluid is insufficient to balance the patient's intake, and fluid retention results. The diagnosis is suggested by urinalysis showing cells and casts as well as the signs and symptoms of chronic renal failure, such as azotemia, hyperphosphatemia, anemia, hypertension, and often, small kidneys demonstrable by x-ray or ultrasound.

D. Idiopathic Edema

Patients with idiopathic edema formation do not fall into a single group characterized by a uniform abnormality in salt and water regulation. These patients exhibit edema despite normal cardiovascular and hepatic function and, when measured, normal colloid oncotic pressure in the intravascular space. At least some patients seem to exhibit an increase in transcapillary movement of salt and water, and the edema formation thus could be explicable on the basis of subtle contraction of "effective" intravascular volume. Other patients, however, appear to accumulate edema without the translocation of intravascular volume into the interstitial fluid being the primary event. The reasons why the latter patients form edema in the first place and fail to "escape" more readily and exhibit a spontaneous diuresis are obscure.

1. Cyclic Edema

There is a syndrome characterized by periodic episodes of edema without obvious cause. It has been observed most commonly (but not exclusively) in women, and there appears to be some relationship to the menstrual cycle—hence, the name cyclic edema. The fact that most cases are seen in women may be due, in part, to the unfortunate cosmetic consequences of facial edema, which are more likely to disturb women than men. Frequently, large diurnal alterations in weight occur, so that the patient may weigh several pounds more in the evening than in the morning after having been in the upright posture during the day. The large diurnal weight change suggests the possibility that patients may well have increased capillary permeability in general which is exaggerated by the upright posture and the consequent increased hydrostatic pressure in the dependent vessels.

2. Oral Contraceptives

As in cyclic edema, the weight gain and edema that occurs in some women prior to their menstrual periods is not well understood. Women taking oral contraceptives also have increased fluid retention, suggesting that estrogens and progesterone may be causative. Careful history establishes the diagnosis.

E. Drugs

The administration of drugs occasionally results in detectable edema. When glucocorticoids or mineralocorticoids are given, fluid accumulation occurs for a short period, usually about 3 days. After that time, however, vascular volume expansion increases the stimuli for tubular rejection of salt and water, with urine volume and salt concentration increasing as a consequence (the so-called escape phenomenon). With chronic glucocorticoid administration, some degree of edema may be present.

General Considerations in the Differential Diagnosis of Edema

In addition to the criteria already mentioned, certain findings may help elicit the cause of edema. The distribution of edema is of diagnostic importance. Edema of only one extremity is usually the result of vascular or lymphatic obstruction. Generalized edema is most likely the result of hypoproteinemia, but this edema may be especially evident in the eyelids and face and tends to be more pronounced in the morning because of the recumbent posture assumed during the night. However, while the edema of congestive heart failure is also generalized, edema tends to be more extensive in the legs and to be accentuated in the evening, a feature also determined largely by posture. Certain patients with cardiac disease but no orthopnea (tricuspid stenosis, constrictive pericarditis) may prefer the recumbent posture, and the factor of gravity may result in the presence of facial edema. Other common causes of facial edema include trichinosis, allergic reactions, and myxedema.

Considerations of the color, thickness, and sensitivity of the skin may be of help. Local tenderness and increase in temperature suggest inflammation. Local cyanosis may signify venous obstruction. Venous pressure is important in evaluating edema. Elevation of this measurement in an isolated part of the body usually reflects venous obstruction. In congestive heart failure, generalized elevation of venous pressure is observed. Determination of the concentration of serum proteins, particularly albumin, clearly differentiates those patients in whom edema is caused, entirely or in part, by diminished intravascular colloid osmotic pressure. It should be emphasized that edema may originate from a variety of abnormal states; it is not, therefore, necessarily a consequence of only one of the disorders enumerated above. For example, in a diabetic patient, edema may be the result of hypoalbuminemia associated with the nephrotic syndrome due to intercapillary glomerulosclerosis or increased venous pressure associated with congestive heart failure due to atherosclerotic and hypertensive heart disease and the anemia consequent to uremia.

Clinical Problem

T. S., a 10-year-old white male, was well until the summer of 1976. His parents noted the gradual and intermittent occurrence of periorbital edema, but it was not until he fell asleep in the bathtub one day that they noted that he also had scrotal edema.

The patient was admitted to the hospital, at which time he weighed 32.3 kg, his usual weight being 25 kg. His blood pressure was 120/90, and he had generalized edema with his eyes nearly swollen shut, a fluid wave in the abdomen with shifting dullness, scrotal edema, and pitting edema to the knees. Placement of the stethoscope on the chest left an indentation.

Laboratory findings were as follows: Urinalysis showed 4+ protein by dipstick and 10 to 12 red blood cells per high-power field. Total serum protein value was 4.3 gm/dl; and serum albumin concentration, 1.9 gm/dl. Serum cholesterol value was 732 mg/dl, and quantitation of the urinary protein excretion was 12 gm/24 hours, with the volume of urine 325 ml/24 hours. BUN level was 23 mg/dl; serum creatinine, 1.1 mg/dl. The chest x-ray revealed a small asthenic heart shadow with small pleural effusions bilaterally.

The patient was placed at strict bed rest and was given a dietary allowance of 1 gm of sodium chloride per day. He was restricted to 500 ml of fluid per day. When the laboratory values returned, prednisone therapy, 60 mg/day orally, was begun.

Questions

1. What is the most likely cause of edema in this patient?

2. What is the most likely cause of the nephrotic syndrome in this setting?

Discussion

The presence of heavy proteinuria (12 gm/24 hours), hypoproteinemia with hypoalbuminemia, hypercholesterolemia, and edema makes the diagnosis of the nephrotic syndrome. In childhood the most common cause of the nephrotic syndrome is "nil disease" or minimal change nephrotic syndrome (see Chapter 2 on proteinuria). Children with this disease usually respond to prednisone therapy with a decrease in urinary protein excretion, a rise in serum albumin, and a diuresis.

After 14 days of prednisone, the daily urinary volume began to increase and over the next 6 days averaged 1200 ml/day. Three days after the onset of diuresis the urine became protein-free. The BUN level dropped to 15 mg/dl and the serum creatinine level to 0.7 mg/dl. Ten days from the onset of diuresis, the prednisone was changed to a dose of 60 mg every other day, and the patient was discharged.

Over the next 6 weeks the alternate-day prednisone was decreased gradually, and at the end of that time the patient developed an upper respiratory infection. In 2 days' time, he again had generalized edema and was again admitted to the hospital. The clinical and laboratory findings were similar, and again he was placed on the same supportive regimen in association with daily prednisone. Again, he sustained a diuresis and lost his proteinuria, but this time when the prednisone dosage was changed to alternate days, the patient again developed proteinuria. Because of his age, the presence of microscopic hematuria, and the frequency of relapse with poor late response, the patient underwent percutaneous renal biopsy. Light microscopic sections revealed focal segmental sclerosis in many of the glomeruli.

When there was no further response to prednisone therapy, chlorambucil was added. With increasing fluid retention the patient was referred to Children's Hospital. While prednisone and chlorambucil were continued, the patient was placed at bed rest and on strict fluid and dietary sodium restrictions. With the exception of the excess fluid intake he ingested while taking showers, he slowly lost weight. After 6 weeks of daily medication, the proteinuria was the same, and the patient was still grossly edematous. In addition, his BUN was 52 mg/dl and his serum creatinine was 3.5 mg/dl. Since it appeared that response of his nephrotic syndrome was going to be delayed, if it occurred at all, and to allow the patient to be managed at home, he underwent "artificial diuresis." To accomplish this, spironolactone, an aldosterone antagonist, was given orally. When it had been given for 3 days, low sodium albumin, 1 gm/kg body weight, was administered intravenously daily for 5 days. Each daily infusion was given over a 1-hour period, and midway through the infusion and again at the end of infusion, furosemide, 1 mg/kg body weight, was given intravenously. The urine volume rose from 250–375 ml/day to 1200–1600 ml/day; after the 5 days of albumin administration the patient weighed 25.5 kg, and a small volume of ascites was the only remaining manifestation of his anasarca. The patient is being managed at home on salt and fluid restriction and continued spironolactone administration. Furosemide is required in small daily doses to keep the patient edema-free. His renal function has returned to normal with a BUN level of 10 mg and a serum creatinine level of 0.5 mg/dl.

References

Dirks, J., Seely, J., and Levy, M. "Control of extracellular fluid volume and the pathophysiology of edema formation." *In:* The Kidney, B. Brenner and F. Rector (eds.). W. B. Saunders, Philadelphia, pp. 495–552, 1976.

Wedeen, R. P., Goldstein, M., and Levitt, M. F. "Mechanisms of edema and the use of diuretics." Pediatr. Clin. North Am. *18:* 561–576, 1971.

Welt, L. G. "Edema." *In:* Harrison's Principles of Internal Medicine, 6th ed., M. M. Wintrobe et al. (eds.). McGraw-Hill, New York, pp. 213–217, 1970.

Welt, L. G. "Disorders of fluids and electrolytes." *In:* Harrison's Principles of Internal Medicine, 6th ed., M. M. Wintrobe et al. (eds.). McGraw-Hill, New York, pp. 1357–1371, 1970.

Weston, R. E. "Pathogenesis and treatment of edemas with special reference to the use of diuretics." *In:* Clinical Disorders of Fluid and Electrolyte Metabolism, 2nd ed., M. H. Maxwell and C. R. Kleeman (eds.). McGraw-Hill, New York, pp. 163–178, 1972.

Chapter 10

Polyuria

General Considerations

In the broadest sense, polyuria may be defined as "an increase in the rate of urine excretion above what would be expected in normal individuals." In practice, the physician is likely to be confronted with polyuria in two different settings. In the office, where a patient will come to him complaining of an increase in urine output, careful questioning will virtually always identify the associated symptom, a marked increase in the ingestion of water (polydipsia). The symptom of polydipsia is essential in establishing the complaint as polyuria rather than urgency or frequency resulting from inflammation of the lower urinary tract. With the exception of fatigue and concern, these patients are usually in a state of relatively good health. On the other hand, a more serious situation is seen in hospitalized patients where the signs of profound negative water balance (i.e., dehydration, hypotension, and hypernatremia or hyponatremia) may be the presenting problem, and polyuria may be discovered only after careful examination of the hospital records.

Polyuria, in its simplest terms, reflects a decrease in the renal tubular reabsorption of water that may or may not be appropriate for the individual's water intake. It may result not only from a decrease in reabsorption of water per se but may also be secondary to a reduction in the renal tubular reabsorption of solute (e.g., urea, sodium chloride, glucose).

An absolute upper limit for normal urine output is difficult to define. In Table 10-1, data obtained from 24-hour water balance studies in humans are shown. Under normal conditions the nitrogenous end products, resulting from protein breakdown, excreted in the urine are equal to 600 mOsm/day. If the maximal urine osmolality is 850 mOsm/kg, then the total urine volume required per 24 hours to excrete this osmolar load would be approximately 700 ml. This volume of urine is frequently referred to as the *obligatory* urinary volume. It is apparent from these simple calculations that this component of urine will depend on the protein intake and catabolic state of the individual in question. From Table 10-1, it can be seen that humans usually exceed the obligatory urine volume by an additional liter of so-called facultative urine and, under normal circumstances, urine volume will approach 1700 ml/24 hours. Therefore, in absolute terms, polyuria may be defined as urine flow rates in excess of 1700 ml/24 hours. In practical terms, 2 liters/day places the patient in a polyuric state. The exception to this rule is a condition where urine output may be less than 2 liters but exceeds water intake, and a state of *relative* polyuria is then said to exist.

Renal Regulation of Water Excretion

If the GFR of normal man is approximately 120 ml/min, then roughly 173 liters of water are filtered in a 24-hour period. Of this amount, less than 2 liters of urine, or approximately 1% of the amount filtered, is excreted. For any individual the fraction of filtered

Table 10-1

A Rounded-off, 24-Hour Water Balance Statement for a Normal Male at 15°C and 40% Relative Humidity, Based on a Particular 3000-Calorie Diet and Energy Expenditure

The diet contained 98.8 gm of protein, 163.3 gm of fat, and 294.3 gm of carbohydrate, yielding 377.6 gm of oxidative and 755.6 gm of preformed water in "solid" food (1910.8 gm of preformed water if fluid foods such as orange juice, milk, etc., have been considered). The pulmonary water loss is based upon the assumptions that oxygen extraction in the lungs is 6% and that expired air is saturated at 35°C.

	Water Intake (grams)			Water Output (grams)	
	Obligatory	Facultative		Obligatory	Facultative
Drink	650	1000	Urine	700	1000
Preformed	750		Skin	500	
Oxidative	350		Lungs	400	
			Feces	150	
Subtotals	1750	1000	Subtotals	1750	1000
Total	2750		Total	2750	

Source: Reprinted by permission from Wolf, A. V., Thirst. Charles C Thomas, Springfield, Ill., 1958.

water (FE_{H_2O}) excreted per unit time may be easily calculated by taking the reciprocal of the U/P creatinine (Cr) ratio and multiplying it by 100. The expression can be derived in the following manner.

$$FE_{H_2O} = \frac{V}{GFR} \times 100 = \frac{V}{\frac{U_{Cr}V}{P_{Cr}}} \times 100 = \frac{100}{\frac{U}{P}Cr} = \frac{P}{U}Cr \times 100$$

With the exception of setting an upper limit for the absolute amount of water that can be excreted per unit time, the GFR is not involved in the regulation of water excretion. This upper limit achieves importance only under conditions where the GFR is profoundly reduced, as in acute oliguric renal failure and end-stage chronic renal disease. In a normal setting the tubule plays the most important role in the renal regulation of water excretion.

The reabsorption of water is not an active process but is always the result of passive diffusion of water down its concentration gradient into a region of higher osmolality.

In the *proximal tubule,* this gradient is established in the lateral and basilar intercellular spaces and is a consequence of active transport of sodium out of the tubular lumen—and ultimately into these spaces. Water follows rapidly through this highly water-permeable segment of the renal tubule, and as a consequence, tubular fluid osmolality is not different from plasma. Hence, reabsorption of water in the proximal tubule is said to be *iso-osmotic.* Further, it is frequently termed *obligatory* reabsorption, since in the presence of such high water permeability, water must follow sodium out of the tubular lumen. It is estimated that nearly 60% of the filtered water is reabsorbed by the end of the proximal tubule. The control of water reabsorption in this segment is intimately related to those factors that control the reabsorption of sodium. These factors are discussed in Chapters 9 and 11 and therefore will only be mentioned briefly in this section in relation to resultant polyuric states.

Beyond the proximal tubule, this relationship between water and the reabsorption of sodium is lost. The movement of water out of these segments is by passive diffusion into an interstitium that is hypertonic with respect to tubular fluid. Such movement is, to a large extent, independent of the concomitant reabsorption of solute and is therefore frequently referred to as the reabsorption of solute-free water or simply *free water.*

The reabsorption of free water is largely dependent on the interrelationship of four factors.

1. The concentration of solute in the interstitium through which the renal tubule passes.
2. The concentration of solute in the tubular fluid.
3. The permeability of the renal tubule to water and solute.
4. The levels of circulating antidiuretic hormone.

It is well known that the concentration of solute or osmolality of renal tissue progressively increases from the corticomedullary junction to the tip of the renal papilla. In the cortex, the interstitial osmolality is equal to that of plasma, while near the tip of the papilla, tissue osmolality may be four times greater. This progressive rise is the result of the deposition of solute, chiefly NaCl and urea, in the renal interstitium and occurs as a consequence of countercurrent multiplication.

Countercurrent multiplication is graphically depicted in Figure 10-1. It is apparent from this illustration that three factors are essential for the mechanism to function. First, there must be flow through two channels in opposing directions (countercurrent flow). Second, there has to be a force (frequently referred to as the "single effect") that will result in the net movement of solute out of the tubular lumen of the limb leaving this environment. And, finally, this segment must be relatively impermeable to water, while the limb by which fluid enters this area must be freely permeable to water or solute or both. The net effect is the establishment of a progressive increase in interstitial osmolality and the production of an effluent that is hypotonic with respect to the fluid entering.

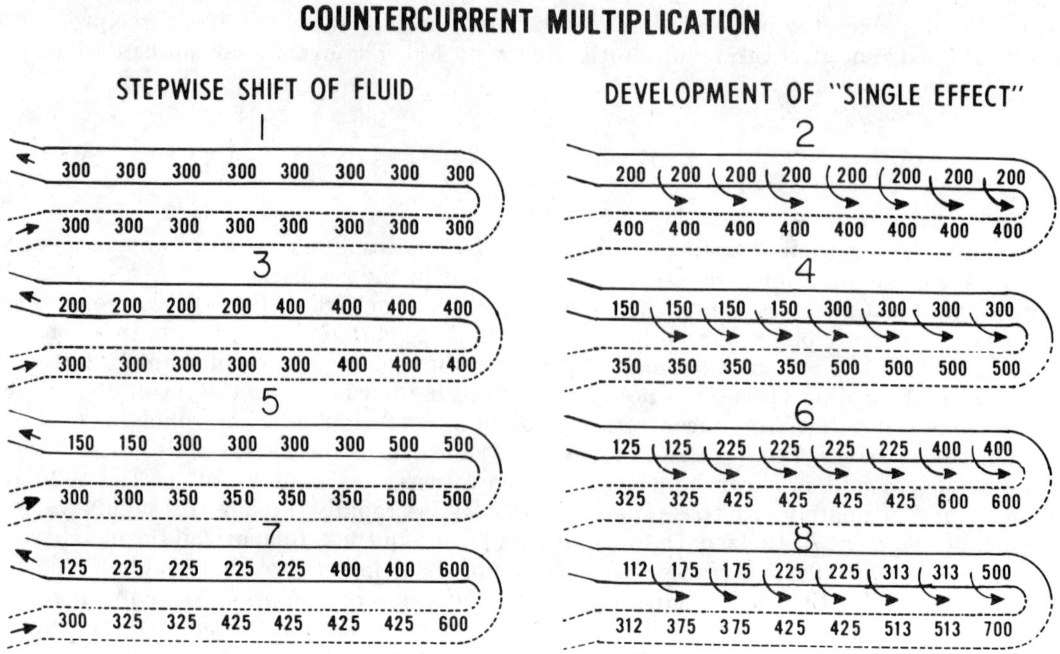

Fig. 10-1.

The principle of countercurrent multiplication of concentration, based on the assumption that, at any level along the loop of Henle, a gradient of 200 mOsm/liter can be established between ascending and descending limbs by active transport of ions. (From Pitts, R. F., The Physiology of the Kidney and Body Fluids, 3rd ed., 1974 Yearbook Medical Publishers, Chicago, by permission.)

In man, nephrons whose glomeruli are located at the corticomedullary junction, called juxtamedullary nephrons, are responsible for countercurrent multiplication. These nephrons are morphologically distinct from nephrons whose glomeruli lie just below the cortical surface, called cortical nephrons (Figure 10-2). One important difference is that juxtamedullary nephrons possess long, thin loops of Henle which extend deep into the inner zone of the medulla. Cortical nephrons have only short, thin, descending limbs which extend only into the outer medullary areas. The thin descending and ascending limbs of juxtamedullary nephrons lie in close proximity to each other as they enter and leave the medulla—hence flow through them is countercurrent. Further, the limbs of the loop of Henle are functionally distinct. The descending limb is highly permeable to water. It is probably only slightly permeable to urea and highly impermeable to sodium. On the other hand, the thin ascending limb is highly permeable to sodium, moderately permeable to urea, but *not* at all permeable to water (Fig. 10-2). The osmolality in the ascending limb gradually decreases, becoming hypotonic with respect to interstitium and the descending limb. Hence, solute is being extracted from the thin ascending limb in excess of water. The mechanism responsible for this decline, that is, the single effect, is not clear. It is thought by some that the decline in osmolality is due to the active reabsorption of sodium or chloride by this water-impermeable segment. Others have suggested that the dilution of fluid in the thin ascending limb is the result of differences in the permeability of this segment to sodium and urea. They have proposed that the sodium concentration in fluid entering the ascending limb is greater than that of the papillary interstitium; hence, sodium would diffuse passively out of this segment. On the other hand, the concentration of urea in the tubular fluid is lower than that of the papillary interstitium for reasons that will be discussed later. Thus, there is a tendency for urea to move into the tubular lumen, but at a rate slower than the efflux of sodium, since this segment is considerably less permeable to urea than to sodium. The net effect would be an increase in the solute content of the medulla and the production of tubular fluid that is hypotonic with respect to the surrounding interstitium.

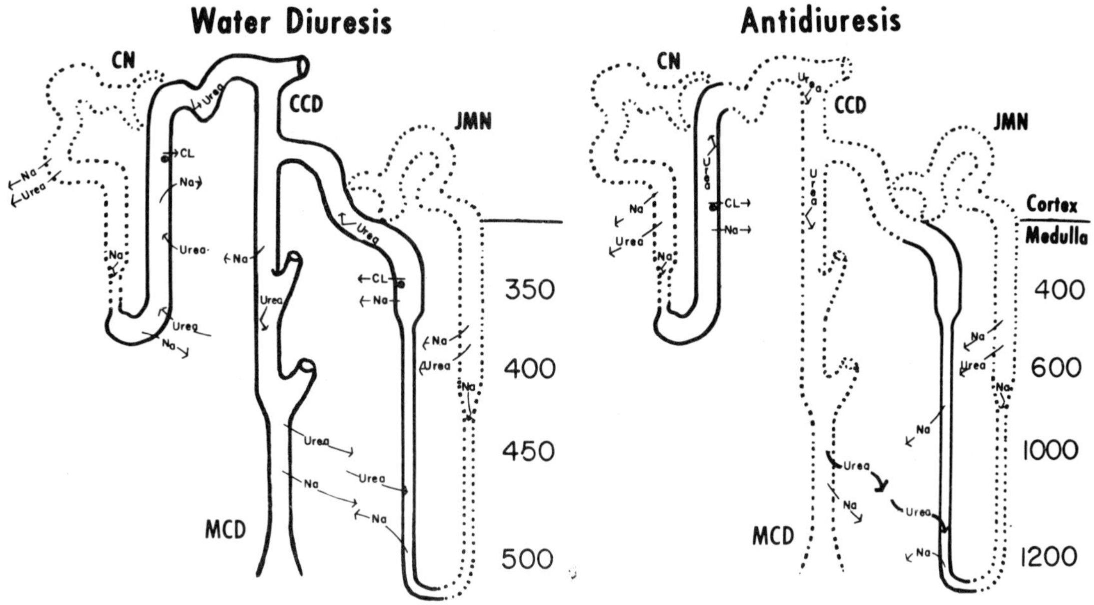

Fig. 10-2.

Here is depicted the movement of sodium (Na) and urea out of the highly water-permeable (-----) proximal tubule of both cortical (CN) and juxtamedullary nephrons (JMN) but no movement of Na out of the equally water-permeable thin descending limb of the loop of Henle. At the bend of the loop of Henle the characteristics of the epithelium change. The thick and thin ascending limbs are impermeable to water (——) but highly permeable to sodium. Sodium moves out of this segment into the interstitium, and to a lesser extent, urea moves into the tubular fluid and hypertonic medullary interstitium. The outward movement of sodium is potentiated by active chloride transport (♂→ Cl) in the thick ascending limb of the loop of Henle. In the absence of antidiuretic hormone the distal tubule, the cortical collecting duct (CCD), and the medullary collecting duct (MCD) are only slightly permeable to water, and the free water formed is excreted in the urine (water diuresis). In the presence of ADH (antidiuresis), part of the distal tubule and the cortical collecting duct are rendered highly permeable to water. Permeability of these segments to urea is not significantly altered, but the medullary collecting duct is rendered highly permeable to both water and urea.

The process of tubular fluid dilution continues in the thick ascending limb of both cortical and juxtamedullary nephrons. As in the thin, ascending limb, this segment is permeable to NaCl but not to water. In addition, the thick ascending limb actively reabsorbs chloride, thus enhancing the rate of tubular fluid dilution. The production of hypotonic tubular fluid is frequently referred to as the formation of solute-free water (or simply free water) and is said to occur wherever solute reabsorption exceeds that of water. In the absence of antidiuretic hormone (ADH), free water formation continues along the distal tubule and throughout the length of the collecting duct. These sites of free water formation are collectively referred to as the diluting segment (Figure 10-3). The amount of free water excreted per minute is called free water clearance (C_{H_2O}) and may be calculated by the following formula:

$$C_{H_2O} = V - C_{Osm}$$

where V is the urine flow per unit time and C_{Osm} is the osmolar clearance $\left(\frac{U_{Osm} \times V}{P_{Osm}}\right)$ which is equal to the fraction of urine produced required to excrete the solute cleared from the plasma in an isotonic state. From this statement it is clear that in order for free water to be excreted, the osmolality and, therefore, the solute concentration of the urine must be below that of the plasma. In humans, maximal free water clearance approaches 18 ml/min or 25 liters/day. This is roughly 15% of the filtered water. It is clear from these figures that

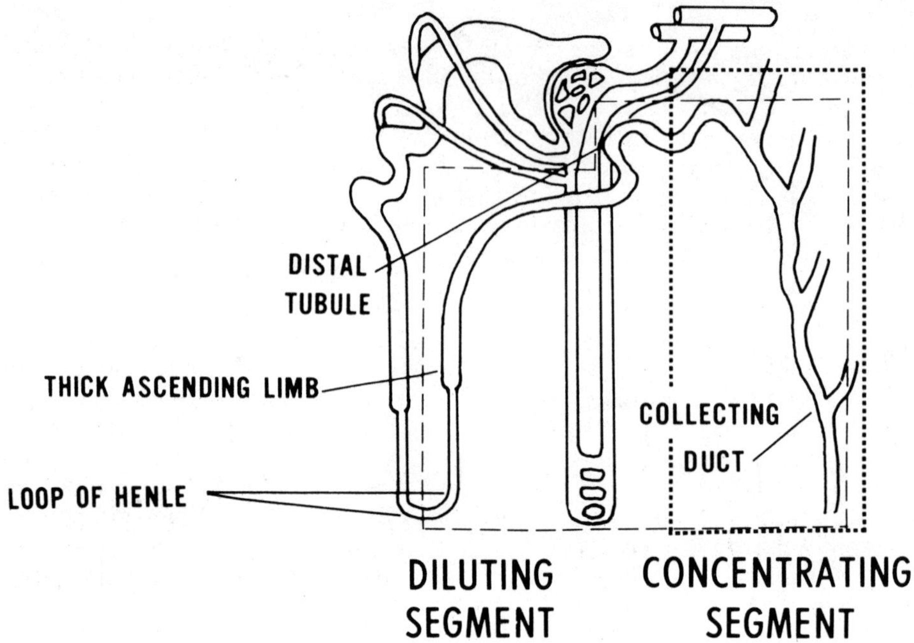

Fig. 10-3.

Illustrated here is the nephron and part of the collecting duct system. Those portions that contribute to the production of free water (diluting segment) are circumscribed by the thin broken line (-----) and that part responsible for the reabsorption of free water (concentrating segment) is outlined by the thicker line (----). Note that collecting duct and distal tubule are involved in both processes.

the ability of humans to excrete excess water ingested far exceeds the normal intake. Further, patients with impaired renal function are not likely to have difficulty with the excretion of excess free water until their GFR falls below 10 ml/min.

The capacity to reabsorb the free water formed is largely dependent upon circulating levels of arginine vasopressin. The antidiuretic hormone is stored in the neurohypophysis and produced by the supraoptic nuclei of the hypothalamus. The release of ADH is controlled primarily by the plasma osmolality and to a lesser extent by intravascular volume. Alterations in plasma osmolality affect osmoreceptors, which govern the release of ADH. These receptors are extremely sensitive and respond to changes of approximately 1% in plasma osmolality or 2.9 mOsm/kg H_2O). An essential part of the homeostatic mechanisms involved in the control of cellular osmolality is the presence of hypothalamic centers near these osmoreceptors that control thirst. These centers respond to similar changes in osmolality and volume.

In the presence of ADH, the distal tubule and collecting duct system become highly permeable to water, which will then diffuse into the interstitium (Fig. 10-2). As a result, the tubular fluid becomes iso-osmotic with respect to the surrounding interstitium. This process of equilibration is complete by the end of the distal tubule. That is, the fluid at the end of the distal tubule is iso-osmotic with respect to the renal cortex and therefore to plasma. This change in osmolality from approximately 60 to 280 mOsm/kg reflects the reabsorption of nearly 80% of the free water formed. The remaining free water will be extracted as fluid passes through the medulla where the osmolality of the interstitium progressively rises. From these observations, it is readily apparent that the bulk of free water is reabsorbed in the distal tubule and cortical collecting ducts and is therefore not dependent on the production of a hypertonic renal medulla.

The efficiency with which the remaining 20% of the free water formed is extracted from the lumen will be dependent on the degree to which solute is concentrated in the medullary interstitium. Besides the presence of normally functioning juxtamedullary nephrons, two other factors are involved in the generation of high solute concentrations in the renal medulla.

One is the manner in which urea is handled by the distal tubule and collecting duct system. Unlike water, the permeability of the distal tubule and cortical collecting duct to urea is only slightly increased by ADH; hence the concentration of urea in these segments rises as water is extracted in the antidiuretic state. On the other hand, the medullary collecting duct is rendered much more permeable to urea by ADH. Thus the high concentrations of urea generated in the cortical segments result in the deposition of urea in the medullary interstitium and a total increase in the osmolality of the medulla.

The second factor is medullary blood flow. The blood supply to the medulla is brought through long loops of the vasa recta. They function not only to supply nutrients to the medullary structures but also to carry off water that has been reabsorbed. Their configuration is such that they tend to preserve the osmolality generated by the loops of Henle, and they are frequently referred to as countercurrent *exchangers*. An increase in medullary blood flow would result in an increase in the rate of removal of both sodium chloride and urea from the medulla and ultimately to the dissipation of the osmotic gradient established by countercurrent multiplication.

Those structures involved in the extraction of free water from the tubular lumen are collectively referred to as the concentrating segment (Fig. 10-3). The capacity of this segment to reabsorb free water in an antidiuretic state (TC_{H_2O}) can be quantitated with the formula for C_{H_2O}.

$$TC_{H_2O} = V - C_{Osm}$$

Under such conditions, C_{H_2O} will be a negative number.

Differential Diagnosis of Polyuric States

It is apparent that a polyuric state can result from alterations in the reabsorption of water by one of the two mechanisms discussed previously. It could be the consequence of a decrease in the reabsorption of sodium in any segment of the tubule, but particularly in the proximal tubule. This polyuria would be *secondary* to an increase in solute excretion. On the other hand, an increase in urine flow could be the result of a decrease in the reabsorption of free water, a state that may be referred to as *primary* polyuria. Table 10-2 is an incomplete list of the conditions known to produce these polyuric states.

I. Increased Excretion of Solute and Obligate Water Loss (Secondary Polyuria)

A. Increased Solute Load

1. Osmotic Diuretics

An important cause of secondary polyuria is the glomerular filtration of high concentrations of small molecular-sized particles that are not reabsorbed by the renal tubule. Such molecules exert an intraluminal osmotic force. One example is the osmotic diuretic, mannitol.

a. Mannitol. Mannitol is freely filtered at the glomerulus but not reabsorbed by the renal tubule. It is of small molecular size (mol wt=180) and as such will exert an osmotic force in high concentrations. Such an effect will tend to reduce the iso-osmotic movement of water out of the proximal tubule. Thus, as sodium and water are reabsorbed along the proximal tubule, the concentration of mannitol will rise, increasing the osmotic force it ex-

Table 10-2

Factors Involved in the Production of Polyuric States

I. Increased excretion of solute and obligate water loss (secondary polyuria)
  A. Increased solute load
    1. Osmotic diuretics
      a. Mannitol
      b. Angiographic dyes
    2. Glycosuria—diabetes mellitus
    3. Urea
      a. Recovery phase of acute oliguric renal failure
      b. Gastric tube feeding of high protein intake
      c. Postobstructive diuresis
  B. Impaired renal tubular reabsorption of NaCl
    1. Nonoliguric renal failure
    2. Diuretic therapy
    3. Interstitial disease, e.g., pyelonephritis

II. Impaired reabsorption of free water (primary polyuria)
  A. Vasopressin deficiency (vasopressin-deficient diabetes insipidus)
    1. Idiopathic
    2. Posthypophysectomy
      a. Surgical
      b. Traumatic
    3. Tumor
      a. Metastatic
      b. Primary
    4. Miscellaneous
      a. Granuloma
      b. Histiocytosis
      c. Vascular
      d. Infection
  B. Renal defect (vasopressin-resistant diabetes insipidus)
    1. Congenital
    2. Acquired
      a. Renal tubular damage
        i. Chronic interstitial/infiltrative disease
          (a) Amyloid
          (b) Multiple myloma
          (c) Pyelonephritis
          (d) Sjogren's syndrome
        ii. Distal tubular and/or collecting duct defects
          (a) Sickle cell trait/disease
          (b) Nephrocalcinosis
          (c) Chronic obstructive uropathy
          (d) Hypokalemic nephropathy
          (e) Medullary cystic diseases
          (f) Polycystic diseases
      b. Hormone interference at receptor site
        i. Drugs
          (a) Demeclocycline
          (b) Lithium carbonate
          (c) Methoxyflurane
          (d) Dextropropoxyphene
        ii. Hypercalciuria

III. Increased intake of free water
  A. Primary polydipsia
    1. Psychogenic
    2. Postencephalitic
  B. Intravenous therapy

erts and decreasing the movement of water out of this segment. At first, sodium reabsorption will continue, and there will be a progressive decline in the concentration of sodium in tubular fluid. When the concentration of sodium falls below 100 mEq/liter, the back flux of sodium will equal its active reabsorption, and the net movement of sodium out of the proximal tubule will cease. Hence, the presence of a nonreabsorbable solute, such as mannitol, not only impairs water reabsorption in the proximal tubule but also reduces the amount of sodium reabsorbed by this segment. This is graphically illustrated in Figure 10-4. This effect may suppress proximal tubular reabsorption of filtered sodium and water by as much as 10% and 20%, respectively.

In the presence of a nonreabsorbable solute, the movement of water out of the descending limb of loop of Henle is impaired because of a decrease in the osmolality of the medullary interstitium. This decline in medullary osmolality results from a number of factors. One factor is that the concentration of sodium in luminal fluid may be reduced by as much as 50 mEq/liter. Thus the concentration gradient favoring the movement of sodium out of the loop is significantly decreased, and the mechanism of countercurrent multiplication will be impaired to the extent that this driving force is reduced. Second, medullary blood flow is increased, perhaps as a result of the direct effect of mannitol on blood vessels but also because of an increase in the amount of water reabsorbed in terminal collecting duct segments. This seemingly paradoxical increase in the reabsorption of water by these segments probably results from the presence of high levels of circulating antidiuretic hormone, which is the result of the hypernatremic state produced by excess water loss. As a consequence the terminal collecting duct permeability would be enhanced in the face of a fourfold to fivefold increase in delivery of water to this segment. Thus the reabsorption of water by this segment would be increased, and the resultant removal of this fluid from the medulla would necessarily increase renal blood flow and tend to dissipate the osmotic gradient established by countercurrent multiplication.

It would appear that active reabsorption of sodium chloride out of the thick ascending

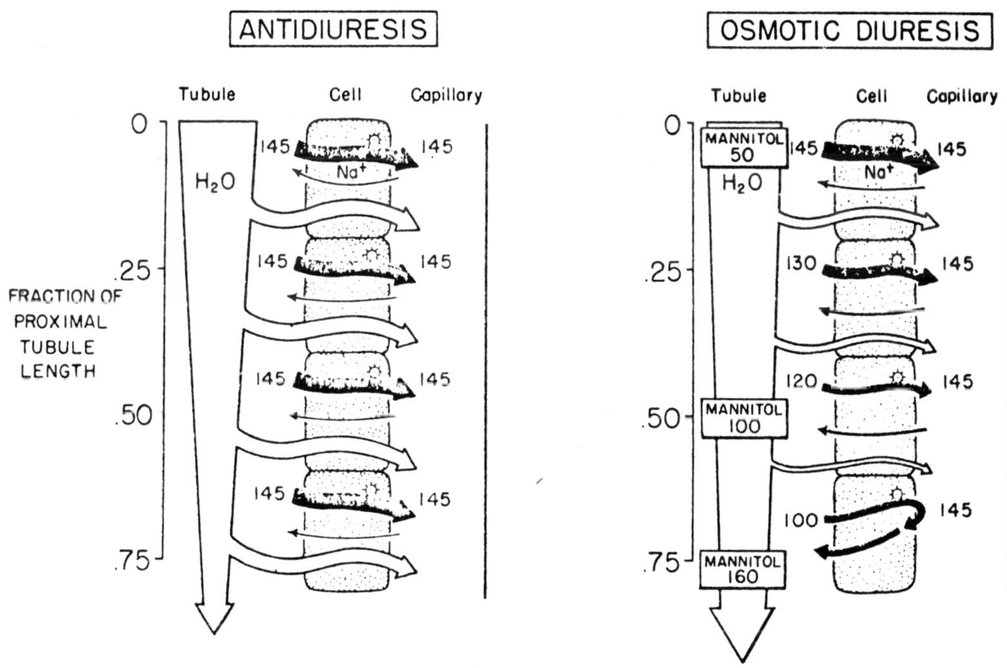

Fig. 10-4.

Schematic representation of sodium and water reabsorption in the proximal tubule during antidiuresis and osmotic diuresis. During antidiuresis, the concentration of sodium in the tubular fluid does not change; during osmotic diuresis, the presence of mannitol in the filtrate (50 millimol/liter) reduces water reabsorption, and thus as sodium reabsorption proceeds, tubular fluid sodium concentration falls progressively. (From N. Engl. J. Med. *291:* 714, 1974, by permission.)

limb is not impaired. The concentration of sodium will fall below 100 mEq/liter in this segment as free water is formed. However, as in the proximal tubule, the reabsorption of water in the distal tubule and cortical collecting duct is impaired by the presence of the osmotically active mannitol. Most of the free water formed in the thick ascending limb is reabsorbed in this segment, but the water obligated by the presence of mannitol is not recaptured. Since the early result of increasing the delivery of water to the medullary collecting duct is a dissipation of the osmotic gradient in this segment, urinary osmolality will be only slightly higher or equal to that of plasma.

b. Angiographic Dyes. Similar results can be seen in patients who have been subjected to procedures involving the intravenous use of large doses of radiographic contrast materials. These dyes are of small molecular size and not reabsorbed by the renal tubule. Such patients may develop a solute diuresis, especially in studies where the radiopaque dye is injected directly into the renal artery, and are likely to become dehydrated and hypotensive if they are on diets where salt and water are restricted.

2. *Glycosuria*

While the infusion of mannitol is the best example of an osmotic diuresis, it is not a frequent cause of secondary polyuria. Probably the most common cause is the development of glycosuria in patients with poorly controlled diabetes mellitus. In this setting the amount of glucose filtered through the glomerulus per unit time (i.e., the filtered load of glucose) exceeds the reabsorptive capacity of the renal tubule. As in the case of mannitol, the unreabsorbed glucose impedes the iso-osmotic movement of water out of the proximal tubule and can result in a significant reduction in the proximal tubular reabsorption of sodium and water.

3. *Urea*

Urea is another small molecule that is not well reabsorbed in the proximal tubule. Therefore, high concentrations of urea in the blood can give rise to an increase in the loss of obligate water. One example of this may be seen in patients who are in the *recovery phase of acute oliguric renal failure* and who have been treated conservatively (i.e., without dialysis) and are likely to have a markedly elevated BUN level. Such patients may move rapidly from an oliguric to the polyuric phase and go into a state of negative water balance. Another example can be seen in patients who are *fed high-protein diets by gastric tube.* These patients will excrete a greater than normal load of urea and therefore obligate water loss may increase markedly. It also is thought that part of the polyuric state that follows relief of urinary tract obstruction *(postobstructive diuresis)* is due to high plasma levels of urea that accumulate in the antecedent period of anuria. Although it is likely that this state is also the result of other factors that are not well characterized but that have been shown to directly suppress the reabsorption of sodium at some unknown site in the renal tubule.

B. Impaired Renal Tubular Reabsorption of Sodium Chloride

It naturally follows that any factor that impairs sodium reabsorption at any point in the nephron will give rise to an increase in the excretion of water. The urine produced will be similar to that seen in a state of osmotic diuresis, except that fractional sodium excretion will be somewhat higher. Such a decrease in the reabsorption of sodium may be the result of direct tubular injury. One such example is *nonoliguric renal failure* where it appears that renal tubular injury exceeds injury to the glomerulus, and while filtration continues at a reduced rate, renal tubular function is impaired to an even greater extent. A similar state is occasionally seen in patients who are in the *early phases of chronic renal disease* and where the major lesion is *tubular or interstitial.* Similarly, it is important in evaluating polyuric states to establish whether the patient is on *diuretic therapy*, surreptitious or otherwise.

Diagnosis of Polyuric States Caused by Increased Solute Excretion

From the above discussion, it is apparent that the diagnosis of secondary polyuria can be established rather easily. A careful history and physical examination with special attention to family or past history of diabetes mellitus is essential. Knowledge of the types of medications utilized by the patient is important. If hospitalized, close inspection of the clinical records for recent diagnostic procedures and types of medications given the patient must be sought. Afterwards, some simple studies should be performed on a simultaneously collected plasma and urine sample. The plasma sample should be analyzed for sodium, osmolality, creatinine, and the two likely causes of osmotically induced polyuria, glucose and urea nitrogen. The urine sample should be tested for glucose and analyzed for osmolality, creatinine, urea, and sodium. In almost all cases, the urine osmolality will be slightly higher or equal to that of plasma. The concentration of sodium will be in the range of 50–70 mEq/liter, but more important, the fraction of the filtered load of sodium excreted (FE_{Na}) will be greater than the normal value of less than 1.0% and may exceed 10%. This value may be quickly calculated by utilizing the following formula:

$$FE_{Na} = \frac{\frac{U}{P} Na}{\frac{U}{P} Cr} \times 100$$

II. Impaired Reabsorption of Free Water (Primary Polyuria)

As stated previously, primary polyuria is a condition in which the excretion of free water is increased. The magnitude of this increase is quite variable and is not particularly related to the cause. By definition, such patients will produce hypotonic urine. The extent of the hypotonicity will depend largely on the degree of impairment in the concentrating segment. But in most cases, urinary osmolality will fall below 200 mOsm/kg H_2O. In contrast to secondary polyuria, sodium excretion will be in the normal range, that is, less than 1.0% of the amount filtered. Obviously, the concentration of sodium in the urine will also depend on the rate of urine flow but in all cases will be relatively low.

Listed in Table 10-2 (Parts II and III) are the conditions known to produce an increase in the excretion of free water or primary polyuria. These conditions are easily divided into two categories. One group consists of those cases in which an increase in the ingestion of water is the *primary* event and the resultant polyuric state is simply the normal physiologic response to a state of positive free water balance. The second group includes those patients whose ability to reabsorb free water is impaired. This decrease in the reabsorption of free water can either be the result of low circulating or absent levels of ADH, referred to as vasopressin-*deficient* diabetes insipidus, or a defect in the concentrating segment which, as a consequence, does not respond to ADH and is termed vasopressin-*resistant* or nephrogenic diabetes insipidus.

A. Vasopressin-Deficient Diabetes Insipidus

Vasopressin-deficient diabetes insipidus is characterized by inappropriately low levels of circulating ADH (a partial defect) or by a complete absence of the hormone. The causes for vasopressin-deficient diabetes insipidus appear to be nearly equally distributed among the first three groups listed in Table 10-2. Although, in recent years with the development of hypophysectomy for the treatment of diabetic retinopathy and the increased incidence of traumatic injury in auto accidents, it is likely that the *posthypophysectomy category* is becoming the most frequent cause.

While the diagnosis in this group may be readily apparent from the beginning, management immediately following *surgical* or *traumatic hypophysectomy* may be complicated. The reason for this is that the urine output in these patients may exhibit a triphasic pattern that is characterized by an initial marked increase in urine output followed in hours to days by a period during which urine output falls to normal and urinary osmolality markedly increases. This *interphase* is transient, lasting several days, and is probably the result of a release of arginine vasopressin from degenerating nerve fibers located in the hypothalamic stalk. Hence the level of ADH in plasma during the interphase period is not under any physiologic control. Careful management is essential in this period, since such patients are prone to develop acute water intoxication if water intake is not reduced appropriately.

Craniopharyngioma is the tumor most frequently associated with diabetes insipidus, with considerably fewer cases being the result of gliomas and vascular tumors. *Metastatic tumor* is rarely a cause, but when it is, carcinoma of the breast is the most likely primary tumor. It is important to emphasize that *pituitary tumors* rarely cause diabetes insipidus unless they extend beyond the sella turcica and either invade the hypothalamus or destroy the supraoptic nuclei by pressure. In less than 10% of patients the cause will be found to be an infiltrative lesion like *histiocytosis, sarcoid,* or *tuberculosis.*

Approximately 30% of patients who present with vasopressin-deficient diabetes insipidus will have no known etiology. The bulk of patients with *idiopathic diabetes insipidus* are young adult females who give a history of an abrupt onset of polyuria that may exceed 10 liters/day. Aside from the annoyance of the polyuric state, a profound increase in thirst, and a particular craving for cold water, such patients will be relatively healthy. However, those patients with long-standing symptoms may develop marked bladder and ureteral dilation that occasionally leads to impairment in renal function. Less than 3% of these patients have a familial incidence. And, as a group, patients with *congenital diabetes insipidus* differ from the majority in that the onset of polyuria always occurs during infancy or early childhood.

B. Vasopressin-Resistant Diabetes Insipidus

The causes of nephrogenic diabetes insipidus (NDI) are divided into a small but interesting group of patients who possess an inherited defect in collecting duct function and a much larger group who acquire a resistance to ADH as a consequence of a wide variety of factors.

1. Congenital

Congenital NDI is a rare hereditary disease that appears to be sex linked and of dominant inheritance. In its complete form, it is seen in only the male offspring but may be variably present in female carriers. If the child is to survive normally, the diagnosis must be made shortly after birth. Frequent failure to make an early diagnosis is likely to expose the child to multiple episodes of profound hypovolemia and hypernatremia when the intake of water is restricted. It is felt that such exposure is the explanation for the high incidence of mental retardation in these children. The defect in collecting duct function in these individuals appears to be the result of failure to produce cyclic AMP in response to circulating ADH. This intermediary is essential in the action of vasopressin on the collecting duct. As in those patients with long-standing vasopressin-deficient diabetes insipidus, these patients frequently develop hydronephrosis, which can result in a decrease in renal function.

2. Acquired

As stated previously there are a great number of causes for acquired NDI. Those renal diseases that preferentially affect the distal tubule and the collecting duct segments of the nephron, such as *medullary cystic disease, chronic obstructive uropathy, nephrocalcinosis,* and *polycystic kidney disease,* are virtually always associated with some degree of unresponsiveness to vasopressin. In addition, prolonged and *profound hypokalemia* impairs the renal response to ADH. This state is not immediately improved by potassium repletion, but improvement seems more related to resolution of the lesions found in distal tubules.

The concentrating defect seen in patients with *sickle cell trait* or *disease* is likely the result of impaired medullary collecting duct function. In this instance the relative hypoxia of the medulla is thought to be the primary event. It is proposed that this relative decrease in oxygen content results in sickling of erythrocytes. Medullary blood flow is therefore reduced, and oxygen content falls even further. Eventually, sludging of erythrocytes occurs and gives rise to tissue anoxia and ultimate destruction of medullary structures. Such changes are said to be the pathogenesis of papillary necrosis in these patients. It is interesting to note that while such patients frequently cannot maximally concentrate their urine, when $^{T}C_{H_2O}$ is measured, it is in the normal range. This observation reemphasizes the statement made previously. That is, that in the presence of ADH, the bulk of the free water formed is reabsorbed by the distal tubule and cortical segments of the collecting duct that are not as likely to be affected by this process.

In a broader sense, a relative impairment in concentrating ability is likely to be seen in any *chronic renal disease that preferentially affects tubular or medullary structures.* Thus, *chronic interstitial diseases* like *pyelonephritis* or infiltrative diseases like *amyloid* are likely to be associated with some degree of polyuria. However, the magnitude of the polyuric state in these diseases seldom reaches massive proportions and is usually limited by the concomitant decline in the GFR. Its recognition is only important in terms of providing adequate fluid intake to those patients where intake may be independent of the individual's thirst mechanism, such as patients who are comatose or who, following surgery, are not allowed to drink but are receiving fluids intravenously.

In recent years, a number of pharmacologic agents have been shown to impair the response of the concentrating segment to arginine vasopressin. This effect is usually reversible shortly after removal of the offending agent. It has been shown in animal studies that both *lithium carbonate* and *demeclocyclene* impair cyclic AMP production by the collecting duct. It is not known how *propoxyphene* or *methoxyflurane* interferes with the response of the collecting duct to ADH.

Marked increases in the urinary excretion of calcium can result in a vasopressin-resistant polyuria. The effects of *acute hypercalciuria* are thought to be the consequence of both impaired cyclic AMP production in response to circulating arginine vasopressin and alterations of the polar structure of water. Methoxyflurane produces a marked increase in the excretion of calcium oxalate. It has been postulated that the NDI seen after Penthrane anesthesia is a consequence of this hypercalciuria. Such effects are frequently reversible. On the other hand, chronic hypercalciuria may result in irreversible damage to the distal tubule and collecting duct and the development of nephrocalcinosis.

III. Increased Intake of Free Water

By far, the most common cause of increased intake of free water or polyuria secondary to increased thirst is *psychogenic* in origin. The severity of the affliction varies widely from patients who are profoundly disturbed and may present with the symptoms of acute water intoxication to those whose symptoms may only be detected after careful questioning. Although in recent years a significant number of cases have been reported in infants and young children, in most instances the patients are neurotic women above the age of 40. In most cases, there is usually a long past history of frequent hospitalizations for a variety of vague complaints, many of which are hysterical in nature. Many cases have a past history of psychiatric hospitalizations for symptoms ranging from depression to schizophrenic behavior. In all cases the polydipsia and the subsequent polyuria are intermittent and frequently associated with periods of increased stress. The onset is usually gradual.

Primary polydipsia can also result from an organic lesion near the thirst center and has been reported as a sequela to *viral encephalitis,* but these occurrences are extremely rare and in most cases such lesions inhibit thirst. Increased thirst is reported to also occur in patients who have *hypercalcemia* or who are *potassium depleted;* however, it is nearly impossible to differentiate such an effect from an increase in thirst resulting from the defect in concentrating ability known to be present in these patients.

By definition, patients with psychogenic polydipsia are in a state of positive water balance. As a consequence, plasma osmolality falls and the secretion of ADH is suppressed. Figure 10-5 illustrates the osmolality of plasma obtained from patients with primary polydipsia, normal individuals, and patients with vasopressin-deficient diabetes insipidus several hours after they had been warned of the fact that a blood sample would be taken. Although there is considerable overlap with controls and patients with diabetes insipidus, it is apparent that as a group, patients with primary polydipsia have a decrease in plasma osmolality. This overlap would be even greater if the patients with primary polydipsia had not been told in advance of the test, since such a warning was likely to have provoked many of these patients to increase their intake of water. Hence, plasma osmolality alone will not differentiate primary polydipsia from other causes of primary polyuria.

Diagnosis of Polyuric States with Impaired Reabsorption of Water

It is apparent that while the diagnosis of primary polyuria may be established relatively easily, it may be considerably more difficult to determine its cause. A careful history is essential and should include the nature of the polyuric state, how it began, and whether it was associated with stressful situations. Obviously, knowledge of the types of medications used by the patient are important. A past history of mental disturbances should alert one to the possibilities that the polyuric state might be secondary to an increase in drinking or that part of the patient's therapy may include lithium carbonate. A past medical history of heart disease or hypertension should suggest the possible use of diuretics in the patient's therapeutic regimen and the possibility of potassium depletion. A history of visual defects, headaches, or head trauma is of obvious importance.

Routine laboratory studies should include measurements of osmolality, calcium, and

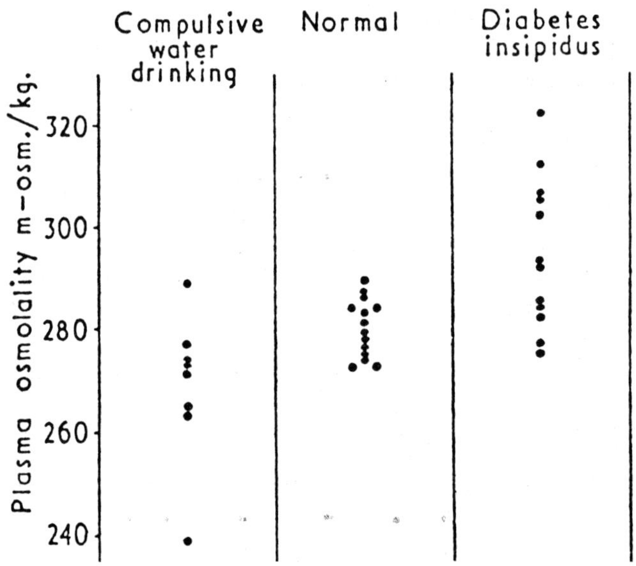

Fig. 10-5.

The plasma osmolality in compulsive water drinking, in normal subjects, and in diabetes insipidus. (From Q. J. Med. *28:* 235, 1959, by permission.)

potassium, and black patients should be screened for sickle cell trait. Renal function should be assessed with at least a creatinine clearance, which should be followed by an intravenous pyelogram if the GFR is reduced or if, at a later juncture, the diagnosis of nephrogenic diabetes insipidus is suspected. On the other hand, if later studies lead to the diagnosis of vasopressin-deficient diabetes insipidus, radiologic studies of the skull are essential. A physical examination is important in determining the state of hydration of the individual and should include a careful neurological evaluation.

Once these preliminary studies have been performed and the obvious causes have been ruled out, the diagnosis may still be unclear. This is particularly true when trying to differentiate primary polydipsia from idiopathic vasopressin-deficient diabetes or where NDI is suspected but no agent has been found.

The best and most accepted approach in the differential diagnosis of the remaining patients is fluid deprivation followed by the administration of vasopressin. The first part of the test is designed to dehydrate the patient and to maximally stimulate the endogenous production of arginine vasopressin. At the onset of the test, urine and plasma osmolalities are measured. Then the urine osmolality should be determined hourly until the change in osmolality is less than 30 mOsm/kg per hour. This usually requires 12 to 16 hours of water deprivation. It is essential that the patients be monitored carefully during this interval for two reasons. First, subjects who have psychogenic polyuria tend not to be reliable and will drink if not continually watched. Second, those individuals with vasopressin-deficient or vasopressin-resistant diabetes insipidus may become profoundly dehydrated. Hence, this part of the test should be discontinued when a patient has lost 3% to 5% of body weight. Once urine osmolality has stabilized or weight loss is significant, a blood sample should be obtained for plasma osmolality after which 5 units of aqueous vasopressin should be administered subcutaneously. Another plasma and urine sample should be obtained in 60 minutes. When this test is administered to normal subjects, maximal urine osmolality is achieved in 16 to 18 hours and ranges from 850–1440 mOsm/kg. In addition, the plasma osmolality is likely to increase slightly. After the administration of ADH, urine osmolality will either fall slightly or not change. The reason for this is that maximal stimulation of endogenous ADH release brings the final urine into equilibrium with the papillary interstitium; hence, additional amounts of vasopressin will have no effect. The magnitude of the change in normal individuals is usually less than 5%.

Patients with primary polydipsia will behave in a similar fashion, and urine produced always becomes hypertonic with respect to plasma. As in normal patients, the increase in urine osmolality after the administration of ADH will be less than 5%. However, maximal urine osmolalities may be considerably less than normal, usually averaging around 700 mOsm. This diminished ability to maximally concentrate the urine is temporary. It may be the result of an increase in renal medullary blood flow with dissipation of the osmotic gradient. The reasons for this increase in medullary blood flow are not clear. It may be partly related to increased delivery of water to the medullary collecting ducts. Although this segment is less permeable to water in the absence of ADH, water is reabsorbed. Hence, in conditions where delivery of water to this segment is increased severalfold, more water could be reabsorbed, and as a consequence, blood flow would increase and the solute gradient would be dissipated. A note of caution should be made at this juncture. Since the *primary* problem in this group is increased thirst, it is essential that patients with primary polydipsia be watched closely after vasopressin is administered. Continued drinking could easily lead to acute water intoxication and death.

Urinary osmolality will seldom rise above plasma osmolality after fluid deprivation in individuals with vasopressin-deficient diabetes insipidus. In most instances the maximal urinary osmolality will be less than 200 mOsm/kg H_2O. On the other hand, there will be a striking rise in plasma osmolality, frequently above 300 mOsm/kg H_2O. After vasopressin, the urine osmolality will rise significantly. For reasons discussed previously, the osmolality of urine will not be as great as in normal subjects. More importantly, the increase in urine osmolality after ADH in vasopressin-deficient diabetes insipidus is likely to be greater than 180% of baseline values contrasted to the less than 5% increase seen in normal individuals or patients with primary polydipsia. In patients with a partial defect in ADH secretion, dehydration will produce an increase in urine osmolality perhaps to 400 mOsm/kg,

Table 10-3

Systematic Approach to the Differential Diagnosis of Polyuric States

Polyuric State	PAV*	U_{Osm}	FE_{Na}	P_{Osm}	U_{Osm} after H_2O deprivation	
					Before ADH	*After* ADH
Secondary polyuria (obligate water loss)	↑	↑ or = P_{Osm}	10–15%	↑		
Primary polyuria			> 1.0%			
Primary polydipsia	↓	↓↓ P_{Osm}		↓	↑	NC
Secondary polydipsia						
ADH-deficient	↓	↓↓ P_{Osm}		↑	NC	↑
ADH-resistant	↑	↓↓ P_{Osm}		↑	NC	NC

Note: PAV, plasma arginine vasopressin; U_{Osm}, urine osmolality; FE_{Na}, fraction of filtered sodium excreted; P_{Osm}, plasma osmolality; NC, no change.

but unlike patients with primary polydipsia, these patients will usually have a further increase in urinary osmolality after ADH administration. However, the magnitude of the increase is considerably less than in those patients with complete absence of ADH and an increase in urine osmolality of 25% after ADH is thought to be diagnostic of a partial defect.

As would be predicted, patients with vasopressin-resistant diabetes insipidus continue to produce a hypotonic urine after prolonged water deprivation and will not produce a hypertonic urine after the administration of vasopressin.

Other tests have been used to differentiate between these three causes of primary polyuria. However, a number of factors that might alter the patient's response are involved and frequently make these tests difficult to interpret. One such test is the use of nicotine inhalation to further stimulate the release of endogenous vasopressin. Such a test may frequently be associated with profound nausea and vomiting, which may in turn alter renal blood flow and GFR. The infusion of hypertonic saline will also increase ADH production but poses a danger to patients with borderline compensated cardiovascular status. Further, in well-hydrated patients, the urine flow may actually increase. Therefore, in this study $^{T}C_{H_2O}$ must also be measured.

Probably the most helpful diagnostic tool becoming available is the radioimmunoassay for measurement of plasma arginine vasopressin. Such measurements will obviously be important in differentiating between partial defects in ADH production and release from those individuals with mild degrees of nephrogenic diabetes insipidus.

As is depicted in Table 10-3 using these studies and other measurements previously mentioned, the symptom of polyuria may be approached systematically and the site of impaired water reabsorption can be ascertained. In some instances, it will be necessary, through additional studies, to determine which of the specific causes listed in Table 10-2 is the reason for the resultant polyuria.

Clinical Problem

An 18-year-old white female was referred to Washington University Medical Center for evaluation of increased thirst and polyuria. The patient had consumed large quantities of water since age 7 days, when it was noted that she preferred to drink rather than eat. Such drinking habits continued unaltered throughout her childhood. During this period, her normal intake of water exceeded 6–8 liters/day. She had considerable difficulty in school because of the frequent interruptions for drinking and urination. In a recent hospitalization for gastroenteritis characterized by nausea, vomiting, and watery diarrhea, the patient was reported to have been 16 pounds below her normal weight, with physical signs of severe dehydration but with a urine specific gravity of 1.001. The patient gives a history of being continually thirsty. She states that frequently she will drink cold water from a fountain until she is nearly sick. She relates no history of headaches or blurred or double vision. She has no past history of hospitalizations other than for evaluation of polyuria. There is no family history of diabetes mellitus or of polyuria. She denies urgency, frequency, or dysuria. At present, she awakes to pass urine only once during the night.

A careful physical exam revealed an essentially normal white female with no evidence of neurological abnormalities. A random urine was negative for glucose and hypotonic (U_{OSM} = 60 mOsm/kg). Routine laboratory studies including BUN, serum calcium, and creatinine levels were all within the normal range.

The patient was hospitalized and further studies were performed. During the initial evaluation, the patient's urine output was reported to be greater than 11 liters/day. During this time, she was observed to void 1500 ml of urine at one time. Again, urine osmolality was usually in the range of 60 mOsm/kg. Sodium concentration in the urine was found to be 22 mEq/liter on one occasion, and Fe_{Na} was calculated to be 0.89%. Creatinine clearance was 134 ml/min. An intravenous pyelogram was interpreted as normal with the exception of widely dilated ureters and bladder. A radiologic skull series was normal.

After 12 hours of fluid deprivation, the patient had lost nearly 6 pounds. On standing, her blood pressure fell from 130/70 to 90/60. A urine and plasma osmolality obtained at this time was 290 and 297 mOsm/kg, respectively. Ten units of aqueous vasopressin was then given subcutaneously, and 60 minutes later, repeat urine osmolality was 530 mOsm/kg. Subsequently, blood samples collected shortly before the administration of vasopressin were found to contain no measurable levels of arginine vasopressin by radioimmunoassay.

Questions

1. What is particularly unusual about the patient's history?
2. Does this patient have primary or secondary polyuria? Can this be determined from the studies done prior to the fluid deprivation test?
3. Based on the data at hand, can a diagnosis be made?
4. What is the significance of the levels of vasopressin?

Discussion

This young girl most likely has a form of vasopressin-deficient diabetes. She is a rare case in that it is extremely unusual for the onset of the polyuria to begin in infancy. The remainder of the history is completely compatible with this diagnosis. The fact that she complains of unrelenting thirst, particularly for cold water, which is not worse under conditions of stress, is typical of patients with diabetes insipidus. The history of a 16 pound weight loss during a mild viral illness where fluid intake was reduced and gastrointestinal losses were increased is evidence that strongly suggests that the primary mechanism is polyuria. It is initially disturbing that the patient voids only once during the night, but when the patient's record indicates that she voids large amounts of urine at one time and the IVP reveals a markedly dilated ureteral system and increased bladder size, it is clear that polyuria is a constant phenomenon.

The low urinary osmolality, fractional sodium excretion, and the absence of glucose in the urine establishes the fact that her daily urine output of 11 liters is the result of an increase in the excretion of free water and, hence, that she has primary polyuria.

The water deprivation test confirms the initial observations that thirst is a consequence rather than a cause of the polyuria, since after 12 hours she continues to put out large amounts of hypotonic urine, has lost over 6 pounds, and has developed postural hypotension.

The increase in urinary osmolality from 60 to 290 mOsm shows that the patient has some capacity to concentrate the urine, although it is certainly insufficient to maintain plasma osmolality within the normal range. The administration of vasopressin confirms this, since U_{Osm} rises nearly 100%. At this juncture, psychogenic polydipsia has been eliminated as a cause, as has vasopressin-resistant diabetes insipidus. Thus the most likely diagnosis is a partial defect in vasopressin production or release and, in the absence of any positive physical or radiologic findings, must be classified as idiopathic.

The measurement of arginine vasopressin levels in the blood confirms the diagnosis as vasopressin-deficient diabetes insipidus but does not eliminate a partial defect, since the levels may be too low to measure with the assays available.

References

Barlow, E., and DeWardener, H. "Compulsive water drinking." Q. J. Med. *28:* 235–258, 1959.

Berl, T., Anderson, R., McDonald, K., and Schrier, R. "Clinical disorders of water metabolism." Kidney Int. *10:* 117–132, 1976.

Gennari, F., and Kassirer, J. "Osmotic diuresis." N. Engl. J. Med. *291:* 714–720, 1974.

Hays, R., and Levine, S. "Pathophysiology of water metabolism." *In:* The Kidney, B. M. Brenner and F. C. Rector, Jr. (eds.). W. B. Saunders, Philadelphia, pp. 553–614, 1976.

Jamison, R. "Urinary concentration and dilution." *In:* The Kidney, B. M. Brenner and F. C. Rector, Jr. (eds.). W. B. Saunders, Philadelphia, pp. 391–441, 1976.

Miller, M., Dalakos, T., Moses, A., Fellerman, H., and Streeten, D. "Recognition of partial defects in antidiuretic hormone secretion." Ann. Intern. Med. *73:* 721–729, 1970.

Chapter 11

Alterations in Serum Sodium Concentration

General Considerations

The clinical significance of changes in the serum sodium concentration is often the cause of unnecessary confusion. This frequently results from a failure to remember that the *concentration* of sodium reflects the amounts of both sodium and water in the extracellular fluid compartment and that changes in the serum sodium concentration do not necessarily indicate comparable changes in the total body sodium *content* or even sodium content of the ECF space. Thus, hyponatremia (serum Na <130 mEq/liter) may result from the addition of water to the ECF, from loss of sodium from this compartment, or from a combination of changes that result in there being *relatively* more water than sodium in the ECF. As a consequence, hyponatremia may be observed when the sodium content of the ECF is either low, normal, or even increased. Conversely, hypernatremia (serum sodium concentration of >150 mEq/liter) indicates relatively more sodium than water in the ECF and occurs with either the addition of sodium or loss of water from this space or from a combination of these changes.

Under normal circumstances, serum sodium concentration is maintained within a relatively narrow range (135–145 mEq/liter) despite large daily and minute-to-minute variations in intake of sodium and water. This is accomplished by a complex series of interrelated physiologic regulatory mechanisms. Before discussing the diseases associated with changes in sodium concentrations, it is appropriate to review briefly the physiologic mechanisms responsible for the normal regulation of sodium and water balances.

Sodium

Total body sodium approximates 58 mEq/kg body weight (e.g., over 4000 mEq in a 70 kg man), of which 40 mEq/kg is in the exchangeable sodium pool. Sodium is the principal extracellular cation and represents the major solute responsible for osmolality of the ECF. In contrast, intracellular sodium concentrations are low, and intracellular sodium content amounts to less than 2.4% of total body sodium (1.4 mEq/kg). It is now widely recognized that almost 43% of total body sodium is in bone, so that the sodium content of the ECF space totals only 40% of the total body sodium. This is comprised of 6.5 mEq/kg of sodium (11.2% total body sodium) and 16.8 mEq/kg of sodium (29.0% total body sodium), respectively, in the plasma sodium pool and interstitial fluid.

Intake

Since some patients with salt-losing diseases experience salt craving, there may be a regulatory mechanism for sodium intake. However, at best, this mechanism appears to be poorly developed, especially when compared to that for water. In general, sodium intake varies according to cultural customs; the average American diet provides an intake of approximately 100–170 mEq of sodium per day. To remain in sodium balance the healthy adult must excrete sodium in an amount equal to that ingested.

Excretion

Sodium is excreted in sweat, in stools, and in urine. Sweat sodium concentrations normally range between 25 and 30 mEq/liter, with the usual losses by this route amounting to approximately 5 mEq/day. Although sweat sodium concentrations vary in different disease states and are affected by the adrenal secretion of aldosterone, there is little evidence to suggest that this is a route for regulating sodium balance. Similarly, loss of sodium in normal stools is small compared to the average daily intake and does not appear to provide a regulatory pathway for sodium balance.

The principal organ responsible for regulating sodium balance is the kidney, which acts under a variety of extrarenal influences. Under normal conditions each day the kidney filters an amount of sodium—22,000 mEq—equal to five times total body sodium. Since only 100–170 mEq are excreted in the urine, it is apparent that more than 99% of the sodium filtered through the glomeruli must be reabsorbed by the renal tubules. The bulk of this reabsorption—approximately 60%—occurs in the proximal convoluted tubule where water and solute are reabsorbed in proportion to one another. The second major transport site for sodium is the thick ascending limb of the loop of Henle where progressive dilution of the urine occurs. Although the exact proportion of filtered sodium reabsorbed at this site remains to be delineated, micropuncture studies indicate that between 25% and 40% of filtered sodium is reabsorbed between the end of the accessible portion of the proximal tubule and the earlier accessible portion of the distal tubule. The distal convoluted tubule probably reabsorbs 10% of filtered sodium and the collecting ducts 5%, so that less than 1% is excreted in the urine under normal hydropenic conditions.

Multiple factors have been found to modify renal sodium excretion. The first of these regulating factors is the GFR. Changes in the filtered load of sodium, consequent upon even small changes in the GFR, are large in relation to urinary sodium excretion rates and have the potential of greatly modifying sodium excretion. The secretion of mineralocorticoids is the second factor known to regulate sodium excretion. Aldosterone secretion decreases urinary sodium excretion by increasing sodium reabsorption in the distal convoluted tubule. It may also modify sodium absorption in the proximal convoluted tubule and in the collecting duct. The existence of a third factor—possibly a natriuretic agent—has been suggested by a variety of studies, although direct evidence for such a natriuretic agent has not been obtained. Other factors that have been implicated in modifying renal sodium handling and urinary excretion of sodium include changes in peritubular oncotic pressure, alterations in the intrarenal distribution of renal blood flow, angiotensin, prostaglandins, kinins, several of the steroid hormones, and neural stimuli, especially sympathetic nervous activity.

Water

Water comprises 60% of body weight in the male (55% in the female). Of this, two thirds is intracellular and one third is extracellular fluid. The ECF is composed of intravascular or plasma water (4.5% to 5% body weight) and interstitial fluids (15% body weight) consisting of bone water, connective tissue water, and other interstitial fluids.

Distribution of water between the intracellular and extracellular spaces is maintained by osmotic forces acting across the cell membranes. Although intracellular composition varies markedly from that of ECF, the osmotic pressure in the two compartments of body water are similar, the cell walls appearing to act as semipermeable membranes and thus permitting movement of water if an osmotic gradient develops across the cell wall. If comparable changes in intracellular and extracellular osmolalities occur, there is no net fluid movement across the cell wall. However, a relative increase in ECF osmolality compared to that inside the cells results in fluid movement out of the cells into the ECF and reduction in cell size. Conversely, a relative decrease in ECF osmolality will result in cellular swelling. If there is interference with the normal active transport of cations across the cell wall, that is, sodium out of and potassium into the cell, cellular swelling consequent upon an increase in intracellular osmotic pressure usually occurs. Although the transport across the cell walls of these two cations is linked, it is not on a one-to-one basis, and cell wall permeabilities for sodium and potassium differ. As a consequence, a decrease in active transport results in the accumulation of osmotically active solutes inside the cell.

Vascular volume is maintained by the oncotic pressure of the blood, that is, the osmotic pressure exerted by proteins and other macromolecules confined to the vascular space. A decrease in plasma oncotic pressure results in net movement of fluid into the interstitial space and to a decreased blood volume. Sodium and other small molecules equilibrate across the capillary bed. Thus the concentrations of these components of crystalloid osmotic pressure are not changed by a fluid shift from vascular to interstitial fluid spaces per se. If changes in composition do occur, they are more usually the consequence of compensatory mechanisms or therapy.

Intake

In contrast to sodium, water balance is controlled by regulation of both intake and excretion. *Intake* of water is stimulated by the sensation of thirst and is a major defense against fluid depletion, evidence indicating that one or more centers regulating thirst exist in the hypothalamus. Although the stimulation of thirst and decrease of water losses through release of ADH frequently are interrelated, it would appear that at least some of the thirst centers are separated functionally and physically from those involved in ADH release.

Thirst occurs either when plasma osmolality increases—by as little as 1% to 2%—or when ECF is depleted by blood loss, by sodium depletion, or by other mechanisms. Changes in osmolality are monitored by receptors in the lateral preoptic area of the hypothalamus. It is proposed that an increase in ECF osmolality results in dehydration of these osmoreceptors which trigger the thirst mechanism. Osmoreceptors for thirst may also be present in the pancreas and in the hepatic portal vein.

The mechanisms by which volume depletion produces thirst are less well understood. It has been suggested that baroreceptors in the atria and elsewhere in the vascular bed may be involved; however, more investigation is required before this hypothesis can be confirmed. More recently, a third stimulus to thirst—angiotensin—has been demonstrated. Recent studies indicate that the injection of angiotensin II or its precursors will induce thirst. In addition, preliminary data indicate that the kidney may be involved in regulating water intake, perhaps through the renin-angiotensin system. Although these new observations are exciting, much work is required before these pathways and their interrelationships are fully understood.

Excretion

The usual adult daily intake of water—as fluids and as water of oxidation from food — normally amounts to between 2 and 2.5 liters/day. To maintain balance, fluid losses must equal intake. Evaporative losses of about 800 ml occur through the lungs and as sweat. Small amounts of fluid are lost in the feces. An additional 500 ml/day is obligated for the excretion of solute through the kidney. None of these losses, however, can be used to regulate water balance.

Regulation of the excretion of the remaining fluid and indeed of fluid balance in general is the responsibility of the kidney acting under the influence of ADH. Release of this cyclic octopeptide into the circulation results in several changes, one of the principal ones being an increase in the permeability of the collecting duct to water, with cyclic AMP acting as an intermediary in the cells of this segment of the nephron. As a consequence, there is an increased reabsorption of filtered water from the collecting duct into the hypertonic renal medulla, decreasing urine output and conserving water. Human ADH (arginine vasopressin) is synthesized in the supraoptic nuclei, transported down axons in the supraopticohypophyseal tracts and is stored in the posterior pituitary. Release, by exocytosis, occurs in response to stimuli from the hypothalamus. As with thirst, ADH release occurs in response to increased osmolality of the ECF or to volume depletion or to both. Receptors, similar or identical to those described for thirst, monitor these changes and regulate ADH release. It has now been shown that ADH release has a threshold of approximately 280 mOsm/kg. Levels of this hormone also increase significantly after 8% volume depletion and rise exponentially with more marked dehydration.

In addition to the physiologic pathways described, ADH release may be stimulated by pain, emotional stress, cholinergic and beta-adrenergic drugs, demerol, barbiturates and morphine, nicotine, and prostaglandins. Its release is inhibited by diphenylhydantoin and possibly by glucocorticoids.

Although osmotic and volume controls are interdependent, physiologic regulation appears designed to minimize changes, especially rapid changes, in osmolality even at the expense of volume changes. This is achieved by modulating water balance—a change that can be accomplished quickly. Correction of changes in volume and sodium *content* of the ECF occur more slowly.

Hyponatremia

General Considerations

By definition, a patient with a serum sodium concentration reduced below the lower limit of normal (135 mEq/liter) is hyponatremic. However, it is important to emphasize again that this does not necessarily indicate a decreased sodium *content* either in the ECF or the total body. Since the concentration of sodium is dependent on the relative amounts of sodium and water in the ECF, all that a low serum sodium concentration indicates is that there is relatively more water than sodium in this space. This may occur when ECF sodium content is decreased, for example, with diarrhea where there are losses of both sodium and water, but the sodium losses are greater than those of water; when ECF content of sodium is normal, for example, with excess administration of water; or when ECF sodium content is increased, for example, with edema when there are increases in both sodium and water contents.

Keeping these considerations in mind, the diseases most commonly associated with hyponatremia have been classified in Table 11-1 according to the basic abnormality responsible for this alteration in electrolyte concentration. The diseases are subdivided further according to the mechanisms responsible for these abnormalities. In most situations the primary mechanism is obvious, but when multiple abnormalities coexist, the disease is listed according to the principal cause. This classification helps to develop a logical approach in determining the cause of hyponatremia and designing the appropriate management for the patient.

Differential Diagnosis of Hyponatremia

I. Expansion of Extracellular Fluid by Water

A. Excessive Intake of Water

The ability of the kidney to excrete free water often exceeds 10 ml/min/100 ml GFR. Thus, it is rare for a high rate of fluid administration per se to cause hyponatremia, since

Table 11-1

Differential Diagnosis of Hyponatremia

I. Expansion of extracellular fluid by water
   A. Excessive intake of water (output not increased)
      1. Oral: compulsive polydipsia; acute psychosis
      2. Parenteral: excessive amounts of fluids such as 5% glucose in water
      3. Other: tap-water enemas; postoperative irrigation of prostatic bed with hyponatremic solutions
   B. Reduced output of water (intake normal)
      1. Renal
         a. Intrinsic diseases: glomerulonephritis; nephrotic syndrome; acute tubular necrosis, etc.
         b. Extrinsic factors: syndrome of inappropriate secretion of antidiuretic hormone; congestive heart failure; following cardiovascular surgery; cirrhosis
      2. Extrarenal
         a. Lungs and skin: infants in high humidity environment
   C. Redistribution of water
      1. Acute hyperglycemia, e.g., diabetic ketoacidosis
      2. Mannitol administration

II. Extracellular deficit of sodium
   A. Reduced intake of sodium
      1. Low-salt diet
      2. Prolonged intravenous therapy, e.g., with 5% glucose in water
   B. Excessive loss of sodium
      1. Renal
         a. Intrinsic diseases: "salt-losing nephritis;" diuretic phase of acute tubular necrosis or nephrotic syndrome; postobstructive diuresis; Bartter's syndrome
         b. Extrinsic factors: diuretics; hypoadrenalism; myxedema; central nervous system disease; ventricular shunts; sickle cell disease
      2. Extrarenal losses
         a. Gastrointestinal tract: vomiting; diarrhea; gastric or pancreatic drainage
         b. Skin: excessive sweating; abnormal sweat, e.g., cystic fibrosis or adrenal insufficiency; burns
      3. Other: "third-spacing;" thoracentesis; paracentesis
   C. Redistribution of sodium
      1. Sick-cell syndrome
      2. Potassium deficiency
      3. Severe malnutrition

III. Pseudohyponatremia
   A. Hyperlipidemia or hypoproteinemia

IV. Other causes
   A. Resetting of "osmostat"
   B. Artifact
      1. Intravenous therapy in vein distal to site of venipuncture
      2. Laboratory dilutional error

the kidney is able to handle the water load presented and maintain fluid balance. More often, hyponatremia occurs when a high fluid load is combined with some other factor, for example, secretion of antidiuretic hormone, which limits the ability of the kidney to excrete the water. However, patients with the psychogenic disorder of compulsive polydipsia may ingest so much water that it results in hemodilution and a decreased serum sodium. Urine output is high, with the urine being dilute (e.g., specific gravity 1.001 and osmolality below 100 mOsm/kg). The diagnosis should not be difficult, but patients with diabetes insipidus or nephrogenic diabetes insipidus may be confused with those with compulsive polydipsia because they too have a high urine flow rate and dilute urine. In diabetes insipidus, however, polydipsia is secondary to a renal inability to conserve water and, consequently, serum sodium and plasma osmolalities tend to be elevated rather than reduced from normal. In compulsive polydipsia, fluid deprivation should result in an increase in the concentration of the urine above that of plasma, whereas patients with diabetes insipidus are unable to achieve this concentration unless their lesion is a partial one. A more detailed discussion of this separation is presented in the chapters on hypernatremia and polyuria.

Recently, an interesting group of patients has been described in whom an acute or chronic psychosis appears to stimulate both polydipsia and ADH secretion. These patients develop hyponatremia as a consequence.

The excessive parenteral administration of fluids, such as 5% dextrose in water, may also result in hemodilution and hyponatremia. This occurs more frequently in patients who have a reduction in the GFR and who, as a result, are less able to handle a water load. Thus, hyponatremia may be seen in the very young, the elderly, after blood loss, or postoperatively. Not infrequently, additional circumstances compound the primary problem. For example, infants may be nursed in a high humidity environment, decreasing their extrarenal losses of water, or postoperative patients may have received drugs known to stimulate the release of or potentiate the action of ADH (see below). The diagnosis is usually made by identifying the clinical situation that caused the hyponatremia and documenting a positive fluid balance and a significant weight gain from the patient's chart. The diagnosis is confirmed if the serum sodium and the patient's weight return to normal when the rate of fluid administration is reduced.

Other situations in which an excess fluid load has resulted in hyponatremia include the frequent use of tap-water enemas in megacolon and irrigation of the prostatic bed with a hyponatremic solution in patients during and following prostatectomy. Under both circumstances, large volumes of water appear to be absorbed from these solutions, and this, combined with other factors such as reduction in the GFR, results in hemodilution. Diagnosis consists of being aware of these complications and recognizing them when they occur.

B. Reduced Output of Water

1. Renal

a. Intrinsic Diseases. The majority of patients with renal diseases can regulate sodium and water excretion, albeit over a reduced range from normal, and therefore maintain a normal serum sodium concentration. However, hyponatremia may occasionally be seen. This is usually the consequence of a decreased GFR, which limits the ability of the patient to excrete free water. As a result, the patient is unable to excrete a water load that would have been handled easily by a subject with normal renal function. The existence of renal disease as a cause of hyponatremia is suggested by an elevated BUN or serum creatinine level, especially in the absence of clinical evidence of dehydration. It is also suggested by the presence of proteinuria or by urinary sediment abnormalities such as granular casts.

b. Extrinsic Factors. The *syndrome of inappropriate antidiuretic hormone secretion (SIADH)* has been recognized only relatively recently but now tends to be overdiagnosed, especially if the diagnostic criteria outlined below are not strictly followed. Until an assay for serum ADH becomes readily available for routine clinical use, the diagnosis must be based on a series of clinical criteria, including:

1. The presence of hyponatremia with a decreased plasma osmolality.
2. A urine that is less than maximally dilute. The urine osmolality is inappropriately high for the plasma osmolality and frequently is greater than that of the plasma.
3. Despite hyponatremia, there is continued renal excretion of sodium; indeed the urine sodium often reflects the dietary sodium intake. This is in contrast to patients with hyponatremia from other causes, such as salt depletion, in whom urine sodium concentration is low.
4. There should be no evidence of fluid volume depletion. Since blood volume also regulates ADH secretion, ADH secretion in

a patient with hyponatremia but with a decreased blood volume may be appropriate rather than inappropriate.

5. Renal function should be normal. Chronic renal disease may limit the ability of the kidney to excrete water and is often associated with a high fractional excretion of sodium in the urine. Thus, one must be sure of the diagnosis before attributing hyponatremia to SIADH in the presence of chronic renal disease.
6. The patient should not be receiving diuretics. The clinical features of SIADH may be mimicked during diuretic administration in the overloaded patient.
7. Adrenal function should be normal. Primary or secondary adrenal insufficiency may be difficult to differentiate from SIADH. The presence of hyperkalemia and volume contraction would suggest adrenal insufficiency to be the correct diagnosis, but a definitive diagnosis depends on measurement of urinary steroids, aldosterone excretion rates, and plasma cortisol levels.

Having established that SIADH is present, one must then determine its cause (Table 11-2). For convenience the causes can be classified into five major categories. The first is ectopic production of ADH by malignancies. The most frequent lesion responsible for this form of SIADH is bronchogenic carcinoma of the oat cell type. It has been shown by immunoassay that ADH or ADH-like material frequently is present in these tumors or their metastases and that slices of tumors are capable of synthesizing ADH from amino acid precursors. The second group of diseases causing SIADH is chronic pulmonary infections due to tuberculosis and other agents. Although the mechanism responsible for the increased ADH levels in these diseases is not fully understood, it is postulated that they may interfere with stretch receptors in the atria and ventricles. As indicated in Table 11-2, many diseases involving the CNS have been associated with SIADH, presumably as a result of stimulation of endogenous ADH release. In some of these patients the lesion in the CNS may also stimulate the patient to drink large amounts of fluid, thus potentiating the development of hyponatremia. The fourth group of diseases resulting in SIADH are all associated with stress, which is known to stimulate ADH release. Thus, hyponatremia seen in the postoperative patient may result in part from ADH release secondary to the stress of the anesthetic, pain, or the surgical procedure itself. Finally, the use of a variety of drugs has been found to be complicated by the development of hyponatremia. These drugs may act

Table 11-2

Disease States Associated with SIADH

A. Ectopic production of ADH by malignant tumors
   Bronchogenic carcinoma; adenocarcinomas of pancreas and duodenum; lymphoma and Hodgkin's disease
B. Pulmonary diseases
   Bacterial pneumonia; chronic chest infections; lung abscess; tuberculosis; aspergillosis
C. Neurological diseases
   1. Central nervous system
      Brain tumors, aneurysms, abscesses; subarachnoid hemorrhage; bacterial and tuberculous meningitis; herpes simplex encephalitis; head injury
   2. Other
      Guillain-Barré syndrome; acute intermittent porphyria; systemic lupus erythematosus
D. Stress
   Postoperative; anesthesia; pain; assisted respiration
E. Drugs
   Sulfonylureas (chlorpropamide, tolbutamide); polymyxin B; vincristine

either by stimulating ADH release or by increasing the renal sensitivity to this hormone (Table 11-3), reducing the ability of the kidney to excrete free water.

In all these diseases the ectopic production, increased endogenous release, or potentiation of the action of ADH per se will not produce hyponatremia but will only limit the ability of the kidney to excrete free water. When one of these lesions is combined with a continued high intake of water, dilutional hyponatremia will be the consequence. Because of this, the diagnosis of SIADH should not be made without evidence of positive fluid balance and an increase in body weight. When the presence of the syndrome has been confirmed, the underlying cause should be sought by reviewing the list of drugs the patient is taking and by performing chest and skull roentgenograms, brain scans, and other appropriate studies.

Hyponatremia is a common finding in patients with *congestive heart failure*. Originally it was proposed that this was a complication of a low-salt diet combined with diuretic therapy with resulting sodium depletion. However, this view has not been supported by measurements of total body sodium, which have shown that patients with congestive heart failure have an increased rather than a decreased total body sodium concentration.

It is now thought that a multiplicity of factors contribute to the hyponatremia, the primary abnormality being a decreased cardiac output secondary to the heart failure. This results in a fall in renal blood flow, a reduced GFR, and an associated increase in fractional reabsorption of sodium and water by the nephron. In consequence the urine volume is reduced and the urine concentration of sodium is low. The alteration in renal hemodynamics may also modify intrarenal distribution of blood flow, with preferential perfusion of the juxtamedullary nephrons resulting in a decreased excretion of sodium in the urine. In addition, there is increased secretion of renin, presumably in response to the changes in renal function or to a decreased perfusion pressure in the renal artery. Aldosterone secretion is stimulated by this renin release through the formation of angiotensin II and provides a further mechanism for sodium retention. Aldosterone secretion may be stimulated further if the patient has developed hypovolemia in response to the use of diuretics.

Although those mechanisms result in sodium retention, much of the retained sodium is contained in the accumulating edema, so that total blood volume may not be as markedly increased as one might expect. Because of the decreased cardiac output, any increase in blood volume will be predominantly on the venous side of the circulation, the effective arterial blood volume being decreased. It is argued that this decrease in arterial volume or altered stimulation of the left atrial stretch receptors stimulates ADH release. Thus, patients with congestive heart failure not only have stimulation of sodium retention but also have a strong stimulus for water retention. If they drink or are given a high fluid intake, they will retain the water and will become hyponatremic despite an increase in total body sodium.

Table 11-3

Effect of Drugs on Antidiuretic Hormone

Drug	Augments ADH Action	Releases ADH
Chlorpropamide	+	+
Tolbutamide	?+	
Diguanide	+	
Vincristine		+
Cyclophosphamide	?	?
Carbamazepine		+
Clofibrate		+
Acetaminophen	+	+

Source: From Bay, W. H., and Ferris, T. F., Geriatrics, August 1976, p. 63 (©1976 by Harcourt Brace Jovanovich, Inc.).

The diagnosis of congestive heart failure can usually be made clinically. Symptoms include fatigue, a reduced exercise tolerance, anorexia, and orthopnea. Classically, there is dependent pitting edema, an increase in central venous pressure detected by distention of the external jugular veins, and hepatomegaly. In patients with left ventricular failure, there is evidence of increased fluid in the lungs, with moist sounds heard at both lung bases. There may be a gallop rhythm and heart murmurs. The presence of the above findings, especially in the appropriate clinical setting, usually establishes the diagnosis. A chest roentgenogram may show increased heart size, an altered cardiac configuration, evidence of pulmonary congestion with a "bat's wing" appearance in the hilar regions, or increased pulmonary fluid with Kerley lines. An electrocardiogram and serum transaminase levels may provide evidence of the underlying pathology such as a myocardial infarction. Arterial pO_2 is usually reduced, hypokalemia should be checked for, BUN concentrations may be mildly elevated, and urine volume is low, with urine sodium concentrations often being below 10 mEq/liter.

Cirrhosis: Patients with cirrhosis are often found to be hyponatremic, especially if they are volume expanded or if they have had a large amount of ascitic fluid removed. Although the explanation for the hyponatremia is not fully understood, patients with cirrhosis may have an inappropriately concentrated urine even after water loading. Many of the mechanisms discussed under congestive heart failure may be operative, since cirrhotics may also have a decrease in effective arterial blood volume.

The diagnosis may be suspected if there are ascites and clinical evidence of portal hypertension—splenomegaly, "caput medusae," esophageal varices, and hemorrhoids —especially in the presence of reduced liver size. Asterixis and constructional apraxia may herald the onset of hepatic coma or precoma. Biochemical evidence of the disease includes elevated levels of serum transaminases and alkaline phosphatase. Characteristically, the serum albumin level is reduced and globulins increased. Bromsulfalein excretion may be impaired and prothrombin time prolonged. Evidence of more advanced liver failure includes elevation of serum bilirubin and blood ammonia levels. The serum potassium concentration should always be measured, since hypokalemia is often associated with the development of hepatic precoma. When a diagnosis of cirrhosis is established, the underlying cause may not be apparent without a liver biopsy.

2. Extrarenal

When planning fluid therapy, it is important to take into account insensible fluid losses through the *lungs and skin.* However, if the amount of these losses is overestimated, the excess water administered may result in ECF expansion and hyponatremia, especially if there is a limited renal ability to excrete this extra fluid. This situation may be observed in the premature or full-term neonate who is being nursed in an incubator with a high humidity environment or in an older child or adult treated by mist tent therapy.

C. Redistribution of Water

In most situations hyponatremia is associated with a decrease in plasma osmolality. However, diabetics with a high blood glucose may develop hyponatremia but have an increased plasma osmolality due to the elevated blood glucose concentration. Since this increase in plasma osmolality is not accompanied by a comparable increase in intracellular osmolality, it results in an osmotic gradient increasing water movement from the intracellular to the extracellular compartment. It is this dilution of the ECF space that results in hyponatremia. An increase in blood glucose of 180 mg% will increase plasma osmolality by 10 mOsm/kg, and this will result in sufficient movement of water into the ECF to reduce the sodium concentration by approximately 5 mEq/liter. A similar situation may be seen transiently after the infusion of large amounts of mannitol given in an attempt to reduce cerebral edema.

The diagnosis of this cause for hyponatremia should not be difficult. The finding of glycosuria will suggest the presence of hyperglycemia, which can be confirmed by measuring the blood glucose concentration. Alternatively, there may be a history of recent administration of mannitol.

II. Extracellular Fluid Deficit of Sodium

A. Reduced Intake of Sodium

It is rare for a reduced sodium intake *alone* to result in hyponatremia. The kidney has a remarkable ability to conserve sodium and, although a low sodium intake will result in a negative sodium balance, water losses are adjusted so that isonatremia is maintained. In a classic series of experiments, R. A. McCance (1936) produced negative sodium balance in himself and healthy volunteers by ingesting a virtually salt-free diet combined with increased sweating. Free access to water was permitted. Total body sodium losses of up to 800 mEq and body weight losses of 2–3 kg were observed. However, hyponatremia occurred only after sodium losses exceeded 300 mEq. Until these losses were achieved, isonatremia was maintained.

When a low or absent sodium intake is combined with continuing generous fluid intake, for example, in a patient requiring prolonged intravenous therapy given 5% dextrose in water, hyponatremia may develop.

B. Excessive Losses of Sodium

Volume depletion consequent upon excessive losses of sodium and water either by renal or extrarenal routes may result in hyponatremia if there is persisting water intake. With volume depletion the GFR tends to fall, and sodium and water reabsorption in the proximal tubule increase. Thus, there is a decreased delivery of filtrate to the distal nephron and a decreased potential for maximal free water clearance. Indeed, it has been shown that in such circumstances urine that is either isotonic or even hypertonic in relation to the plasma may be generated in the absence of ADH. If volume depletion stimulates the release of ADH, the ability to excrete free water is diminished further, increasing the likelihood of hyponatremia developing.

1. Renal

a. Intrinsic Diseases. Patients with certain forms of chronic glomerulonephritis—sometimes referred to in the past as having "salt-losing nephritis"—may excrete large amounts of sodium in their urine and become hyponatremic. Although this salt loss and the resultant dehydration and reduced delivery of filtrate to the diluting segments of the nephron is one mechanism contributing to the hyponatremia in these patients, another important factor is the decreased GFR due to nephron loss. It has been shown that in chronic renal failure, excretion of free water per unit of GFR is well maintained, but the decreased levels of GFR are accompanied by concomitant decreases in absolute values for free water clearance. Thus the patient's ability to excrete a water load is reduced and the risk of developing hyponatremia increased.

The presence of chronic glomerulonephritis may be suggested by a past history of acute glomerulonephritis or of nocturia, by proteinuria or an abnormal urinary sediment, or by an elevation of BUN or serum creatinine level. However, even if the presence of chronic renal failure is established, the clinician should try to determine whether the hyponatremia resulted principally from excess fluid administration or from sodium loss, since the treatment varies in these two circumstances. This differentiation is usually possible by review of the patient's previous intake and output and from any changes in body weight. Measurement of urinary sodium levels and rates of excretion may also help.

During the diuretic phase of *acute tubular necrosis* and *minimal change nephrotic syndrome* and after relief of *obstructive uropathy,* urine losses of water and electrolytes may be massive and can result in dehydration and hyponatremia if correct management of the patient is not employed.

Not infrequently, patients with *Bartter's syndrome* are hyponatremic and hypochloremic. The syndrome is characterized by hypokalemic alkalosis. Peripheral vein renin levels are markedly elevated, and aldosterone secretion and excretion rates are increased. Despite the elevated renin levels, the patients are normotensive and do not show the usual pressor response to exogenous angiotensin. On renal biopsy, juxtaglomerular cell hyperplasia with increased renin granules in these cells is seen. The urinary excretion of both sodium and potassium is inappropriately high. Family members may have an incomplete form of the syndrome. Recent studies have suggested that the primary defect in this disease is increased production of renal prostaglandins. The response of patients with Bartter's syndrome to indomethacin or aspirin supports this view.

b. Extrinsic Factors. Addison's disease results in hyponatremia as a consequence of increased urinary losses of sodium, volume depletion, and nonosmotic stimulation of ADH release. In young children, in whom this disease usually results from adrenal hypoplasia or a defect in steroidogenesis, it is characterized by failure to thrive, vomiting, lethargy, anorexia, dehydration, and if not recognized early, by circulatory collapse and death. In older patients the symptoms consist of lassitude, muscle weakness, anorexia, loss of weight, wasting, and a low blood pressure. In primary Addison's disease, increased skin pigmentation due to elevated ACTH and MSH levels may be obvious, and pigmentation of the buccal mucosa is virtually pathognomonic. If adrenal crisis develops, clinical evidence of ECF volume depletion becomes obvious with a weak, rapid pulse, a cold skin, and cyanosis. Later the blood pressure falls precipitously, and rapid, labored respirations develop.

In addition to hyponatremia and hypochloremia, laboratory studies reveal hyperkalemia, hypoglycemia, and an increase in the eosinophil count. BUN level is increased if there is volume contraction. A chest roentgenogram characteristically shows a small, narrow heart shadow, and abdominal roentgenograms may show adrenal calcification. Urinary sodium and chloride levels are high, while that of potassium is low. The diagnosis is established by measurement of plasma or urinary levels of corticosteroids. Urinary excretion of 17-ketosteroids and 17-hydroxycorticosteroids and response of the patient to corticotropin administration may help to establish a more definitive diagnosis.

Hyponatremia may be seen in patients with *myxedema,* especially in those with myxedema coma. Although the mechanism remains to be determined, abnormalities in these patients' renal handling of salt and water have been described. The possibility of myxedema as a cause of hyponatremia should always be borne in mind, since the serum electrolytes return to normal rapidly with thyroid hormone replacement. The diagnosis may be suspected if the typical clinical features—coarse, scanty hair; loss of eyebrows; characteristic facies; large tongue; hoarse or croaking voice; preference for warm weather; slow pulse; low blood pressure; and thick scaly skin—are present. Laboratory abnormalities include an elevated level of serum cholesterol and low or borderline levels of serum T3 and T4.

The use of *diuretics,* especially those that act on the ascending limb of Henle's loop (i.e., ethacrynic acid or furosemide or the thiazide diuretics) may result in hyponatremia. Not only can they result in salt depletion but they may also result in a decrease in free water clearance, both mechanisms being potential causes for hyponatremia. Before attributing hyponatremia to the use of a diuretic, one should check whether or not the appearance of this electrolyte abnormality preceded the use of the diuretic, since the hyponatremia could have been the consequence of the disease for which the diuretics were prescribed (e.g., heart failure) rather than being a complication of drug treatment.

Patients with a variety of diseases involving the *central nervous system* may develop hyponatremia. In these patients, urinary sodium excretion has been found to be high, and the term "cerebral salt wasting" has been coined to describe this entity. The original patients reported with cerebral salt wasting were clinically dehydrated and usually had a self-limited disease. More recently, there has been some confusion in separating such patients from those who also have hyponatremia and CNS disease but who are volume expanded.

As discussed previously, it is now recognized that many of these latter patients have SIADH.

Patients with *sickle cell disease* are prone to develop hyponatremia, especially during a crisis. Originally this was attributed to treatment involving the administration of excessive amounts of water. However, recent studies have suggested that it may be the consequence of excessive losses of sodium in the urine for an as yet undetermined reason.

2. Extrarenal Losses

Increased losses from the *gastrointestinal tract,* such as those seen with vomiting, diarrhea, and gastric pancreatic drainage, may result in hyponatremia. Although the sodium concentrations in these fluids are less than that in the plasma, such losses do not result in hypernatremia in the majority of patients. This is because there is usually concomitant replacement of some of the sodium and water losses, the replacement of water loss usually being relatively greater than that of sodium. Thus, of all patients admitted to hospital with diarrhea and dehydration, only 10% to 15% are hypernatremic; approximately 70% are isonatremic, and the remaining 10% to 15% are hyponatremic. In these hyponatremic patients, there is usually a history of considerable intake of low electrolyte or electrolyte-free fluids, either by mouth or intravenously, occurring during the period of gastrointestinal fluid losses.

Increased sodium losses through the *skin* can result in negative sodium balance and hyponatremia. More often, though, these losses are associated with a normal serum sodium level unless there has been a concomitant intake of large amounts of water. Patients with *cystic fibrosis* are an exception and are prone to develop hyponatremia, especially during warm weather. Concentration of sodium in the sweat of these patients is increased, classically being 60 mEq/liter or higher. This loss of large amounts of sodium, combined with the inability of patients with cystic fibrosis to excrete free water maximally through the kidneys, the frequent use of mist tents that reduce extrarenal losses of water, and treatment regimens that often include large amounts of intravenous fluids, contributes to the hyponatremia. The diagnosis of cystic fibrosis should be suspected in any patient with failure to thrive or with recurrent pulmonary infections. The finding of elevated concentrations of sodium and chloride (above 60 mEq/liter) in the sweat, evidence of chronic pulmonary infections on chest roentgenogram, a malabsorption syndrome, and a family history of cystic fibrosis confirm the diagnosis.

An increased loss of sodium in the sweat is postulated as one of the mechanisms that results in hyponatremia in patients with *adrenal insufficiency.* Similarly in patients with *burns,* loss of sodium through the burned skin may be one of the contributing factors if hyponatremia develops.

3. Other

Additional routes of sodium losses include removal of fluid by *thoracentesis* or *paracentesis.* Similarly, *"third-spacing"* of ECF, for example, into the gastrointestinal tract in ileus, may result in considerable fluid losses from the ECF. If there is resulting contraction of the ECF from any of these causes and if the patient drinks large volumes of water in response to thirst or if the patient is treated by the administration of large amounts of hyponatremic solutions, a decreased serum sodium concentration may result. On occasion, patients on *hemodialysis* may develop hyponatremia. This is usually the consequence of incorrect preparation of the dialysis bath water or of malfunction of the machine's proportionating pump.

C. Redistribution of Sodium

A low serum sodium concentration occurs frequently in *seriously ill* patients regardless of the nature of the underlying illness. Usually there is no evidence of either external sodium losses or of water retention, for example, from SIADH, in these patients. Since intracellular sodium levels are increased in the cells of patients with grave illnesses, it has been proposed that their hyponatremia results from a shift of sodium ions from the extracellular into the intracellular compartment. However, this alone should not result in hyponatremia, since such a movement of sodium should be accompanied by an equivalent movement of water to maintain osmolality in the intracellular and extracellular fluid compartments. Thus, it has been suggested that in severe illnesses, an increase in permeability of cell membranes permits increased *exchange* of intracellular and extracellular ions. This would not stimulate significant movement of water into the cells and would result in hyponatremia. Because of the proposed etiology for the hyponatremia in severe illness, it has come to be called the *sick-cell syndrome.* The diagnosis is one of exclusion and should be considered in any severely ill patient in whom other causes for hyponatremia are not apparent.

The serum sodium concentration is dependent not only on total body sodium and water but also on total body potassium levels. Potassium is the principal intracellular cation, and significant body *potassium depletion* may be accompanied by hyponatremia, probably as a result of redistribution of sodium secondary to the decreased intracellular potassium. This diagnosis may be apparent from measurements of serum potassium. However, an electrocardiogram should be performed to look for the classical changes of hypokalemia, since serum potassium levels are notoriously poor indicators of intracellular potassium levels.

A variety of abnormalities in the renal handling of sodium and water have been described in patients with *severe malnutrition.* However, it has been suggested that the hyponatremia sometimes seen in these patients is most likely the consequence of redistribution of body sodium, perhaps on a similar basis described in patients with the sick-cell syndrome.

III. Pseudohyponatremia

Measurements of serum sodium concentrations in patients with hyperlipidemia or hyperproteinemia may suggest that the patient is hyponatremic when, in fact, there is no disturbance of sodium or water metabolism. Since these patients have a normal sodium concentration in their plasma (or serum) water, this form of hyponatremia is referred to as pseudohyponatremia. The important sodium concentration is that in the serum water, but when a considerable portion of serum volume is occupied by a non-sodium-containing solute such as protein or lipid, the sodium in the serum water appears to be distributed over a much larger volume, resulting in apparent hyponatremia.

One can calculate the water content of serum (Ws) from the following formula:

$$\text{Ws} = 99.1 - 1.03\ \text{Ls} - 0.73\ \text{Ps}$$

where 99.1 = volume of serum minus crystalloids, i.e., the nonlipid, nonprotein solids
Ls = total lipid concentration (gm/100 ml serum)
Ps = total protein concentration (gm/100 ml serum)

The sodium concentration (in milliequivalents per liter) in serum water can then be calculated:

$$\frac{100 \times \text{observed serum sodium}}{\text{Ws}}$$

Normal values range from 148 to 163 mEq/liter, with an average normal of 156 mEq/liter (the same concentration as normal saline).

However, an easier way to determine whether a low serum sodium concentration represents true or pseudohyponatremia is to measure serum osmolality. This measurement, which indicates the solute content of the serum water, is reduced in true hyponatremia but remains normal in pseudohyponatremia. The importance of recognizing pseudohyponatremia is that, once diagnosed, it can save one a frustrating search for other causes of low serum sodium concentration, apparent sodium concentration remaining low in pseudohyponatremia despite all therapeutic efforts to bring it into the normal range.

IV. Other Causes

A. Resetting of "Osmostat"

Recent reports have suggested that some patients may have hyponatremia as a result of resetting of their osmostat. Such patients respond appropriately to variations in sodium intake, can dilute their urine, and can excrete a water load, but they maintain their serum sodium concentrations in the hyponatremic range, for example, 125 mEq/liter in one instance. This entity has been associated with chronic illnesses such as tuberculosis or alcoholism or with a massive cerebrovascular accident.

B. Artifact

Occasionally, an apparently low serum sodium concentration may result from artifact. Most often, this is the consequence of obtaining the blood sample from a vein into which a hyponatremic solution is infusing more distally. Other causes include putting the blood sample into a tube that already contains fluid with a low sodium concentration, wrongly identifying results from two patients, or a laboratory diluting error.

Diagnostic Approach

Whenever possible the cause of hyponatremia should be established. However, if this cannot be accomplished, it is important to try to determine whether the principal cause of the electrolyte disturbance is water retention with expansion of the ECF or sodium depletion of this space, the management of the two forms of hyponatremia being radically different. Increasing sodium intake in a patient with hyponatremia resulting from water intoxication is often remarkably ineffective and may aggravate the situation or the disease that resulted in the hyponatremia. Conversely, restriction of fluid in a patient with hyponatremia secondary to a deficit of sodium in the ECF is inappropriate and may cause deterioration of the patient's course.

The symptoms of hyponatremia per se include confusion, anorexia, lethargy, nausea, vomiting, coma, and seizures. They rarely occur until the serum sodium concentration has fallen to below 120 mEq/liter and, when present, do not help to identify whether the electrolyte disturbance resulted from water excess or from sodium depletion. Indeed, it would appear that symptoms are related to the relative net increase in brain water and loss of brain electrolytes, this being determined in large part by the rate of development of hyponatremia rather than by its underlying cause. Thus, patients with hyponatremia occurring over a 3-day period have fewer symptoms than those with comparable levels of serum sodium developing in less than 12 hours.

This does not, however, imply that the cause of hyponatremia is necessarily difficult to determine. Using a systematic approach such as that presented in Tables 11-1 and 11-4, one can usually identify the cause of hyponatremia relatively easily and without performing an enormous battery of tests. Indeed, most of the important information can be obtained from a good history, a careful physical examination, and a detailed review of the patient's medical records. A step-by-step approach to establish the cause of hyponatremia is presented below.

Step 1. Could the low serum sodium have resulted from artifact? Was fluid being infused into the vein from which the blood sample was obtained? Was sample handling and labeling correct? Has the laboratory had problems with other serum sodium determina-

Table 11-4

Data Required When Calculating Sodium and Water Balance

I. Intake during period of illness
  A. Quantity by each route
    1. Oral: as fluids, in food, water of oxidation from foods
    2. Intravenous
    3. Other routes: clysis; in peritoneal dialysis, etc.
  B. Composition of each fluid
    1. Electrolyte content
    2. Protein content
II. Output during same period
  A. Sensible
    1. Quantities
    2. Kind—urine, vomitus, diarrhea, drainage, etc.
    3. Compositions—either measured or estimated
  B. Insensible
    This must be estimated-modified by fever, tachypnea, ambient temperature, and humidity
III. Observed balance
  A. Weight changes—these may be misleading if the patient has "third-spaced"

tions that day? If there are any doubts about the validity of the measurement, it is worth measuring the serum sodium concentration again.

Step 2. Could hyponatremia represent pseudohyponatremia? Does the patient have hyperproteinemia or hyperlipidemia or evidence of a disease associated with either of these biochemical changes?

Step 3. Obtain a detailed history. In this history, determine whether the patient has had any excessive losses of fluid and electrolytes from causes such as diarrhea, vomiting, or excessive sweating. If so, what was the patient's concurrent intake of water and sodium in the food and as other fluids? In the absence of a history of excessive losses, try to obtain some idea of the patient's normal dietary habits so that an estimate of normal sodium and water intakes can be obtained. Is the patient taking drugs known to be associated with hyponatremia, for example, those inducing SIADH, those that modify action of ADH, or diuretics? If the hyponatremia was developed in hospital, is the patient postoperative or have there been enema treatments or administration of mannitol? Is there a past history to suggest a previous episode of nephritis, a disease predisposing to congestive heart failure, the existence of cystic fibrosis, adrenal insufficiency, or diabetes mellitus?

Step 4. Perform a careful physical examination. Look for clinical evidence of diseases associated with hyponatremia, for example, chronic glomerulonephritis, adrenal insufficiency, myxedema, Bartter's syndrome, or cystic fibrosis. Determine whether the patient is clinically dehydrated, overhydrated, or euhydrated. In hyponatremic dehydration, ECF volume is markedly decreased, but ICF volume may be somewhat increased. This is reflected in the physical findings, which in severe cases show a cold, clammy skin with a gray appearance and poor tissue turgor illustrated by "tenting of the skin." The pulse is rapid, and the blood pressure markedly reduced. The eyeball tension is reduced, the mucous membranes dry, and in the infant the fontanelle is sunken. The psyche is characterized by coma in the more severe cases. Although these findings do not necessarily help to delineate the cause of hyponatremia, they help to distinguish hyponatremic from hypernatremic dehydration where water is lost from both the ECF and the ICF. Thus, in hypernatremic dehydration, for any given degree of dehydration the degree of ECF contraction is less marked, so that shock occurs less frequently and tissue turgor is better preserved.

Step 5. Carefully calculate the patient's sodium and water balance for the preceding several days or for the period of the illness (see Table 11-4). Check the patient's weight changes. Do these determinations indicate a positive water balance or a negative sodium balance? Are they supported by an appropriate change in body weight and by your clinical estimation of the degree of hydration?

Very often at this stage the cause of the hyponatremia is apparent or the basic mechanism for this electrolyte disturbance, for example, water retention or sodium depletion, has been elucidated. If the diagnosis is still in doubt, the answer can often be obtained from a few simple laboratory tests.

Step 6. Measure urine sodium concentration and calculate the urine-to-serum creatinine concentration ratio from measurements of creatinine in this urine and a serum sample obtained as near the midpoint of the urine collection as possible. If the urine sodium concentration is less than 20 mEq/liter, go to step 7; if greater than 20 mEq/liter, go to step 8.

Step 7. A low urine sodium concentration of below 20 mEq/liter, and especially below 10 mEq/liter, usually results from diseases that either (1) result in dehydration and volume contraction (e.g., sodium loss from diarrhea, sweating, "third-spacing," etc.) or (2) reduce "effective arterial blood volume" and decrease renal perfusion (e.g., congestive heart failure, cirrhosis, nephrotic syndrome with marked edema, and chronic illness) or (3) cause an acute reduction in the GFR such as seen in acute glomerulonephritis. In most of these situations, renal tubular fractional reabsorption of water filtered at the glomerulus is high. This is reflected by a high urine-to-serum creatinine concentration ratio. In these diseases the ratio should be greater than 20 and may exceed 100. These diseases can usually be separated from one another with relative ease by laboratory studies of the serum and urine.

Step 8. If the urine sodium concentration exceeds 20 mEq/liter, one should try to determine whether the patient has any evidence of renal disease by reviewing the results of the patient's BUN and serum creatinine values, GFR (creatinine clearance), urinalyses, and intravenous pyelogram if one is available. If there is evidence of kidney disease, proceed to step 9; if not, go to step 10.

Step 9. If there is evidence of renal disease, one should consider the possibility of chronic glomerulonephritis, chronic pyelonephritis, renal cystic disease, partial obstruction, renal tubular diseases, or renal toxins, the exact diagnosis being confirmed by the appropriate studies. Further evidence in support of one of these diseases is provided by a urine-to-serum creatinine concentration ratio of less than 20, indicating reduced fractional reabsorption of water by the renal tubules.

Step 10. If there is no evidence of renal disease, consider (1) SIADH; (2) diuretic administration (e.g., thiazides, furosemide, etc.) or use of diuretic substances such as glucose, mannitol, or roentgenographic contrast agents; and (3) adrenal insufficiency. These entities can usually be separated from one another without difficulty.

Clinical Problem

You are called to see a patient who was found to have a serum sodium concentration of 105 mEq/liter when admitted to hospital. The patient, a 6.5-month-old white female infant, was the product of a normal delivery following an uneventful pregnancy. Labor had lasted 3 hours, and following delivery the patient's Apgar score was 10. On the third day of life, she was noted to have streaks of blood in her stools. Studies at this time failed to reveal a cause, and the patient was discharged home on the tenth day of life after the bleeding had ceased.

At home, she thrived normally for approximately 5 weeks, when she began to spit up small amounts of milk after feeding. However, the mother, who had reared two other children, was not unduly concerned by this symptom. Two weeks before admission the infant had become irritable. One week later, vomiting increased in amount and frequency, and both bile and blood were noted in the vomitus. Up to this time the child had been breastfed, but the mother was now concerned about the child's intake and added formula to her diet. There was still no improvement and 3 days later she was taken to her pediatrician, who found that in a 5-week period the child's weight had fallen from 6.4 to 5.8 kg. This latter weight was in the third percentile for her age. Despite the weight loss, the patient was not in any acute distress and did not appear to be markedly dehydrated. Changing the infant's formula failed to stop the vomiting, and she was admitted to hospital 4 days later when her weight had fallen further to 5.4 kg.

There was no history of diarrhea. The patient had continued to urinate with a normal frequency throughout the illness until the day of admittance to hospital, when the mother noted she had had to change the diaper on only one occasion. The patient had not received any drugs. Family history was unremarkable.

When the patient was admitted to hospital, she looked chronically ill. There was loss of skin turgor, and her anterior fontanelle was depressed. It was estimated that she was 10% dehydrated. Her pulse rate was 148 beats per minute, but she was not in shock, her blood pressure being slightly increased to 100/80. She was afebrile (temperature 36.0° C). Neurological examination was normal; she was awake and alert, her neck was supple and the fundi were normal with sharp disc margins. Examination showed that her ears, nose, throat, heart, and lungs were all normal. When first seen, her bladder was palpable, almost up to her umbilicus, but she subsequently voided, and then the bladder was no longer palpable. There was an indistinct mass palpable in the left flank, the significance of this being questioned by some observers. The patient had normal female genitalia; there was no increase in skin pigmentation and no edema.

Laboratory values obtained shortly after admittance to hospital were as follows: *Blood count:* hemoglobin level, 10.4 gm%; hematocrit reading, 30%; the indices indicated a hypochromic microcytic anemia, and this was confirmed on smear; WBC, 25,500/mm^3. *Urinalysis:* specific gravity, 1.014; pH, 6.0; proteinuria, 2+. The urinary sediment contained 10 to 15 red blood cells, more than 100 white blood cells, and numerous bacteria per high-power field (urine sample centrifuged before examination). *Electrolytes:* sodium concentration, 105 mEq/liter; potassium, 7.5 mEq/liter; chloride, 59 mEq/liter; and bicarbonate, 18 mEq/liter. A second blood sample gave similar values except for the potassium concentration, which was 6.2 mEq/liter. *Other studies:* BUN level, 68 mg/dl; a blood glucose obtained after treatment had been started so that 5% dextrose was being administered into another vein at the time of sampling was 227 mg/dl. 2+ glycosuria was found at the same time.

Questions

1. What causes of hyponatremia should be considered in this patient?
2. What would be your immediate treatment of the patient?
3. What studies would you undertake in an attempt to define the cause of the patient's illness, and how would you manage the patient on a long-term basis?

Discussion

Diagnosis of Hyponatremia

The recent weight loss, as well as the absence of a history of excessive fluid ingestion, suggests that the patient's hyponatremia resulted from excess sodium losses rather than from water retention. It is tempting to view the patient's fluid and electrolyte disturbances as a consequence of her vomiting. However, this is unlikely to be the correct interpretation. Although the vomiting may have contributed to her illness, there are several pieces of evidence that suggest that another disease (or diseases) was the primary problem.

First, the magnitude of the losses by vomiting do not appear to have been sufficiently great to account for the entire clinical picture. It is unusual for vomiting alone to result in moderate or severe dehydration; most often, this occurs as a consequence of both vomiting and diarrhea. Patients with pyloric stenosis may develop dehydration from vomiting alone, but the magnitude of losses by vomitus is impressive, and vomiting is usually projectile in nature. Such a history was not present in the patient under discussion. Moreover, patients with pyloric stenosis typically are hypochloremic and alkalotic when seen. The patient under discussion had marked hypochloremia, but her serum bicarbonate concentration was reduced to 18 mEq/liter, and her anion gap was increased.

Second, patients with dehydration from gastrointestinal losses most often have isonatremic dehydration. In such patients, hyponatremia is the consequence of partial replacement of the water losses but little, if any, replacement of sodium losses. There was no history of high rates of fluid replacement at any stage of the illness in the patient under discussion. Thus, an alternate source of sodium loss had to be considered.

Third, the patient was remarkably asymptomatic despite marked dehydration and severe hyponatremia. Although symptoms of hyponatremia rarely occur until the serum sodium concentration falls to below 120 mEq/liter, to tolerate a serum sodium concentration of 105 mEq/liter with remarkably few symtoms is surprising. Thus the absence of symptoms in the presence of severe hyponatremia suggests that the disease process was a chronic one and that the hyponatremia and dehydration developed slowly over a period of weeks or months rather than hours or days. Thus, an underlying cause other than the recent increase in vomiting is more likely.

Fourth, there were several pieces of evidence to indicate that the patient has renal disease. A typical, dehydrated patient is oliguric. This was not the case in the present patient. Despite marked dehydration, she continued to have an apparently normal urine output. Furthermore the urine specific gravity was low (1.014) before rehydration was started, demonstrating the presence of a renal concentrating defect. The abnormal urinary sediment also indicated renal disease, and these findings were interpreted as being those of urinary tract infection.

There were several other findings that supported the diagnosis of renal disease, but their presence alone must not be overinterpreted, since they could be produced by nonrenal mechanisms. The urine pH of 6.0 was inappropriately high if the patient was acidotic as suggested by her serum bicarbonate concentration of 18 mEq/liter. This does not necessarily imply a renal acidification defect. The presence of infection in the urinary tract might have resulted in the inappropriately high urine pH if the infecting organism was urea-splitting as most gram-negative organisms are. Thus, as a result of bacterial urease, some of the urine urea would have been hydrolyzed. Similarly, urine standing at room temperature for any length of time will become progressively more alkaline as a result of contaminating bacteria breaking down urea. The proteinuria may have resulted from many causes, including the presence of a urinary tract infection. However, proteinuria may be seen in many dehydrated patients and does not necessarily indicate primary renal disease. The elevated BUN concentration could have resulted from dehydration and does not necessarily indicate renal disease. If the patient's dietary intake in the preceding weeks had been poor, as suggested by the history, then correction of the dehydration might be expected to reduce the BUN concentration to below normal levels (i.e., less than 10 mg/dl) if renal function is normal. In such circumstances, a fall in BUN concentration to approximately 15 mg/dl does not exclude the presence of renal disease. The mild anemia could have been the consequence of chronic renal disease but could equally well have resulted from other causes, such as chronic blood loss from the gastrointestinal tract, a poor iron intake as a consequence of the vomiting, or the anemia often seen with chronic infection. Indeed, one of these latter causes is more likely, since the anemia was hypochromic and normocytic. The glycosuria does not necessarily indicate the presence of a renal tubular disease. It was thought to be the consequence of glucose administration in the intravenous fluids. However, the possibility of other causes of hyperglycemia was reconsidered later in the patient's course.

The diagnosis of adrenal insufficiency should be considered in any patient with a serum sodium concentration as low as 105 mEq/liter. In this patient the presence of hyperkalemia is consistent with this diagnosis, whereas the absence of hypotension and increased skin pigmentation are evidence against it. Hypoglycemia is a feature of adrenal insufficiency, but the elevated blood glucose level in the patient was of questionable significance, and hypoglycemia could have been present before the 5% glucose was administered. A further consideration in the patient was whether she might have one of the forms of the adrenogenital syndrome associated with salt loss. The more common of these entities is the complete form of 21-hydroxylase deficiency, the rarer entity being the 3-β-hydroxysteroid dehydrogenase defect. Typically, both are associated with virilization, so that the presence of normal female genitalia in the patient would make either diagnosis unlikely. A third alternative is that there could have been an isolated deficiency of aldosterone production due to a defect in either the 18-hydroxylation of corticosterone or the dehydrogenation of 18-hydroxycorticosterone. The principal manifestations of these defects are primarily those of salt loss.

Immediate Management

The primary goal of the initial phase of treatment was to reexpand the ECF space and minimize the risk of the patient developing shock. This was accomplished using an isonatremic solution—5% glucose in lactated Ringer's; 20 ml/kg body weight was given as rapidly as possible and followed by an infusion rate to provide 60 ml/kg body weight over the next 8 hours. The patient had very few symptoms attributable to the hyponatremia per se; thus it was decided not to use a more concentrated sodium solution. The physicians responsible for the patient's care were uncertain as to whether she had adrenal insufficiency and decided to administer Doca, 1 mg, and Decadron, 1 mg, by intramuscular injection. It was argued that although the diagnosis of adrenal insufficiency was not established, the use of these drugs would not harm the infant. However, her blood pressure was monitored carefully to detect the possible development of hypertension.

The patient responded well to this treatment, and 14 hours later her serum sodium concentration had risen to 128 mEq/liter, with her serum potassium concentration falling to 3.4 mEq/liter. Her body weight increased by almost 7%.

Long-term Management

The sodium concentration in the urine, obtained before treatment was started, was 30 mEq/liter. This high value, obtained at a time when the patient was dehydrated and had a serum sodium concentration of 105 mEq/liter, confirmed that the renal handling of sodium was abnormal and that there must have been significant and inappropriate urinary losses of sodium contributing to the dehydration and hyponatremia. This could have resulted from intrinsic renal disease or from external influences such as a deficiency of mineralocorticosteroids.

After the patient responded to the initial treatment, studies were undertaken to determine the cause of the illness. The diagnosis of a urinary tract infection, suggested by the urinalysis, was confirmed when *Pseudomonas aeruginosa* was cultured from a clean-voided sample of urine. When pyuria and bacteriuria had been found, the patient had been started on ampicillin. She failed to show any improvement on this drug and, when the urine culture and sensitivity results demonstrated that the organism was resistant to it, it was discontinued and gentamicin substituted. By the time the patient had responded to antibiotics and to parenteral fluids, her BUN level had fallen to 5 mg/dl and her serum sodium concentration stabilized at 139 mEq/liter. At this time, an intravenous pyelogram was performed and demonstrated a normal right kidney but a markedly hydronephrotic left kidney. This was thought to be due to obstruction at the ureterovesical junction. A cystogram demonstrated no ureteral reflux. When it was apparent that no functioning tissue in the left kidney could be saved, the kidney was removed.

Because of the history of vomiting and the previous history of blood in the stools, the existence of a lesion in the gastrointestinal tract was considered. However, an abdominal roentgenogram demonstrated a normal bowel gas pattern, and stool guiacs were normal.

It was not clear whether the use of steroids contributed to the rapid return of the patient's serum sodium concentration to normal. A cortrosyn stimulation test was performed and demonstrated a normal steroid response. On the basis of this test, exogenous steroids were discontinued. The patient's serum sodium concentrations remained normal.

Summary

The following sequence of events is proposed. The primary abnormality was unilateral obstructive uropathy at the left ureterovesical junction. Being unilateral, this produced no problems in the early weeks of life but soon predisposed the patient to infection in the left kidney. The presence of chronic or recurrent infections caused the patient's vomiting for several weeks prior to admission to hospital. The pyelonephritic changes in the left kidney resulted in sodium wasting in the urine. Under normal circumstances the patient could have compensated for this if sodium intake had been adequate, but as a consequence of vomiting, her sodium intake was reduced well below normal. Her rapid deterioration before admission to hospital was probably precipitated by an exacerbation of the infection, perhaps with the *Pseudomonas*. Not only could this have increased the vomiting but it could also have increased sodium losses through increased sweating associated with fevers. Thus, by the time medical advice was sought, recent sodium losses, in addition to the chronic deficits, resulted in the severe abnormalities found. The question remains whether there was adrenal insufficiency. If there was a deficit, it must have been transient and most probably affected aldosterone production alone at the level of 18-hydroxylation or dehydrogenation.

Hypernatremia

General Considerations

As with hyponatremia, disturbances of either sodium or water metabolism may result in an elevated serum sodium concentration (Table 11-5). Thus, hypernatremia (serum sodium concentration greater than 150 mEq/liter) can result when normal fluid losses from the body are not replaced, when there are excessive fluid losses, and when there are both water and sodium losses but the water losses exceed the sodium losses. Hypernatremia may also be the consequence of excessive administration or retention of sodium. In addition, there is a small group of patients in whom none of these mechanisms explain the increased serum sodium concentration; this condition is referred to as essential hypernatremia.

Since sodium and chloride are the principal osmotically active solutes in the serum, hypernatremia is always accompanied by an increased serum osmolality. However, the converse is not always true, so that an elevated serum osmolality does not always indicate an elevated serum sodium concentration. For example, elevated concentrations of either blood glucose or blood urea nitrogen will result in hypertonicity without serum sodium concentrations necessarily being altered. A useful rule of thumb is to remember that serum osmolality equals

$$2\,[\text{serum sodium (mEq/liter)}] + \frac{\text{Plasma glucose (mg\%)}}{18} + \frac{\text{BUN (mg\%)}}{2.8}$$

Differential Diagnosis of Hypernatremia

The differential diagnosis of hypernatremia is listed in Table 11-5 and discussed below.

Table 11-5

Differential Diagnosis of Hypernatremia

I. Loss of water in excess of sodium loss
 A. Normal fluid losses—inadequate replacement
  1. Interference with water intake: nausea, vomiting; inability to swallow; adipsia
  2. Patients dependent on others for fluid intake: stuporous, comatose, or senile patients; patients with strokes; infants
  3. Unavailability of fluids
 B. Excess fluid losses
  1. From gastrointestinal tract: diarrhea, vomiting; gastric drainage; hypertonic enemas
  2. From kidney:
   a. Diabetes insipidus; nephrogenic diabetes insipidus
   b. Osmotic diuresis: urea; mannitol; radiology contrast media; glucose
   c. Diets providing high solute loads: incorrect mixing of powdered milk formulas; infants fed cow's milk; protein supplementation; parenteral hyperalimentation
   d. Chronic renal failure; hypokalemia; hyperkalemia
  3. From skin and lungs: fever; heat stroke; high environmental temperature; overventilation
  4. Other: excess fluid removal by peritoneal dialysis or hemodialysis
II. Excess of sodium
 A. Steroid excess: aldosterone; cortisol
 B. Excess sodium administration or ingestion
  1. Excess saline administration
  2. Excess use of salt tablets
  3. Sea water ingestion
  4. Substitution of salt for sugar in infant formulas
  5. Incorrect preparation of electrolyte powders when treating diarrhea
III. Essential hypernatremia
 A. Defective thirst mechanism
 B. Deranged setting of osmoreceptors
 C. Idiopathic
IV. Artifact
 A. Sampling problem
 B. Drying out of sample

I. Losses of Water in Excess of Sodium Loss

A. Normal Fluid Losses with Inadequate Replacement

The obligatory fluid losses—evaporative losses through the lungs and skin plus the amount necessary to excrete the renal solute load with a maximally concentrated urine—amount to about 1300 ml/day or approximately 10% of ECF volume. Obligatory sodium losses are much smaller. As indicated earlier, daily losses of sodium in sweat and feces normally total less than 10 mEq. Urine sodium concentration can be reduced to below 5 mEq/liter, so that sodium loss can be reduced if necessary to an amount equal to less than 1% of the sodium pool in the ECF. If these daily losses of sodium and water are not replaced, the negative water balance exceeds that for sodium, and the sodium concentration in the ECF will increase progressively. If the patient has a fever, pneumonia, or is in a high environmental temperature, the situation will be aggravated, since all these conditions increase evaporative water losses more than sodium loss.

There are several situations in which this mechanism may be responsible for hypernatremia. Patients with nausea, vomiting, or dysphagia experience thirst consequent upon the hypernatremia but are unable to increase their fluid intake appropriately. Comatose patients or those with strokes may not be aware of thirst or may not be able to communicate their needs. Such patients are dependent on others for adequate fluid intake, and a failure on the part of their attendants to recognize the magnitude of the required fluid replacement will result in dehydration and hypernatremia. Infants are particularly susceptible to this problem. Their surface area per unit of body mass is much greater than that of the adult, so their evaporative water losses are greater. In addition, their ability to concentrate their urine is incompletely developed, increasing obligatory urinary losses. Thus the normal daily fluid turnover in infants amounts to almost half their ECF volume, as compared to adults, in whom the turnover is only one sixth of their ECF. This must be remembered when planning fluid intake for infants. Finally, water may not be available to fulfill a person's fluid requirements.

The underlying cause for hypernatremia in these situations usually is not difficult to diagnose, the clinical picture frequently indicating the correct diagnosis. Careful calculation of the patient's sodium and fluid balances, making adequate allowances for insensible losses, will indicate a negative fluid balance, and this should be accompanied by a progressive decline in body weight of more than 0.5 kg/day (in the adult). Signs of hypertonic dehydration (see below) may be apparent, and severe dehydration may be accompanied by a fever (which will aggravate fluid losses).

In addition to hypernatremia, laboratory studies will show evidence of hemoconcentration with an increasing hematocrit reading, hemoglobin value (unless blood sampling has been excessive), and serum protein concentration. BUN and serum creatinine concentrations may be somewhat elevated. Unless the patient has coexisting renal disease, urine output will be low (approximately 500 ml/day) and the urine will be concentrated but with a low urine sodium concentration.

B. Excessive Fluid Losses

1. Gastrointestinal Tract

a. Diarrhea. Diarrhea is the most common cause of hypernatremia in a pediatric population, especially in infancy, although adult patients with severe or protracted diarrhea may also become dehydrated and hypernatremic. Among the reasons for the propensity of infants to develop dehydration with diarrhea is their high rate of water turnover in relation to body water and their inability to obtain water in response to thirst unless it is made available by others. The fever accompanying dehydration contributes by increasing fluid losses through the skin as a result of the increased rate of sweating and through the lungs as the consequence of hyperventilation. Renal immaturity prevents maximal conservation of water by the kidney. The use of oral or parenteral electrolyte replacement fluids with a too-high sodium concentration also contributes to hypernatremia, as does the use of skim milk or other fluids that provide a high solute load. Warming of skim milk results in greater evaporative water losses than might be anticipated and unexpected high sodium concentration. This, or the well-intentioned but erroneous addition of salt to skim milk, also contributes to hypernatremia.

The sodium concentration of diarrhea fluid is normally less than that of serum, characteristically being about 40 mEq/liter. Thus, it would be reasonable to expect that diarrhea would most often result in hypernatremic dehydration. This is not the case, however, and hypernatremia is seen in less than 25% of patients admitted to hospital because of diarrhea and dehydration. The remainder of the patients have normal or even reduced serum sodium levels because a larger proportion of fluid than sodium losses are replaced in the period prior to the patient receiving medical care. Indeed the incidence of hypernatremia is found to increase dramatically with increasing sophistication of the lay population and the use of homemade electrolyte solutions—a questionable development since the prognosis for hypernatremic dehydration is worse than for its hyponatremic counterpart.

The cause of hypernatremia is usually obvious with the history of the passage of copious water stools either with or without vomiting. The concurrent intake of a homemade electrolyte solution or of skim milk would increase the possibility of the development of hypernatremia. Physical examination will reveal the features of hypernatremic dehydration. The loss of potassium and bicarbonate in the stools, in addition to sodium, chloride, and water, results in a systemic metabolic acidosis with a reduced blood pH, serum bicarbonate, and pCO_2, the latter being the consequence of respiratory compensation. Total body potassium is reduced but is not necessarily reflected by a reduced serum potassium level, especially if there is a marked systemic acidosis. Here, increased intracellular movement of hydrogen ion results in movement of potassium out of the cells into the ECF, maintaining ECF potassium concentration. Severe dehydration results in a decrease in renal function with increases in BUN and serum creatinine levels. On occasion the BUN level may rise in excess of 100 mg%, suggesting the concurrent development of acute tubular necrosis. Despite dehydration, hemoconcentration is seen surprisingly infrequently, so that anemia often becomes apparent after rehydration has been completed. Characteristically the urine flow rate is low and the urine is concentrated, although urinary sodium should be low. Albuminuria and granular casts are commonly seen.

b. Vomiting, Gastric Drainage. Extensive and protracted vomiting, such as that seen in pyloric stenosis or other forms of high intestinal obstruction, or prolonged gastric drainage results in losses of sodium, water, potassium, and hydrochloric acid. The relative losses of sodium and water depend on the source of the fluid loss. The sodium concentration of gastric juice is usually between 20 and 80 mEq/liter; that of fluid in the duodenum, 20–133 mEq/liter; whereas small bowel fluid sodium concentration is higher, being in the range of 100–150 mEq/liter. As with diarrhea, the resulting dehydration may be hyponatremic, eunatremic, or hypernatremic, depending on the nature of both the loss and replacement.

The biochemical changes seen in this form of dehydration are characteristic. Hypochloremic alkalosis occurs with associated increases in serum bicarbonate and blood pCO_2 levels. Relatively little potassium is lost from the gastrointestinal tract, but large amounts are lost in the urine as a consequence of the kaliuresis induced by metabolic alkalosis. Thus the majority of patients are hypokalemic or become so during repletion therapy if adequate amounts of potassium are not administered. As with other forms of dehydration, hemoconcentration occurs. Characteristically the urine is alkaline, but if significant potassium depletion has occurred, a paradoxical aciduria results.

The changes in urinary composition have physiologic explanations. Early in the course of the disease, when dehydration is developing, sodium reabsorption from the tubular fluid in the distal convoluted tubule is high, sodium being exchanged preferentially for potassium because of the systemic alkalosis—hence the kaliuresis. As the disease progresses and potassium depletion becomes more marked, sodium reabsorption must continue but now at the expense of hydrogen ion secretion, resulting in a paradoxical aciduria.

c. Hypertonic Enemas. The use of soapsuds enemas has been associated with water intoxication and hyponatremia. Conversely, hypernatremia can occur with the use of commercially available concentrated phosphate enemas (e.g., Fleet or Tudvad enemas). The usual clinical situation in which this occurs concerns the patient with megacolon treated repeatedly with one of these preparations. These enemas have a sodium concentration in excess of 2000 mEq/liter, and their use results in osmotic movement of water into the bowel with some sodium reabsorption. The consequence is hypernatremic dehydration with sodium concentrations as high as 166 mEq/liter having been reported. This may be associated with hypokalemia, probably due to loss of potassium into the fluid in the bowel. In addition the absorption of phosphate may result in hyperphosphatemia, secondary hypocalcemia, and tetany. The risk of tetany is increased if significant amounts of citrate contained in the Tudvad enema preparation are absorbed, resulting in alkalosis. Conversely, systemic acidosis may result if large amounts of monobasic phosphate are absorbed.

The use of diatrizoate (Gastrografin) as an enema in radiology may also result in hypernatremia. Diatrizoate is a nonabsorbable ion and is present in hyperosmotic concentrations in this preparation, causing water movement into the bowel.

2. *Kidney*

a. Diabetes Insipidus and Nephrogenic Diabetes Insipidus. Both of these diseases result in hypernatremia secondary to excessive fluid losses through the kidney. In patients with the complete form of diabetes insipidus (DI), circulating vasopressin cannot be detected in the patient's blood; in patients with the partial form of this disease, circulating levels of vasopressin are inadequate to promote appropriate renal conservation of water. In nephrogenic diabetes insipidus (NDI), circulating levels of vasopressin are appropriate, but the renal tubule fails to respond to circulating vasopressin. All these patients have hemoconcentration in association with their hypernatremia. Urine flow rates are high, frequently exceeding 10 liter/day and occasionally up to 30 liter/day. In complete forms of the diseases the urine is very dilute, with a specific gravity in the range of 1.001–1.005 (osmolality 50–200 mOsm/kg). However, in patients with a less complete form of the disease or in the face of dehydration, urine may be more concentrated but usually remains less concentrated than the plasma, that is, specific gravity <1.010 or osmolality <300 mOsm/kg.

If either diagnosis is suspected, supportive evidence can be obtained from a fluid deprivation test. It is preferable to perform this after hypernatremia has been corrected, but the patient should not be overhydrated at the beginning of the study. The patient is weighed, and all fluids are withheld. Subsequent urine samples are collected, and their volumes and osmolalities (or specific gravities) are determined. A normal response to fluid deprivation consists of urine flow falling to less than 0.5 ml/min and urine concentration increasing to above 850 mOsm/kg after a 16-hour period of deprivation. Patients with DI or NDI maintain a high urine flow, and urine osmolality rarely exceeds 200 mOsm/kg. However, patients with incomplete forms of the lesion may achieve intermediate values for urine concentration, making the diagnosis more difficult. Patients suspected of having DI or NDI should be closely watched during this test, and the study should be terminated if the patient loses more than 3% of body weight.

Some indications of whether a patient has either DI or NDI may be obtained from the history. Many patients have an obvious cause for DI, for example, head trauma or previous neurosurgery. The lesion of NDI may be congenital, being inherited as an X-linked recessive trait. The first affected child may not be diagnosed early in life and may be mentally retarded, possibly as a consequence of periods of severe dehydration. In secondary forms of DI the urine tends to be less dilute and the urine volume not as large as in primary forms or in NDI. However, in many instances this separation can only be made on the basis of determining the patient's response to exogenous ADH. This test is usually carried out after the period of fluid deprivation (see above) and consists of measuring urine osmolalities after the intravenous administration of aqueous Pitressin, 5 milliunits/min over a 1-hour period (this is preferable to the subcutaneous route of administration, since absorption after such an injection is highly variable). Patients with DI should show a prompt response, with urine osmolality increasing above that of plasma. In contrast, patients with NDI are unresponsive to exogenous vasopressin, their urines remaining dilute. Unfortunately there are some patients with partial DI who show an intermediate response, which complicates diagnosis. This dilemma should be resolved when an immunoassay for vasopressin suitable for routine clinical use is developed, since patients with NDI show an increase in circulating vasopressin following fluid deprivation.

A more sensitive measurement of the renal tubules response to vasopressin can be obtained by measuring free water clearance under conditions of water loading before and after administration of exogenous vasopressin. This test is not in routine clinical use, and more details of methodology and interpretation are presented in the references.

Having determined whether the patient has DI or NDI, it is important to attempt to define the underlying cause for these lesions. Differential diagnoses for both entities are presented in Table 11-6. It is beyond the scope of the present discussion to outline how these various entities can be separated from one another, but it is worth stressing that a

Table 11-6

Causes of Diabetes Insipidus and Nephrogenic Diabetes Insipidus

Diabetes Insipidus	Nephrogenic Diabetes Insipidus
Familial	Congenital
Acquired	Acquired
Posthypophysectomy	Obstructive uropathy
Post-traumatic	Amyloidosis
Tumors	Multiple myeloma
Primary, e.g. craniopharyngioma	Sarcoidosis
Secondary, e.g. breast	Sjogren's syndrome
Histiocytoses	Sickle cell disease
Granulomata	Hypokalemic nephropathy
Vascular	Hypercalcemic nephropathy
Aneurysms	Medullary cystic disease
Thrombosis	Chronic renal failure
Postpartum necrosis	Drugs
Infections, e.g. meningitis,	Lithium
encephalitis, Guillain-	Methoxyflurane
Barré syndrome	Demeclocycline
Idiopathic	

careful history from the patient can often suggest the correct diagnosis (see also Chapter 10 on polyuria).

b. Osmotic Diuretics. In an attempt to reduce intracranial pressure, the intravenous injection of large doses of urea or mannitol may result in hypernatremia. The osmotic effects of these agents initially result in movement of water from cells into the ECF, producing hemodilution with a fall in the concentrations of hemoglobin, sodium, chloride, bicarbonate, and so forth. Packed cell volume also falls because of shrinkage of red cells. Subsequently the urea and mannitol are excreted by the kidney, causing an osmotic diuresis. This may result in hypernatremia if the patient is unable to appreciate fluid needs or unable to express those needs because of the underlying neurological lesion.

A similar sequence of events may be seen following the use of radiographic contrast media. The concentration of the agents used for intravenous urography and angiocardiography varies from 50% to 85% (weight/volume) and their osmolalities from approximately 1500 to 2500 mOsm/kg. The effect on serum sodium concentration depends in part on which agent is used. Hypaque 50, Conray 400, and Angioconroy have sodium concentrations of 786, 1088, and 1303 mEq/liter, respectively. The use of these agents is more likely to result in hypernatremia than the use of the contrast media, which are the meglumine salts of iothalamate and diatrizoate, for example, Conray 60, Hypaque-M 60, Renografin 76, and the like.

Patients with nonketotic diabetic coma—a variant of diabetic coma characterized by a high blood glucose, no ketosis, and at worst a mild metabolic acidosis due to lactic acidosis rather than ketoacidosis—have severe hyperosmolality and often develop marked hypernatremia. This is associated with both intracellular and extracellular dehydration and probably is the consequence of the osmotic effects of the elevated blood glucose levels and an osmotic diuresis induced by the high filtered load of glucose in the kidney.

c. Diets Providing High Solute Loads. One of the less well-appreciated causes of hypernatremia is the administration of a diet that provides an excessive solute load. This may be in the form of an obvious solute such as sodium chloride or as a potential solute such as protein, which will result in urea formation. The excretion of these solutes by the kidney will obligate water loss in the urine. If adequate water is not provided in the diet, negative water balance and dehydration with hypernatremia and hemoconcentration will ensue. The patient populations most susceptible to this form of hypernatremia are the young infant and the elderly, since neither of these groups can concentrate their urines to the same extent as older children and young adults. Thus, their basic water requirements are increased.

This problem has been observed in several clinical situations. Low birth weight infants are often fed calorically concentrated formulas in an attempt to induce a more rapid weight gain. However, if the formula is too concentrated, for example, 133 kcal/100 ml (twice the normal), the potential renal solute load may exceed the kidneys' ability to excrete it in the water provided. Infants fed undiluted or inadequately diluted cow's milk may also develop hypernatremic dehydration, since the osmotic load from cow's milk is three times that of human milk. Incorrect reconstitution of powdered milk formulas, the use of either undiluted evaporated or condensed milks, and the use in infants with diarrhea of too concentrated homemade electrolyte solutions or of commercial glucose-electrolyte powders reconstituted in too little water are additional causes.

Parenteral hyperalimentation may provide a very high solute load and produce hypernatremia. In older patients, especially those who are comatose or semicomatose, the use of protein supplements or a high-protein diet fed by nasogastric tube may also result in dehydration and elevated concentrations of serum sodium if inadequate amounts of water are provided. This complication was described 25 years ago but still occurs all too frequently.

Hypernatremia may also be seen in patients with recurrent gastrointestinal bleeding from peptic ulceration or other causes. The blood in the bowel results in increased urea formation and to an increased solute diuresis.

If the clinician remembers excess solute load as a cause of hypernatremia, the correct diagnosis is not difficult and consists of recognizing the underlying error in management. The potential solute load of a diet can be estimated from its electrolyte and protein contents.* One gram of sodium is equivalent to almost 43.5 mEq of sodium and produces an osmotic load in the urine of 87 mOsm when the attendant anions are taken into account (if the diet sodium is expressed in terms of salt equivalency, 1 gm of salt contains approximately 17 mEq of sodium and produces an osmotic load of 34 mOsm). Three grams of protein are catabolized into 1 gm of urea, which results in an osmotic load of 16.7 mOsm. Having calculated potential solute load, one can then determine whether the kidney can excrete this load in the amount of water available for urine formation. This latter figure is calculated by subtracting extrarenal water losses (up to 600 ml/m^2/day under normal circumstances, increasing 12% for every degree Celsius rise in body temperature) from total water intake (as fluids, as water in foodstuffs, and as water of oxidation—each 100 calories generated from food provides 10 ml water). By dividing solute load (milliosmols per day) by water available for urine formation (liters per day), one can determine the urine osmolality necessary to excrete this load.

For example, if a patient is tube fed 100 gm protein, 50 gm glucose, 100 mEq sodium, and 50 mEq potassium each day, using the figures above, the solute load from the protein can be calculated as being approximately 550 mOsm and that from the electrolytes 300 mOsm for a total of 850 mOsm. If the patient's urine could be concentrated to 850 mOsm/kg, a minimum of 1 liter of fluid would be required for urine output. If insensible fluid losses amounted to 700 ml/day, the patient's total *minimum* fluid intake to maintain fluid balance must be 1.7 liter/day. If the patient was elderly and could only concentrate urine to 425 mOsm/kg, the requirements for urine formation would double and the daily intake would have to be 2.7 liters minimum. To provide the patient with less fluid would result in dehydration and hypernatremia.

d. Renal Damage. Patients with chronic renal disease and those with the nephropathies associated with hypokalemia or hypercalcemia are unable to concentrate their urines maximally and may develop hypernatremia if adequate fluid intake is not provided. Hypernatremia has also been observed during the various stages of acute renal failure.

The underlying cause for the electrolyte disturbance with these diseases should not be difficult to determine and is suggested by finding elevated levels of serum urea or

*This calculation does not take into account the small amounts of solute retained for growth in the child.

creatinine, hypokalemia, hypercalcemia, proteinuria, or abnormalities in the urinary sediment.

3. Skin and Lungs

Fever or exposure to a high environmental temperature results in increased losses of water through the lungs and skin, with smaller increments of sodium loss in sweat. For example, insensible fluid loss increases 12% for every degree Celsius rise in body temperature. Under normal circumstances, sweat losses for an adult living in an environment that is temperature and humidity regulated average less than 250 ml/day. If the average ambient temperature increased to 34° C, sweat losses would exceed 2 liter/day. Such losses can cause significant hypernatremia if not replaced. Thus, acclimatized volunteers had serum sodium concentrations ranging from 161 to 173 mEq/liter after a 2-hour march in an environmental temperature of 42° C. A forced water intake during a repeat march prevented hypernatremia.

These losses, especially as a consequence of fever, may contribute to hypernatremia in patients with another primary cause such as diarrhea, since dehydration is frequently accompanied by an increase in body temperature.

4. Other

Serum sodium concentrations are usually normal at the end of dialysis. However, the use of peritoneal dialysis solutions with very high glucose concentrations designed to remove large amounts of fluid from patients with diseases such as heart failure and pulmonary edema may result in hypernatremia due to the removal of amounts of water in excess of sodium.

II. Excess of Sodium

A. Steroid excess

1. Mineralocorticoids

Patients with primary aldosteronism retain sodium and have elevated total body sodium content even though they may have "escaped" and reestablished sodium balance. Although all the original patients described with this entity had elevated levels of serum sodium, it is now recognized that many patients with aldosteronism can have a normal serum sodium concentration.

The clinical features suggesting this diagnosis include the presence of hypertension, polydipsia, polyuria, fatigue, muscle weakness, paresthesias, and, in children, growth retardation. Many of these symptoms are not specific for primary aldosteronism and probably reflect potassium depletion. In addition to the elevated levels of serum sodium, there is hypokalemia and systemic alkalosis with increased serum bicarbonate concentrations. Magnesium levels are decreased. Plasma renin concentrations should be low, separating primary from secondary forms of aldosteronism. Urine pH is either neutral or alkaline, and the kidneys lose their ability to concentrate the urine. Urinary excretion of 17-ketosteroids and 17-hydroxycorticosteroids are normal and that of aldosterone is increased.

2. Glucocorticoids

The administration of glucocorticoid or mineralocorticoid drugs is associated with sodium retention, but plasma sodium concentrations usually remain normal unless excess sodium is administered simultaneously. However, some patients with Cushing's syndrome do have elevation of serum sodium concentrations. The diagnosis may be suggested by the presence of moon facies, increased obesity, a buffalo hump, signs of abnormal masculinization, and hypertension. Laboratory findings suggestive of the diagnosis include polycythemia, lymphopenia, eosinopenia, elevated fasting blood glucose concentrations, a diabetic type of glucose titration curve, and hypokalemia. The plasma cortisol level is increased, but levels may fluctuate, so it is advisable to obtain more than a single value before excluding the diagnosis. Urinary excretion of 17-hydroxycorticosteroids is increased, and urinary 17-ketosteroids may be elevated, especially if the patient is virilized.

B. Excess Sodium Administration

The renal ability to excrete sodium is limited, and hypernatremia will occur if excess sodium is administered, especially if adequate water is not given at the same time. This cause of hypernatremia has been observed in several clinical settings.

1. Normal Saline

The concentration of sodium in normal saline is equivalent to that in plasma water and thus is almost 10% higher (154 mEq/liter) than the normal serum value. Excess administration of this solution may result in elevation of the serum sodium concentration presumably due to greater losses of water than sodium.

One patient population particularly susceptible to this cause of hypernatremia are diabetics in ketoacidosis. If their losses are replaced only by normal saline, many develop hypernatremia. There are two reasons for this. First, with hyperglycemia the urinary losses of glucose produce an osmotic diuresis with continuing water losses through the kidney. Second, as the blood glucose falls in response to treatment with insulin, water returns to the cells, causing increasing concentration of the plasma.

2. Excessive Use of Salt Tablets

Persons working in a hot climate develop severe hypernatremia if they use salt tablets to replace their sodium losses without replacing their water losses or if they ingest an excessive number of salt tablets. Hypernatremia has also been described in a young girl who took large amounts of salt to relieve menstrual cramps. Drinking a saturated salt solution was a traditional Chinese method of suicide.

3. Sea Water Ingestion

The sodium concentration of sea water is 450–500 mEq/liter and its total osmolality 1000–1200 mOsm/kg. Victims of shipwrecks or other persons drinking sea water develop severe hypernatremia in part because of the high sodium intake and in part because of the high solute load, which increases urinary water losses.

4. Accidental Substitution of Salt for Sugar

The substitution of salt in the preparation of infants' formulae has been reported and caused serum sodium elevations of up to 274 mEq/liter.

5. Preparation of Electrolyte Solutions

The use of homemade electrolyte solutions in the treatment of patients with diarrhea has already been referred to. In some instances, these solutions have been used to excess in patients with only mild diarrhea, so that the patients have an excess of sodium in the absence of significant water deficits as a cause of their hypernatremia.

III. Essential Hypernatremia

A group of patients has been described in whom hypernatremia is not due to any of the causes already discussed. They have been labeled as having essential hypernatremia because of the inability of a forced water intake to correct their electrolyte abnormality.

Although a variety of etiologies have been documented to result in essential hypernatremia, the majority of patients share many features in common that may suggest the diagnosis. The hypernatremia is usually sustained, but there are wide fluctuations in the magnitude of elevation of the serum sodium level. Signs of major contraction of the ECF volume and of dehydration are absent. Spontaneous fluid intake is usually 1–2 liter/day or greater, and increasing fluid intake above this does not correct the hypernatremia. Renal functions, including the ability to concentrate the urine, are preserved. The patients' sensorium is not markedly abnormal, but many of the patient's do not complain of thirst even when hypernatremic, and in many there is an impaired antidiuretic response to osmotic stimuli. There may be evidence of dysfunction of the anterior pituitary. Other abnormalities such as obesity or hyperlipidemia may be present to suggest more widespread abnormality of the hypothalamus. In some patients the hypernatremia can be corrected by the administration of exogenous ADH.

In the majority of cases, an underlying neurological lesion such as a tumor or histiocytosis is found, although recognition of this pathological lesion may be delayed for as long as 2 years after hypernatremia is first documented.

Basically, three groups of patients with essential hypernatremia can be identified. They may have a defective thirst mechanism, an apparent resetting of their osmoreceptors, or an idiopathic lesion. Intracranial lesions involving the hypothalamus frequently result in *lack of thirst* and hypernatremia. Since some of the hypothalamic centers involved in thirst are separate from those involved in ADH release, patients may or may not have evidence of abnormal vasopressin secretion. Thus, some patients appear to have a pure defect in thirst, while in others, this may be accompanied by evidence of inadequate ADH production. More recently a further variant has been described. A patient with defective thirst had evidence of increased ADH secretion, hypernatremia occurring when fluid intake was too low or insensible losses were increased by intercurrent illnesses. It deserves reemphasis that a diligent search for an intracranial lesion is warranted in all patients who present with the features of a hypothalamic lesion, since the underlying pathology may not be readily apparent early in the course of the illness. In addition to patients with evidence of a defective thirst mechanism, there are several in whom hypernatremia appears to be the consequence of a *resetting of the osmoreceptors,* a mechanism proposed several years ago. In these patients, plasma osmolality must be elevated pathologically before ADH is released and thirst occurs. In these patients, there is some evidence to suggest that volume and baroreceptors play an increased role in regulating ADH release. Finally there are at least three case reports of patients with hypernatremia who did not have one of the lesions defined above and in whom the cause of the hypernatremia was not obvious. At present these patients must be considered as having *idiopathic* essential hypernatremia.

IV. Artifact

Hypernatremia may be diagnosed incorrectly if a blood sample is obtained from a vein into which normal saline is infusing more distally or if the blood sample is stored incorrectly before analysis, evaporation from the sample causing concentration.

Diagnostic Approach

The principal symptoms from hypernatremia occur irrespective of the cause of this electrolyte abnormality and thus do not help in differentiating the cause. As with hyponatremia the principal symptoms and signs relate to the central nervous system. In contrast to the coma found when the serum sodium concentration is markedly reduced, the hypernatremic patient is lethargic but irritable. Muscular rigidity, tremors, and seizures may be seen, and coma eventually develops. Some patients note muscular weakness, although this symptom is not universally observed. Since hypernatremia results in increased osmolality of the ECF, there is movement of fluid from the intracellular to the extracellular space. Thus, patients with hypernatremic dehydration have better preservation of their ECF volume but more severe depletion of their intracellular volume than do patients with hyponatremic dehydration who have osmotic fluid movements from the ECF into the cells. This accounts, in part, for the differences in physical findings when the two groups of patients are compared. In patients with hyponatremic dehydration, signs of ECF volume depletion dominate and shock occurs more frequently. In hypernatremic dehydration, ECF volume is better preserved, but intracellular contraction is manifested by a small shrunken tongue and a hyperirritable psyche. Although these differences may help the clinician to identify the type of dehydration, again they do not help to define the cause.

However, when confronted by a patient with hypernatremia, it is usually not too difficult to determine the underlying cause if one obtains a careful history and analyzes thoroughly the patient's preceding intake, output, and weight changes (see Table 11-4). Thus, excessive ingestion or administration of salt, a diet providing too high a solute load, excessive fluid losses either obvious or insensible, or inadequate replacement of fluid losses should be apparent. Special emphasis should be paid to the patient's urine output and concentration.

Patients with a dilute urine and polyuria include those with chronic renal failure, hypercalcemia, hypokalemia, diabetes insipidus, or nephrogenic diabetes insipidus. Blood chemistries should help to identify the first three possibilities. The patient's response to exogenous ADH will help to separate pituitary from nephrogenic diabetes insipidus.

Patients with a concentrated or isosmotic urine can be separated into those who are oliguric and those who are polyuric. If the patients are oliguric, it suggests that they have had inadequate replacement of their fluid losses. Conversely, if such patients are polyuric, their hypernatremia may well have resulted from an osmotic diuresis and one should look for the presence of glycosuria or the prior administration of either urea or mannitol.

Clinical Problem

A 6-year-old black male was admitted to hospital from the emergency room with severe vomiting and dehydration. His illness had begun 24 hours earlier when he developed a headache that failed to respond to aspirin. Subsequently he began to vomit, and this precluded him from taking his usual high oral fluid intake. Throughout this illness he had continued to urinate frequently and with large urine volumes, as was normal for him. His mother sought medical advice when he began to feel weak and when she noted his eyes were sunken in appearance.

His past history was of interest. The 8 pound product of a normal pregnancy and delivery, he had thrived well initially. However, even in the first weeks of life his mother noted that he always appeared to be hungry and that he drank more milk or water than infants of a comparable age. Later in life polyuria, nocturia, enuresis, and polydipsia were very apparent. Development during the first year of life appeared normal, but subsequent mental development was delayed. He had been seen by a physician because of hyperactivity and had been treated with Dilantin. His growth was below average. He had had no previous episodes of fever, serious infections, dehydration, or seizures. He had one sister and three brothers who also drank large amounts of fluids, but no other member of the family was affected, this included eight additional siblings who appeared to be normal.

Physical examination revealed a small child whose height and weight were in the 10th percentile. He was dehydrated with soft, sunken eyes; his skin was dry and had poor turgor with marked tenting. His pulse rate was 135 beats per mintue; blood pressure, 96/70 mm Hg; and temperature, 38° C. No other abnormal findings were elicited on physical examination.

After he recovered from this illness his mental age was found to be 2.5 years compared to his chronologic age of 6 years.

Admission laboratory values revealed a hemoglobin value of 13.0 gm/dl, with a hematocrit reading of 39%; WBC was 8700/mm^3. Urinalysis showed a specific gravity of 1.003, a pH of 5.0, proteinuria 1+, and his urinary sediment was normal. Serum sodium concentration was 172 mEq/liter; potassium, 3.8 mEq/liter; chloride, 143 mEq/liter; and bicarbonate, 15.1 mEq/liter. Blood urea nitrogen level was 12.4 mg/dl.

Questions

1. What diagnoses should you consider as a cause of the patient's hypernatremia?
2. What studies would you undertake to establish the diagnosis?
3. How would you manage the patient?
4. Can you relate the patient's mental and growth retardation to the hypernatremia?

Discussion

Diagnosis

Although the illness in the patient was precipitated by vomiting, it would appear unlikely that this was the basic cause of the severe hypernatremic dehydration, since the patient's urine specific gravity was only 1.003 even when he was severely dehydrated. This would suggest that the principal route of water loss was through the kidney, the vomiting preventing him from replacing this water loss. The most likely causes are either diabetes insipidus or nephrogenic diabetes insipidus. A third possibility is that the patient could have had compulsive polydipsia. However, the age of onset of his polydipsia and polyuria make this unlikely, as does the very dilute urine observed in the face of severe dehydration.

Diabetes insipidus may result from any lesion that damages the neurohypophyseal tract. More rarely, it occurs as a hereditary form, autosomal dominant and X-linked recessive modes of transmission having been described. In some instances no cause is obvious, and it is assumed to be a genetic form of the disease.

Patients with diabetes insipidus present in a manner very similar to that seen in the present patient. Because of the age of onset of the polyuria and polydipsia, the lack of clinical evidence of an intracranial lesion, and the family history of siblings with similar problems, the diabetes insipidus would most likely represent one of the hereditary forms.

Unfortunately, there is no way to separate diabetes insipidus from nephrogenic diabetes insipidus by history or physical examination alone. Thus the patient could equally well have nephrogenic diabetes insipidus. This latter entity appears to be inherited as an X-linked recessive with variable degrees of expression in the heterozygote (females). Most patients with this entity descended from a group of Ulster Scots who came to Nova Scotia on the ship *Hopewell*. However, the lesion has now been well described in Negro families with no links to the *Hopewell* settlers. Thus, being a black does not preclude the patient from having nephrogenic diabetes insipidus. The age of onset of symptoms in this patient and his history are classically seen in nephrogenic diabetes insipidus.

The other diagnostic considerations in the patient are either hypokalemia or hypercalcemia resulting in a renal concentrating defect. However, neither appears likely, since the patient has had polyuria almost from the neonatal period and since he has siblings who appear to be affected by a similar problem.

Diagnostic Studies

A fluid deprivation test was probably unnecessary in the patient, since he was severely dehydrated on admission to hospital and his urinary osmolality was consistently below 100 mOsm/kg. However, such a test was undertaken for completeness after his electrolyte disturbance had been corrected. Six hours of water deprivation did not result in any fall in urine output, which exceeded 150 ml/hr throughout the test. His weight fell from 16.6 to 15.9 kg, serum sodium concentration increased from 145 to 155 mEq/liter, and there was an appropriate rise in serum osmolality. However, urine osmolality remained below 90 mOsm/kg, and urine specific gravity below 1.004.

The patient's response to aqueous vasopressin was tested on three occasions with doses of up to 15 units of vasopressin being given. On no occasion did the urine specific gravity increase above 1.005 or urine osmolality exceed 125 mOsm/kg. Urinary excretion of 3′-5′ cyclic AMP was not measured during these tests. A trial of pitressin tannate in oil failed to increase the ability of the kidney to concentrate the urine.

The radioimmunoassay for measuring arginine vasopressin in the patient's blood was not available at the time he was studied.

Studies were performed to ensure that there was no intracranial lesion. Visual fields were normal, as were roentgenograms of the skull which showed a normal sella turcica. Bone age was 7 years. IVP revealed bilateral dilatation of the renal calyces and pelves as well as ureteral dilatation. This was attributed to the persistent diuresis experienced by the patient. A urine sample obtained early in the hospital stay showed generalized aminoaciduria, but a subsequent sample was normal. There was no other evidence of a Fanconi syndrome, that is, no glycosuria, no proteinuria, and a normal tubular reabsorption of phosphorus. Serum calcium, phosphorus, and potassium concentrations were normal throughout.

A diagnosis of nephrogenic diabetes insipidus was made from the results of these tests.

Treatment

Therapy for this patient should be considered in two phases: (1) the initial treatment to return the electrolytes to normal and (2) long-term management.

One of the major concerns in the early phase of treatment is not to lower the serum sodium concentration too rapidly, since such an approach usually results in convulsions. Although the patient was principally fluid depleted, he was rehydrated with a multiple-electrolyte solution containing 40 mEq/liter sodium. This was given at a rate in excess of his urine flow rate, and his serum sodium concentration fell slowly over a period of 3 days from 172 mEq/liter to 140 mEq/liter. The required rate of fluid administration was remarkable, stimulating the house officer to note in the chart that "he is urinating faster than we can replace it." As soon as his nausea resolved, parenteral fluids were supplemented and then replaced by oral fluids.

In an attempt to reduce his urinary losses of water, chlorothiazide therapy was started (approximately 1 gm/m^2/day), and he was placed on dietary salt restriction. This resulted in a decreased urinary output, which had averaged more than 6 liter/day, to a more manageable 4.4 liter/day. His mother was instructed to call for medical advice if intercurrent illnesses prevented the patient from maintaining his normal fluid intake or if he developed other problems such as diarrhea, which would increase fluid losses.

Mental Retardation

Patients with nephrogenic diabetes insipidus not uncommonly have growth and mental retardation. Although the mechanisms for these changes are not completely elucidated, it has been suggested that the patient's dietary intake may be inadequate, since he spends so much time drinking fluids. The mental retardation may be the consequence of periods of transient dehydration and hypernatremia, which develop before the patient's underlying disease is diagnosed and the need for a continuous high fluid intake is appreciated. Once a patient with nephrogenic diabetes insipidus is diagnosed, the same diagnosis should be considered in all subsequent siblings as soon as possible after birth. It is now well established that if the diagnosis is made early and the correct treatment is instituted and maintained, then growth and development appear to progress normally.

References

Arieff, A. I., Llach, F., and Massry, S. G. "Neurological manifestations and morbidity of hyponatremia: Correlation with brain water and electrolytes." Medicine *55:* 121, 1976.

Bartter, F. C. "The syndrome of inappropriate secretion of antidiuretic hormone." Disease-a-Month, November 1973.

DeFronzo, R. A., Goldberg, M., and Agus, Z. "Normal diluting capacity in hyponatremic patients. Reset osmostat or a variant of the syndrome of inappropriate antidiuretic hormone secretion." Ann. Intern. Med. *84:* 538, 1976.

DeRubertis, F. R., Michelis, M. F., and Davis, B. B. "Essential hypernatremia." Arch. Intern. Med. *134:* 889, 1974.

Edelman, I. S., and Liebman, J. "Anatomy of body water and electrolytes." Am. J. Med. *27:* 256, 1959.

Edelman, I. S., Liebman, J., O'Meara, J. P., et al. "Interrelationships between serum sodium concentrations, serum osmolality and total exchangeable potassium and total body water." J. Clin. Invest. *32:* 1236, 1958.

Editorial. "Sick cells and hyponatremia." Lancet *1:* 342, 1974.

Fitzsimmons, J. T. "Thirst." Physiol. Rev. *52:* 468, 1972.

Hays, R. M., and Levine, S. D. "Vasopressin." Kidney Int. *6:* 307, 1974.

Hays, R. M., and Levine, S. D. "Pathophysiology of water metabolism." *In:* The Kidney, B. M. Brenner, and F. C. Rector (eds.). W. B. Saunders, Philadelphia, 1976.

Klahr, S., and Slatopolsky, E. "Renal regulation of sodium excretion in health and edema-forming states." Arch. Intern. Med. *131:* 780, 1973.

Leaf, A. "The clinical and physiologic significance of the serum sodium concentration." N. Engl. J. Med. *267:* 24, 77, 1962.

McCance, R. A. "Experimental sodium chloride deficiency in man." Proc. R. Soc. *119:* 245, 1936.

Moses, A. M., and Miller, M. "Drug-induced dilutional hyponatremia." N. Engl. J. Med. *291:* 1234, 1974.

Ross, E. J., and Christie, S. B. M. "Hypernatremia." Medicine *48:* 441, 1969.

Taclob, L. T., and Needle, M. A. "Hyponatremic syndromes." Med. Clin. North Am. *57:* 1425, 1973.

Waugh, W. W. "Utility of expressing serum sodium per unit of water in assessing hyponatremia." Metabolism *18:* 706, 1969.

Welt, L. G. "Hypo- and hypernatremia." Ann. Intern. Med. *56:* 161, 1962.

Chapter 12

Alterations in Serum Calcium Concentration

General Considerations

Calcium is the most abundant cation of the body and the principal component of the human skeleton. It not only plays a key role in the composition of skeletal tissue but is also involved in a series of regulatory processes that are vital for life. Among the principal functions in which calcium participates are the maintenance and function of cell membranes, neuromuscular excitability, transmission of nerve impulses, enzymatic reactions, regulation of secretion of parathyroid hormone, and activation of 25-hydroxycholecalciferol-1-hydroxylase, the enzyme responsible for the conversion of $25(OH)D_3$ to $1,25(OH)_2D_3$, and so forth. The primary regulatory factor responsible for the maintenance of extracellular calcium balance is parathroid hormone. This hormone acts on a series of organs such as the skeleton, kidney, and small intestine and interrelates with other factors such as vitamin D and perhaps calcitonin to regulate the activity of the above-mentioned organs in order to maintain the extracellular calcium concentration constant.

The skeleton is the most important reservoir of calcium and is in dynamic equilibrium with physicochemically soluble forms of circulating calcium. Thus, alterations in calcium metabolism necessarily lead to derangements in the composition of the skeleton. Unfortunately before the diagnosis of bone disease can be established by roentgenographic studies, serious alterations in bone structure must occur. Thus, an understanding of the normal homeostatic control mechanisms facilitates the selection of specific diagnostic tests to establish a definitive and early diagnosis of alterations in calcium metabolism.

Distribution of Calcium

The adult human body contains 1000–1200 gm of calcium or approximately 20–25 gm/kg of fat-free body tissue. Approximately 99% of the body calcium resides in the skeleton, the remaining 1% being found in blood, extracellular fluid, and intracellular space. In addition, about 1% of the skeletal calcium is freely exchangeable with the extracellular fluid. Calcium in bone exists primarily in the form of small crystals usually considered to be a variant of poorly crystalline hydroxyapatite. Some calcium in bone also exists as amorphous crystals in combination with phosphate. The normal calcium-to-phosphate ratio in bone is 1.5:1.

In humans, total serum calcium concentration is remarkably constant, ranging from 9 to 10 mg/100 ml or 4.5 to 5 mEq/liter, or 2.25 to 2.5 mM/liter. The total serum calcium concentration consists of two major fractions. The first is the ultrafilterable, or diffusible, fraction, which comprises approximately 60% of the total serum calcium. This fraction is composed of two different portions: (1) the ionized calcium, which plays a key role in all of the feedback and enzymatic process and represents roughly 50% of the total serum calcium; and (2) the complex form, in which calcium is complexed with citrate, phosphate, bicarbonate, and the like, which represents approximately 10% of the total serum calcium concentration. The second important fraction is the so-called protein-bound calcium, which constitutes approximately 40% of the total serum calcium concentration. An easy way to remember the concentration of the different fractions of calcium in blood is as follows: ionized calcium, 5 mg/100 ml; complex calcium, 1 mg/100 ml; and protein-bound calcium, 4 mg/100 ml.

Calcium is bound to serum proteins, and 85% to 90% of this calcium is bound to albumin. The binding of calcium by serum proteins obeys the mass law equation for a monovalent association. The relationship between calcium ion and the concentration of protein in blood is represented by the following expression:

$$\frac{(Ca^{++}) \quad (\text{proteinate})}{\text{calcium proteinate}} = K$$

where proteinate equals the concentration of plasma protein. Since K is a constant, the numerator and the denominator must change proportionately. A knowledge of the binding of calcium to plasma proteins is important in the evaluation of serum calcium levels. Low plasma albumin concentrations, which occur in hypoproteinemic states (e.g., the nephrotic syndrome), are accompanied by low values of total serum calcium, while the ionized serum calcium concentration may be normal.

Small amounts of calcium are bound to globulins. It is unusual to see changes in total serum calcium concentration as a result of alterations in the level of serum globulins. However, in some cases of severe hyperglobulinemia, such as multiple myeloma or other similar conditions, elevations in total serum calcium concentration may be observed. One gram of albumin binds approximately 0.7 mg of calcium. An important point that should be emphasized in the analysis of the different components of serum calcium is the acid-base status of the patient. Since the binding of calcium to serum protein increases with a rise in blood pH, a tetanic episode may be precipitated by severe alkalosis due to a decrease in ionized serum calcium levels.

Dietary Calcium

The amount of calcium ingested in the diet plays a key regulatory effect in its overall balance. A series of feedback mechanisms are responsible for the maintenance of calcium balance and absorption from the gastrointestinal tract. Roughly, 1000 mg of calcium per day is ingested in a regular diet. However, this amount varies greatly from patient to patient because of the varying amounts of milk that different people ingest in their diet. Milk is the most important source of calcium and contributes 50% to 60% of the total amount ingested in the diet. Of interest is the fact that in countries like Japan and India, in which the total ingestion of calcium is low (usually less than 500 mg/day), the amount of calcium in the milk is also extremely low. On the other hand, in the United States, 1 liter of milk contains approximately 800–900 mg of calcium. There are some nondairy foods that have a very high calcium content, such as parsley, spinach, and mustard; however, their contribution to the total dietary calcium is extremely small. About 10 mg of calcium per kilogram body weight is the recommended daily intake. However, during the last trimester of pregnancy, there is a greater calcium requirement, since approximately 20–30 gm of calcium enters the fetus. With age, alterations in calcium metabolism, mainly due to a progressive decline in calcium absorption, require an increase in the amount of calcium in the diet.

Calcium Balance

If 1 gm of calcium is ingested in the diet, approximately 30% is absorbed from the intestine. At the same time, endogenous calcium, approximately 200 mg daily, is secreted into the bowel. Thus, of the 1000 mg ingested, approximately 900 mg is excreted in the stool and the remaining 100 mg in the urine. There is a remarkable adaptive mechanism in the gastrointestinal tract that increases the efficiency of calcium absorption in situations in which the requirements for calcium are increased, such as in patients maintained on low-calcium diets. On the other hand, as a protective mechanism, if a patient is placed on a high-calcium diet the percentage of calcium absorbed decreases.

The underlying mechanism responsible for this well-known regulatory function has been recently elucidated. Many studies in animals and humans clearly indicate that vitamin D and its metabolites play a key role in this regulatory process. If a patient is maintained on a low-calcium diet, a mild decrease in ionized calcium will trigger the release of parathyroid hormone, which plays a key role in the conversion of $25(OH)D_3$ to $1,25(OH)_2D_3$. This metabolite is responsible for increasing calcium absorption from the gastrointestinal tract in order to reestablish calcium balance. However, if there is an excess of calcium in the diet the secretion of parathyroid hormone is turned off, the circulating levels of PTH in blood decrease, and the conversion of $25(OH)D_3$ to $1,25(OH)_2D_3$ is greatly diminished. Thus the absorption of calcium decreases and the amount of calcium in the stool increases.

Calcium Absorption

The mechanism by which calcium is transported across the intestinal mucosa is complex and not fully understood. This process involves three steps: (1) the transport of calcium from the intestinal lumen into the cells; (2) the movement of calcium within the cells; and (3) the extrusion of calcium from cells into the interstitial fluid. The movement of calcium from the intestinal lumen across the brush border appears to be an uphill transport process. At the luminal border, a calcium-binding protein, a calcium-dependent ATPase, and an alkaline phosphatase may act together to move calcium into the cell. The movement of calcium into the cell could also be accomplished by a process of facilitated diffusion secondary to changes in the electrical potential produced by the exit of sodium across the serosal side of the cell. The process of intracellular calcium transport is thought to be mediated either by calcium-binding protein or by the uptake and release of calcium by the mitochondria. The extrusion of calcium across the basal lateral membranes requires sodium, and the transport process likely involves a coupling of the sodium-potassium-dependent ATPase to the efflux of calcium across the serosal boundary.

Renal Handling of Calcium

As mentioned before, only 60% of the calcium is ultrafilterable, and this fraction will cross the glomeruli and enter the proximal tubule. Approximately 10 gm of calcium is filtered per day, but usually only 100 mg appears in the urine. Therefore, 99% of the filtered load of calcium is reabsorbed by the kidney. The reabsorption of calcium along the nephron parallels well the reabsorption of sodium. About 50% to 60% of the filtered calcium load is reabsorbed in the proximal tubule, 20% to 30% in the loop of Henle, 10% to 15% in the distal tubule, and 2% to 8% in the collecting ducts.

Many factors are responsible for the renal regulation of calcium. However, the final regulatory control mechanism is located in the distal portion of the nephron. Micropuncture experiments in animals have demonstrated that in the proximal tubule the ratio of tubular fluid calcium to ultrafilterable serum calcium is usually greater than 1. Net calcium reabsorption in the loop of Henle also parallels sodium reabsorption, and a concentration gradient for calcium has been shown from cortex to papilla. Determinations of calcium concentrations in the distal convoluted tubule suggest that further reabsorption of calcium, against a steep concentration gradient, occurs in this segment.

Many factors that modify sodium transport clearly affect calcium reabsorption. ECF volume expansion, a potent stimulus in decreasing sodium transport along the whole length of the nephron, also decreases the reabsorption of calcium. In fact, ECF volume expansion is one of the most important therapeutic maneuvers in the treatment of hypercalcemia.

Similarly, many diuretics such as acetazolamide, ethacrynic acid, and furosemide also block sodium and calcium transport. However, other types of diuretics, such as thiazides, have a dissimilar effect on sodium and calcium excretion. Thiazides produce a large natriuresis and a decrease in urinary calcium excretion. It is possible that this dissociation in sodium and calcium excretion results from the fact that thiazides exert their action in the distal nephron where sodium and calcium transport are independent. It has been postulated that for thiazide administration to result in a decrease in calcium excretion, some degree of ECF volume contraction is necessary as well as the presence of parathyroid hormone. It is believed that one of the mechanisms by which thiazides may decrease urinary calcium excretion is by enhancement of parathyroid hormone activity via inhibition of phosphodiesterase, the enzyme responsible for the conversion of 3′-5′ cyclic AMP to inactive 5-AMP. It is difficult to demonstrate the anticalciuretic effect of thiazides in the absence of parathyroid hormone.

A series of hormones also play a critical role in the regulation of calcium excretion by the kidney. Among these hormones, parathyroid hormone is the most important one. Its effect seems to be different in the proximal as compared to the distal tubule. It has been shown that sodium and calcium reabsorption are greatly diminished in the proximal tubule by the administration of PTH. However, there is a remarkable enhancement in calcium reabsorption in the distal tubule when PTH is given to experimental animals. It is known that patients with hypoparathyroidism, in whom there is a lack of PTH, have a greater amount of calcium in the urine at similar levels of filtered calcium load when compared to normal or hyperparathyroid patients. Thus, it appears that the main action of PTH is to enhance calcium reabsorption in the distal segment of the nephron. Other hormones, such as thyrocalcitonin, growth hormone, thyroid hormone, mineralocorticoids, and glucocorticoids, seem to increase urinary calcium excretion. The relative contribution and role of these individual hormones in the daily regulation of calcium excretion have not been clearly defined.

Another factor that may play a role in the reabsorption of calcium is the acid-base status. Metabolic acidosis decreases renal calcium reabsorption. Several mechanisms have been implicated, including an increase in ionized serum calcium levels with suppression of parathyroid hormone release. However, experiments in parathyroidectomized animals have clearly demonstrated that acidosis per se blocks the reabsorption of calcium independently of the levels of parathyroid hormone.

From the clinical point of view, a condition that is extremely common is immobilization. Patients who are on complete bed rest for prolonged periods of time develop significant hypercalciuria.

Hypercalcemia

General Considerations

The degree and significance of hypercalcemia varies greatly among patients. Some patients may be totally asymptomatic, and mild hypercalcemia may be found during a routine blood chemistry determination; however, the degree of hypercalcemia may be so severe as to produce renal failure, coma, and death. Obviously, between these two extreme conditions, hypercalcemia of moderate degree, in the range of 11–13 mg/100 ml, is responsible for a series of characteristic symptoms.

Many patients with mild hypercalcemia are admitted to psychiatric hospitals because of changes in personality. They may complain of malaise, fatigue, loss of memory, and, if the degree of hypercalcemia is more marked, drowsiness, lethargy, and disorientation.

Commonly they complain of anorexia and sometimes nausea and even vomiting. They feel thirsty and may have polyuria and polydipsia. If hypercalcemia continues for months or years, serious damage to different organs may develop, and nephrocalcinosis, renal stones, and chronic renal insufficiency aggravated by pyelonephritis may be seen. In some patients there is a remarkable degree of vascular calcification with metastatic deposits of calcium in the myocardium. Cardiac arrhythmias may be seen frequently in these patients. If the patients are hypertensive, blood pressure may be more difficult to control in the presence of hypercalcemia. Characteristically, patients with hypercalcemia cannot concentrate the urine and they may become dehydrated and develop prerenal azotemia, which is frequently reversible after volume expansion, providing that the patient does not have severe nephrocalcinosis with pyelonephritis. In addition, patients with hypercalcemia also show a decrease in the GFR and renal plasma flow.

Differential Diagnosis of Hypercalcemia

The most common causes responsible for hypercalcemia are depicted in Table 12-1 and discussed below.

I. Malignancy

Malignancy is the most common cause of hypercalcemia. The mechanism is multifactorial and should be established on an individual basis. Some tumors, such as those localized in the lung, kidney, prostate, and thyroid, frequently produce metastases to bone

Table 12-1

Causes of Hypercalcemia

I. Malignancy
   A. Metastatic
   B. Ectopic PTH
   C. Osteoclastic activator factor (OAF)
   D. Prostaglandin E_2 (PGE_2)
II. Endocrine disorders
   A. Primary hyperparathyroidism
   B. Nonsuppressible (tertiary) hyperparathyroidism
   C. Hyperthyroidism
   D. Multiple endocrine neoplasia
   E. Adrenal insufficiency
III. Vitamin D intoxication
IV. Renal disease
   A. Chronic renal failure
   B. Renal transplant
   C. Diuretic phase of ATN
V. Immobilization
VI. Thiazide diuretics
VII. Milk-alkali syndrome
VIII. Miscellaneous
   A. Hyperglobulinemia
   B. Hemoconcentration
   C. Idiopathic hypercalcemia of infancy
   D. TBC
   E. Sarcoidosis

with characteristic lytic lesions and destruction of vertebrae and other bones leading to the development of pathological fractures. Many of these patients become hypercalcemic. However, there are other types of tumors that secrete a parathyroid hormone-like peptide. The most common tumors in which secretion of a PTH-like peptide have been described are localized in the lung. The material secreted by the cancer biologically behaves like parathyroid hormone, and the patients characteristically present with hypercalcemia and sometimes hypophosphatemia. Immunologically, there are basic differences between this "cancer" peptide and the peptide secreted by the parathyroid glands. Other types of malignancies, such as multiple myeloma, may produce a protein with a molecular weight of roughly 20,000, known as osteoclastic activator factor (OAF), which increases bone resorption by increasing the activity of the osteoclast. In the past it was thought that the lytic bone lesions seen in myeloma were produced by plasma cells. However, it is presently believed that the lytic lesions produced by the plasma cells are mediated by the production of OAF.

Recently several papers have clearly indicated that solid tumors may produce prostaglandins of one PG_2 series that may also be responsible for increasing calcium release from the skeleton with the development of severe hypercalcemia. The patients excrete increased amounts of prostaglandins in the urine, and the hypercalcemia may respond to the administration of inhibitors of prostaglandin synthesis such as aspirin or indomethacin.

II. Endocrine Disorders

A. Primary Hyperparathyroidism

Primary hyperparathyroidism is the most common endocrine disorder responsible for the development of hypercalcemia. This condition is discussed in the chapter on hypophosphatemia.

B. Nonsuppressible Hyperparathyroidism

Nonsuppressible hyperparathyroidism, also known as tertiary hyperparathyroidism, has been reported in patients in whom hypocalcemia was present for a prolonged period of time. Most of these patients have renal insufficiency and have developed severe parathyroid chief-cell hyperplasia. When these patients are treated with vitamin D and calcium to raise serum calcium levels, the secretion of PTH cannot be adequately suppressed because the hyperplasia and hypertrophy are extremely large, and it is difficult in a short period of time to suppress the secretion of hormone by the parathyroid glands.

C. Hyperthyroidism

Several patients with hyperthyroidism have been shown to have mild hypercalcemia. The development of hypercalcemia in patients with hyperthyroidism varies from 10% to 22% in different reports. When parathyroid hormone has been measured in such patients, it has been shown to be normal. It seems that there is a direct effect of thyroxin on bone, resulting in increased bone resorption and mild hypercalcemia. This hypercalcemia may be reversed by antithyroid therapy.

D. Multiple Endocrine Tumors

There are a series of multiple endocrinopathies in which hyperparathyroidism, pituitary tumors, and pheochromocytomas may be associated in the same patients, and hypercalcemia has been one of the manifestations.

E. Adrenal Insufficiency

In some cases of adrenal insufficiency, hypercalcemia has been shown to occur; however, the pathogenesis is not fully understood. It has been suggested that the hypercalcemia is due to an increase in protein-bound calcium that results from volume depletion. Volume depletion may also increase renal calcium reabsorption.

III. Vitamin D Intoxication

As mentioned previously, vitamin D plays a key role in the regulation of calcium absorption from the gastrointestinal tract. Moreover, vitamin D has a direct effect on bone by increasing bone resorption and producing mobilization of calcium from bone into the extracellular fluid. Vitamin D has been used for the treatment of many different pathological conditions such as rickets, osteomalacia, and chronic renal failure. Presently there are very powerful and active metabolites of vitamin D such as 25-hydroxycholecalciferol, 1-alpha-hydroxycholecalciferol, and 1,25-dihydroxycholecalciferol that have the potential risk of producing hypercalcemia. This is especially so with 1,25-dihydroxycholecalciferol, which in very small doses of 2–3 μg has been shown to produce profound hypercalcemia in some cases. If this drug is given to a patient the physician should be extremely careful not to advise the ingestion of large amounts of calcium concomitantly with 1,25 $(OH)_2D_3$. Since the normal feedback mechanism by which dietary calcium controls the production of 1,25 $(OH)_2D_3$ is now bypassed by the use of pharmacologic amounts of 1,25 (OH) D_3, the patients can develop profound hypercalcemia. The serum calcium concentration increases not only because there is increased calcium absorption from the gastrointestinal tract but also because 1,25 $(OH)_2D_3$ has a very potent resorptive action at the level of bone. It has been shown that animals maintained on low calcium diets may develop severe hypercalcemia when receiving pharmacologic doses of 1,25 $(OH)_2D_3$. A careful history should provide clues as to whether or not ingestion of vitamin D or its metabolites is responsible for the hypercalcemia.

IV. Renal Disease

A. Chronic Renal Failure

Hypercalcemia is a rare finding in patients with chronic renal failure. In fact, the majority of patients with renal disease have hypocalcemia, which is responsible for the development of secondary hyperparathyroidism. Nevertheless, a few patients with hypercalcemia have been described.

B. Renal Transplantation

A much more common finding is the development of hypercalcemia after a successful renal transplant. Since the patients who receive transplants usually have severe secondary hyperparathyroidism, when the graft is successful the amount of 1,25 $(OH)_2D_3$ produced by the new kidney may be greatly increased as a result of the excess parathyroid hormone. A synergistic effect of 1,25 $(OH)_2D_3$ and parathyroid hormone will increase the mobilization of calcium from bone with the consequent hypercalcemia. Obviously 1,25 $(OH)_2D_3$ also increases calcium absorption from the gastrointestinal tract. Fortunately this is a rather limited condition that does not require a specific treatment and in most of the cases subsides after 2 or 3 weeks. However, in some patients, specific measures should be taken in order to prevent nephrocalcinosis. ECF volume expansion and diuretics may easily control the mild hypercalcemia. In some patients, the hypercalcemia may be more pronounced and persists for several months and sometimes several years. Occasionally some of these patients require a subtotal parathyroidectomy.

C. Diuretic Phase of Acute Tubular Necrosis

Hypercalcemia also has been reported during the diuretic phase of acute tubular necrosis. This is a rather rare occurrence and most of the cases in which hypercalcemia has been reported have been patients who had rhabdomyolysis with severe hyperphosphatemia and hypocalcemia during the oliguric phase. It seems that there is sequestration of large amounts of calcium in soft tissue during the oliguric phase. During the diuretic phase, part of the calcium is now mobilized entering the extracellular space, and the patient becomes hypercalcemic. Hypercalcemia may also result from alterations in the metabolism of 1,25 $(OH)_2D_3$ during acute renal failure. Again, this hypercalcemia is a rather limited condition that, in most instances, does not require any specific treatment.

V. Immobilization

Immobilization is a frequent and sometimes serious condition that can produce hypercalcemia and severe renal impairment. It has been shown that practically all patients who are immobilized for several days develop some degree of hypercalciuria. However, some patients may develop hypercalcemia. If the patient has an underlying pathological process in which there is an increase in bone turnover, like Paget's disease, severe immobilization could be catastrophic.

VI. Diuretics

Patients taking thiazide diuretics may develop hypercalcemia. The mechanism by which thiazide administration results in hypercalcemia is not fully understood, but it has become apparent that a series of factors are involved. Thiazides decrease urinary calcium excretion, and have been used to treat one of the forms of idiopathic hypercalciuria (see Chapter 5 on renal stones). As mentioned before, for thiazides to reduce urinary calcium excretion, some degree of volume contraction is required as well as the presence of parathyroid hormone. It seems that a synergistic effect of PTH and thiazides occurs not only at the level of the kidney but also at the level of bone, and there is evidence suggesting that when a thiazide is administered together with parathyroid hormone, there is a greater degree of hypercalcemia. There is controversy as to whether or not thiazides per se increase the release of parathyroid hormone. However, most of the evidence indicates that this is not the case.

VII. Milk-Alkali Syndrome

This condition was seen frequently in the past in patients with peptic ulcer disease who ingested large amounts of calcium carbonate. Calcium carbonate has approximately 40% of elemental calcium, and some of these patients ingested up to 10–20 gm of calcium carbonate in 24 hours with the development of severe hypercalcemia.

VIII. Miscellaneous

There are a series of conditions in which hypercalcemia may be seen in a sporadic fashion. Patients with *sarcoidosis* seem to have an increased sensitivity to vitamin D, and it has been postulated that in these patients the amount of calcium absorbed may be a greater proportion of that ingested in the diet. The hypercalcemia of sarcoidosis is mild and usually is seen in no more than 15% to 20% of patients with this disease. Hypercalcemia also may occur in patients with *tuberculosis;* however, the mechanism is unknown. Other conditions, such as *hyperglobulinemia,* have been associated occasionally with hypercalcemia. As mentioned before, serum globulins may bind small amounts of calcium; thus, it is necessary to have severe degrees of hyperglobulinemia before noticeable hypercalcemia occurs. Another condition that has also been responsible for hypercalcemia is the so-called *idiopathic hypercalcemia of infants.*

Factors that Should Be Considered in the Differential Diagnosis of Hypercalcemia

As in any other disorder in medicine, the present illness, the past history, and the physical examination will provide most of the information and clues necessary to establish a definitive diagnosis in patients with hypercalcemia. However, there are situations in which more definitive tests are necessary in order to establish a diagnosis and the right therapy.

When the serum calcium concentration is obtained and found to be abnormally high, serum phosphorus and magnesium concentrations should also be obtained in order to add key factors in the differential diagnosis. Measurements of plasma proteins and total and ionized calcium levels may provide clues as to the cause of the hypercalcemia. If a patient presents with hypercalcemia, a complete medical workup is mandatory to rule out malignancy. If there is no evidence of such a pathological process, the second most common cause of hypercalcemia is primary hyperparathyroidism. If this condition is suspected, then blood should be obtained for parathyroid hormone levels, and if the patient's serum parathyroid hormone levels are high and there are high levels of serum calcium in the absence of a malignant process, the diagnosis of primary hyperparathyroidism could be easily established.

There are a series of other pathological processes that may be easily discarded if one is careful and investigates the ingestion of drugs such as vitamin D, thiazides, and calcium carbonate. Obviously, if a patient has been immobilized in bed or in a cast the diagnosis will be apparent. Some conditions, such as sarcoidosis, hyperglobulinemia, and tuberculosis, should not present a difficult diagnostic problem. There are other conditions that obviously require different types of tests, and if the physician suspects hyperthyroidism, T3 and T4 levels should be determined. If adrenal insufficiency is suspected, plasma cortisol levels and urinary excretion of 17-ketosteroids and hydroxysteroids should also be determined. If a multiple endocrine syndrome is suspected, other studies to rule out adrenal abnormalities, pituitary abnormalities, or pheochromocytoma should be obtained. Finally, if the hypercalcemia occurs in the setting of renal insufficiency, it would be obvious whether or not the patient is in the diuretic phase of ATN or has had a successful renal transplant.

Clinical Problem

M. W., a 34-year-old secretary, was admitted to a psychiatric hospital because of bizarre behavior. The patient was in apparent good health until 6 months prior to admission when she became irritable and forgetful and antagonized members of her family. She also had crying spells and in the 2 months prior to admission became anorectic and had difficulty sleeping. Past history was unremarkable. On physical examination the patient appeared oriented in space and time and in no acute distress. Blood pressure, temperature, and pulse rate were within normal limits, and physical examination was completely unremarkable.

The laboratory data were unremarkable with the exception of an elevated serum calcium concentration of 13.5 mg/dl, a low serum phosphorus concentration of 1.8 mg/dl, and a high alkaline phosphatase level of 350 units (upper limit of normal is 100). Chest roentgenogram revealed bilateral infiltrates and parahilar nodes consistent with the diagnosis of sarcoidosis. Renal function studies were normal; however, a urinalysis revealed 5 red blood cells per high-power field (normal 0-1), trace proteinuria, but no casts. An IVP was obtained and revealed a mass in the upper pole of the right kidney.

Questions

1. What symptoms suggest the presence of hypercalcemia in this patient?
2. The combination of hypercalcemia, hypophosphatemia, and normal renal function greatly simplifies the differential diagnosis of hypercalcemia. Why?
3. The IVP revealed a mass in the right kidney, but the renal function was normal. Is this unexpected?

Discussion

The patient was admitted to the hospital because of psychiatric manifestations; however, the symptoms were all consistent with the finding of hypercalcemia, which was confirmed on several determinations. The patient also had low concentrations of serum phosphorus and high levels of alkaline phosphatase. These findings are consistent with the diagnosis of primary hyperparathyroidism. However, she had two other findings: (1) an abnormal chest roentgenogram that was consistent with the diagnosis of sarcoidosis, and (2) a mass in the right kidney.

Sarcoidosis may be the explanation for the hypercalcemia. However, since the patient also had a low concentration of serum phosphorus, it was thought that sarcoidosis alone could not account for all the biochemical abnormalities found in the patient. Thus, further studies were performed to determine if she had primary hyperparathyroidism or ectopic hyperparathyroidism due to a possible tumor present in the right kidney. Two studies were performed; one was a determination of parathyroid hormone levels that showed mild elevation in peripheral blood and the second, a renal arteriogram that was consistent with the diagnosis of hypernephroma.

The patient was seen by one consultant who, in view of the slight elevation in parathyroid hormone levels, hypercalcemia, and hypophosphatemia, diagnosed hyperparathyroidism and recommended that the patient have a neck exploration. However, the patient was also seen by another consultant who was rather concerned about the possibility of renal carcinoma secreting an ectopic parathyroid hormone-like material. This latter consultant suggested selective neck catheterization to determine the levels of parathyroid hormone in the effluent blood in the thyroid veins as compared to the levels of peripheral blood obtained from both antecubital veins. The rationale used was as follows: If the patient's hypercalcemia was due to primary hyperparathyroidism, the amount of parathyroid hormone present in one of the thyroid veins should be much higher than the levels present in the periphery. However, if the levels were not different, it is possible that the mild elevation of parathyroid hormone observed in peripheral blood was related to poor antigenic cross-reactivity between the parathyroid hormone antibody and a peptide secreted by the renal mass.

The patient's private physician followed the advice given by the second consultant, and the patient had a selective neck vein catheterization. Levels of parathyroid hormone measured in samples obtained from several upper and lower thyroid veins were compared with those of peripheral blood samples. The results clearly indicated that there was no difference in the levels of parathyroid hormone among all the blood samples obtained in this patient. After 6 days in the hospital, the right kidney was removed, and 3 days later the serum calcium and serum phosphorus concentrations returned to normal. This patient illustrates the occurrence of hypercalcemia and hypophosphatemia secondary to ectopic hyperparathyroidism produced by a renal carcinoma.

Hypocalcemia

Differential Diagnosis of Hypocalcemia

Table 12-2 lists the most common causes of hypocalcemia. Most of these disorders already have been considered in the section related to alterations in phosphate metabolism. However, a few points should be reemphasized here.

In addition to clinical syndromes characterized by either a deficiency of parathyroid hormone or an end-organ resistance to parathyroid hormone, hypocalcemia is also observed in uremia, malabsorption, acute pancreatitis, and hypoalbuminemic conditions such as nephrotic syndrome and cirrhosis. The symptoms related to hypocalcemia in patients with low albumin, such as cirrhosis and nephrotic syndrome, are rather mild, since the ionized calcium usually remains within the normal range. However, in those conditions in which ionized calcium is greatly diminished, a series of symptoms may frequently be seen that are attributable to hypocalcemia.

Hypocalcemia with marked irritability and convulsions has been observed in the neonate. Neuromuscular irritability and tetany accompanying hyperventilation have been ascribed to respiratory alkalosis, which causes a remarkable decrease in ionized calcium. The symptoms have already been described in the previous section, but it is important to emphasize that laryngeal stridor, tetany, muscle cramps, and twitching could be fatal if they are not treated adequately. The electrocardiogram may show a prolongation of the S–T interval.

An interesting syndrome, which will be described in detail in the chapter on magnesium metabolism, is the presence of hypocalcemia in patients with profound hypomagnesemia. This syndrome has been seen frequently in patients in whom bypass gastrointestinal procedures have been performed for obesity and who then become hypomagnesemic.

Table 12-2

Causes of Hypocalcemia

I. Renal failure
II. Endocrine disorders
  A. Hypoparathyroidism
  B. Pseudohypoparathyroidism
III. Nutritional and metabolic disorders
  A. Vitamin D deficiency
  B. Magnesium deficiency
  C. Intestinal calcium malabsorption
  D. Hyperphosphatemia
IV. Miscellaneous
  A. Hypoproteinemia
  B. Acute pancreatitis
  C. Drugs

The pathogenesis of hypocalcemia is complex and multifactorial. There are a series of drugs that, in specific circumstances, can or may produce severe hypocalcemia. They are *calcitonin* administered intravenously; the administration of *mytramycin,* a drug used for the treatment of carcinoma of the testes; and administration of *EDTA,* which is a chelating agent.

The most common cause of hypocalcemia is renal insufficiency, which can be easily diagnosed. Providing that renal function is normal, hypomagnesemia should be ruled out. If these two conditions are ruled out and providing that the patient does not have acute pancreatitis and is not ingesting drugs, other tests should be performed to rule out hypoparathyroidism or even pseudohypoparathyroidism. In these two conditions, as is mentioned in Chapter 14, the hypocalcemia will be associated with hyperphosphatemia. However, in hypoparathyroidism the levels of parathyroid hormone will be very low or absent, and in pseudohypoparathyroidism the levels of PTH will be elevated; moreover, the patient will not respond to the administration of exogenous parathyroid hormone. In a child with a diagnosis of vitamin D deficiency suspected, the hypocalcemia also will be associated with hypophosphatemia, and characteristic physical features will clearly indicate the diagnosis.

Clinical Problem

J. P., an 18-year-old male, was admitted to the hospital because of weight loss, anorexia, and multiple hematomas in the lower extremities and right side of his abdomen. On physical examination, he appeared acutely ill, pale, with a temperature of 39.5° C. Blood pressure was 100/70, and respirations were 28 per minute. The pertinent physical findings were pale conjunctiva, multiple hematomas and petechiae, generalized lymphadenopathy, and a palpable spleen. Laboratory data showed a hemoglobin of 6.2 gm/100 ml, hematocrit of 18%; 85,000 WBCs, of which 80% were blasts and 20,000 platelets; serum creatinine of 1.1 mg/100 ml; BUN, 28 mg/100 ml; sodium concentration, 138 mEq/liter; potassium, 5.2 mEq/liter; bicarbonate, 24 mEq/liter; chloride, 99 mEq/liter. Serum phosphorus concentration was 14 mg/100 ml and serum calcium concentration was 6 mg/100 ml. Electrocardiogram was normal. The chest x-ray showed bilateral infiltrates.

Questions

1. What factors are responsible for the maintenance of a normal serum calcium?
2. How does hyperphosphatemia affect the levels of serum calcium?

Discussion

The diagnosis of acute lymphoblastic leukemia was made in this patient, and he was treated accordingly. However, there was a difference of opinion regarding the nature of the hypocalcemia that occurred in the presence of normal renal function and without abnormalities in vitamin D metabolism. The hypocalcemia in the absence of renal disease may have been related to the extremely high levels of serum phosphorus, or the patient may have true hypoparathyroidism. Serum parathyroid hormone was determined and was found to be elevated three times above normal. This indicates a normal response of the parathyroid glands to the hypocalcemic stimulus present. The patient received treatment for his leukemia, he was given phosphate binders with his diet, and after a month of therapy the serum phosphorus concentration returned to 5 mg/100 ml and serum calcium concentration increased to 9.2 mg/100 ml. This patient represents a case of severe hypocalcemia secondary to precipitation of calcium due to severe hyperphosphatemia.

References

Agus, Z. S., Gardner, L. B., Beck, L. H., and Goldberg, M. "Effects of parathyroid hormone on renal tubular reabsorption of calcium, sodium and phosphate." Am. J. Physiol. *224:* 1143, 1973.

Blanchard, B. "Focal hypocalcemic seizures 33 years after thyroidectomy." Arch. Intern. Med. *11:* 382, 1962.

Coburn, J. W., and Massry, S. G. "Changes in serum and urinary calcium during phosphate depletion: Studies on mechanisms." J. Clin. Invest. *49:* 1073, 1970.

Coburn, J. W., Koppel, M. H., Brickman, A. S., and Massry, S. G. "Study of intestinal absorption of calcium in patients with renal failure." Kidney Int. *3:* 264, 1972.

David, S. D., Sakai, S., Brennan, B. L., Riggio, R. A., Stenzel, K. H., Rubin, A. L., and Sherwood, L. M. "Hypercalcemia after renal transplantation." N. Engl. J. Med. *289:* 398, 1973.

Edwards, B. R., Sutton, R. A. L., and Dirks, J. H. "Effect of calcium infusion on renal tubular reabsorption in the dog." Am. J. Physiol. *227:* 13, 1974.

Ginsberg, D. S., Kaplan, E. L., and Katz, A. I. "Hypercalcemia after oral calcium carbonate therapy in patients on chronic hemodialysis." Lancet *1:* 1271, 1973.

Gonda, A., Wong, N., Seely, J. F., and Dirks, J. H. "The role of hemodynamic factors on urinary calcium and magnesium excretion." Can. J. Physiol. Pharmacol. *47:* 619, 1971.

Issekutz, B., Jr., Blizzard, J. J., Birkhead, N. C., and Rodahl, L. "Effect of prolonged bed rest on urinary calcium output." J. Appl. Physiol. *21:* 1013, 1966.

Koffler, A., Friedler, R. M., and Massry, S. G. "Acute renal failure due to nontraumatic rhabdomyolysis." Ann. Intern. Med. *85:* 23, 1976.

Lennon, E. J., and Piering, W. F. "A comparison of the effects of glucose ingestion and NH_4Cl acidosis on urinary calcium and magnesium excretion in man." J. Clin. Invest. *49:* 1458, 1970.

Massry, S. G., and Kleeman, C. R. "Calcium and magnesium excretion during acute rise in glomerular filtration rate." J. Lab. Clin. Med. *80:* 654, 1972.

Massry, S. G., Coburn, J. W., Lee, D. B. N., Jowsey, J., and Kleeman, C. R. "Skeletal resistance to parathyroid hormone in renal failure. Study in 105 human subjects." Ann. Intern. Med. *78:* 357, 1973.

Mundy, G. R., Raisz, L. G., Cooper, R. A., Schechter, G. P., and Salmon, S. E. "Evidence for the secretion of an osteoclast stimulating factor in myeloma." N. Engl. J. Med. *291:* 1041, 1974.

Nusynowitz, M. L., Frame, B., and Kolb, F. O. "The spectrum of the hypoparathyroid states." Medicine *55:* 105, 1976.

Peacock, M., Hodgkinson, A., and Nordin, B. E. C. "Importance of dietary calcium in the definition of hypercalciuria." Br. Med. J. *3:* 469, 1967.

Seyberth, H. W., Segre, G. V., Morgan, J. L., Sweetman, B. J., Potts, J. T., Jr., and Oates, J. A. "Prostaglandins as mediators of hypercalcemia associated with certain neoplasia." N. Engl. J. Med. *293:* 1278, 1975.

Sherwood, L. M., O'Riordan, J. H. L., Aurbach, G. D., and Potts, J. T., Jr. "Production of parathyroid hormone by nonparathyroid tumors." J. Clin. Endocrinol. *27:* 140, 1967.

Walser, M. "Ion association. VII. Dependence of calciuresis on natriuresis during sulfate infusion." Am. J. Physiol. *201:* 769, 1961.

Walser, M. "The separate effects of hyperparathyroidism, hypercalcemia of malignancy, renal failure and acidosis on the state of calcium, phosphate, and other ions in plasma." J. Clin. Invest. *41:* 1454, 1962.

Wang, C. A., Potts, J. T., Jr., and Neer, R. M. "Controversy of parathyroid surgery." *In:* Calcium-regulating Hormones, R. V. Talmage, M. Owen, and J. A. Parsons, (eds.). Excerpta Medica, Amsterdam, p. 82, 1975.

Weeke, E., and Friis, T. H. "Serum fractions of calcium and phosphorus in uremia." Acta. Med. Scand. *189:* 79, 1971.

Chapter 13

Alterations in Serum Magnesium Concentration

General Considerations

Magnesium is the fourth most abundant cation of the body and, after potassium, the second most abundant intracellular cation. Total body magnesium is approximately 2000 mEq, with the skeleton containing about 50% of the total magnesium, the remainder being almost equally distributed between muscle and nonmuscular tissue. Liver and muscle have a high concentration of magnesium, around 15–20 mEq/kg. Red cell magnesium is 5 mEq/liter, and the concentration in normal serum ranges from 1.6 to 2.1 mEq/liter.

Magnesium plays an essential role as a cofactor for a variety of enzymes, most of them utilizing ATP. Approximately 300 mg of magnesium is ingested daily in a normal diet. Roughly one third is eliminated in the urine and the rest in the feces. A large proportion of the magnesium in our diet is provided by the ingestion of green vegetables. A minimum magnesium intake of 0.3 mEq/kg body weight is apparently necessary to maintain magnesium balance in the average person.

Multiple studies have clearly shown that animals fed low-magnesium diets can excrete urine that is practically free of magnesium. However, the gastrointestinal tract continues to secrete small amounts of magnesium, and the animals become magnesium depleted. Most of the magnesium is absorbed in the upper gastrointestinal tract. Magnesium shares with calcium similar pathways for absorption in the intestine, but while most of the evidence suggests that calcium is actively absorbed from the gastrointestinal tract, it seems that magnesium is absorbed mainly by ionic diffusion and solvent "drag" resulting from the bulk flow of water. There is no good evidence to indicate that magnesium is actively transported. Small amounts of magnesium, about 15–25 mg/24 hr, are secreted by the gastrointestinal tract. The factors controlling the absorption of magnesium from the gastrointestinal tract are not fully understood. There is some evidence to suggest that both vitamin D and parathyroid hormone enhance magnesium absorption. Sodium has a similar effect. On the other hand, both calcium and phosphorus seem to decrease the absorption of magnesium from the intestine.

Renal Handling of Magnesium

Approximately 80% of the magnesium present in serum is ultrafilterable; the rest is protein-bound. Most of the ultrafilterable magnesium is present in the ionized form. Approximately 2 gm of magnesium is filtered daily by the kidney, and roughly 100 mg appears in the urine. Thus, approximately 95% of the filtered load of magnesium is reabsorbed, and 5% is excreted in the urine. Recent micropuncture studies have shown some similarities between calcium and magnesium transport and have indicated that the administration of one of these two elements decreases the reabsorption of the other. For example, when large amounts of magnesium are given intravenously, there is a remarkable decrease in the renal reabsorption of calcium and vice versa.

There seem to be some differences in the renal handling of magnesium between dogs and rodents. In the dog, about 60% of the filtered magnesium is reabsorbed in the proximal tubule; in rats, perhaps no more than 30% is reabsorbed in this segment of the nephron. The ascending limb of the loop of Henle seems to play a critical role in the amount of magnesium reabsorbed. The distal tubule also has the capacity to reabsorb magnesium, but in absolute terms the ascending limb of the loop of Henle plays a more important role in the overall reabsorption of magnesium in the nephron. In certain animals, such as the rat, tubular secretion of magnesium can be demonstrated. With mild elevations of serum magnesium levels, on the order of 3 mg/100 ml, a maximum reabsorption for magnesium can be demonstrated, and if the serum magnesium is further increased the amount of magnesium present in the urine may exceed the amount filtered, clearly indicating magnesium secretion. However, when similar studies were performed in other animals, such as dogs, and the serum magnesium level was increased to about 10 mg/100 ml, no clear evidence for magnesium secretion could be demonstrated using clearance methodology. On the other hand, micropuncture studies have demonstrated magnesium secretion in the distal tubule, although this process does not seem to play an important role in the renal regulation of magnesium excretion.

The kidney has the capacity to excrete large amounts of magnesium in the urine; thus the development of hypermagnesemia in clinical medicine is rarely seen in any other conditions except those in which there is severe impairment of renal function or when the patient is receiving large doses of magnesium intravenously. The factors that control the reabsorption of magnesium by the kidney are not fully understood at the present time. It is known that both volume expansion and diuretics decrease magnesium reabsorption. The role of parathyroid hormone in the regulation of magnesium by the kidney is controversial, since studies have shown that PTH may increase, decrease, or produce no change in the reabsorption of magnesium. Also, there is no clear evidence that vitamin D or its metabolites play an important role in the regulation of magnesium excretion.

It is possible that the intracellular concentration of magnesium plays a key role in the renal regulation of this divalent cation. Chronic administration of mineralocorticoids decreases the reabsorption of magnesium. Animals maintained on a low-magnesium diet can excrete a urine that is practically free of magnesium. Urinary magnesium falls to low levels in the first 72 hours of magnesium deprivation, even before plasma magnesium declines.

Alcohol has a clear and distinctive effect on the handling of magnesium by the kidney. A remarkable, short-lived hypermagnesuria is seen after alcohol is given to experimental animals or humans. The administration of glucose intravenously has a similar effect. As mentioned before, calcium and magnesium seem to share some common pathways for reabsorption, and hypercalcemia has a profound inhibitory effect on the distal reabsorption of magnesium, producing a significant increase in urinary magnesium excretion.

Hypomagnesemia

General Considerations

The most common causes of hypomagnesemia are related to pathological processes that involve the small intestine and prevent the absorption of magnesium. Since most of the body magnesium is present inside cells, it is difficult to establish the degree of magnesium depletion from measurements of serum magnesium levels. For a given serum magnesium the degree of magnesium depletion may be mild or extremely profound, so that symptoms and biochemical alterations may vary among patients, despite the fact that they may have similar low serum magnesium levels.

Severe hypomagnesemia is characterized by a series of symptoms that resemble those seen in patients with profound hypocalcemia. Patients may develop mild anorexia and nausea, they may have hyperreflexia, changes in personality, increased irritability, psychotic behavior, carpopedal spasm, and tetany. The electrocardiogram may show prolongation of the Q-T interval and broadening and decreased amplitude of the T waves.

An interesting biochemical abnormality of patients with hypomagnesemia is the development of hypocalcemia. Recent studies have clarified some of the mechanisms responsible for the hypocalcemia observed in patients with profound hypomagnesemia. For many years it was accepted that with hypomagnesemia the skeleton becomes "resistant" to the action of PTH, and the patients develop hypocalcemia due to inability of the osteoclasts to respond normally to PTH. Recently, with the development of the radioimmunoassay for PTH, further knowledge has been obtained regarding the role of magnesium in the regulation of parathyroid secretion. Parathyroid glands incubated in a low magnesium medium demonstrate increased secretion of parathyroid hormone. However, when the glands were incubated in medium with extremely low or no magnesium at all, there was no increase in the release of PTH. Moreover, magnesium does not affect the de novo synthesis of PTH or the conversion of prohormone to parathyroid hormone.

Recent studies also have shown that patients with profound magnesium depletion have low or undetectable levels of PTH in blood. Thus, hypomagnesemia plays a biphasic effect in the secretion of PTH, depending on the degree of magnesium depletion; with mild magnesium depletion and hypomagnesemia, there is an increase in PTH release. However, with profound magnesium depletion and serum magnesium levels below 0.7 mg/dl, there is a state of "true" hypoparathyroidism. Administration of magnesium to these patients has shown that the parathyroid glands may respond rapidly, with an increase in the release of PTH occurring within minutes. What is rather confusing and difficult to explain is the fact that in many patients with profound hypomagnesemia and hypocalcemia the levels of circulating PTH are in the normal range. Obviously, from the physiological point of view, these levels are abnormal, since the hypocalcemia should be able to trigger the release of PTH and increase the levels of the hormone in blood. However, the concentration of PTH in blood should be sufficient, in theory, to activate osteoclasts and mobilize calcium from bones to correct the hypocalcemia, but this is not the case.

The pathogenesis of the hypocalcemia seen in patients with profound magnesium depletion is multiple: (1) there is a decreased release of PTH, but this factor alone cannot explain the hypocalcemia; (2) the skeleton is resistant to the action of PTH. It has been postulated that a physicochemical exchange of ions occurs between the hydration shell of the skeleton and the surrounding medium. In addition to this isoionic exchange of calcium between these compartments, a heteroionic exchange of magnesium for calcium in the hydration shell of the surface of bone has been postulated. This concept has been supported by studies in vitro demonstrating that calcium exchange was less in bone from magnesium-depleted rats than in control animals.

In summary the hypocalcemia of hypomagnesemic animals and humans may result primarily from a decreased heteroionic exchange of magnesium and calcium of the bone surface. In distinction to bone, the kidney responds normally to the action of PTH in the presence of hypomagnesemia. It should also be emphasized that the rat is perhaps the only animal that develops hypercalcemia rather than hypocalcemia in the presence of magnesium depletion; the serum phosphorus level also is decreased, and there is an increased excretion of phosphate in the urine. All these findings in the rat are consistent with the development of secondary hyperparathyroidism, and hypercalcemia may be due, in part, to increased calcium absorption from the gastrointestinal tract. However, in humans, hypercalcemia is practically never seen in patients with hypomagnesemia.

Differential Diagnosis of Hypomagnesemia

Table 13-1 lists the most common causes of hypomagnesemia.

I. Decreased Intestinal Absorption

Diverse pathological entities affecting the small bowel may result in hypomagnesemia. A rough correlation between the degree of steatorrhea and the subnormal levels of serum magnesium has been shown. Magnesium may be lost in the stools, in conditions characterized by steatorrhea, as a result of the formation of insoluble magnesium soaps. Some of these patients have improved their magnesium absorption when placed on a low-fat diet. Hypomagnesemia is especially prominent in patients with idiopathic steatorrhea and diseases affecting the terminal ileum. Hypomagnesemia has been described with increasing frequency in patients undergoing intestinal resections, for the control of obesity, after partial gastric resection, and with biliary fistulas.

A series of patients has been described who may have an isolated defect in gastrointestinal absorption of magnesium. The dietary intake of magnesium in these patients is normal. There seems to be a specific defect for magnesium absorption. The hypomagnesemia can be corrected by markedly increasing the dietary intake of magnesium.

II. Hypomagnesemia Resulting from Decreased Intake

Low magnesium levels have been reported in a large percentage of children with protein-calorie malnutrition. Magnesium depletion in these children presumably results from

Table 13-1

Causes of Hypomagnesemia

- I. Decreased intestinal absorption
  - A. Celiac disease
  - B. Tropical and nontropical sprue
  - C. Invasive and infiltrative process: lymphomas
  - D. Surgical resection
  - E. Intestinal bypass
  - F. Severe diarrhea
  - G. Prolonged gastrointestinal suction
- II. Decreased intake
  - A. Protein-caloric malnutrition
  - B. Starvation
  - C. Prolonged therapy with intravenous fluids lacking magnesium
  - D. Chronic alcoholism
- III. Excessive urinary losses
  - A. Diabetic ketoacidosis
  - B. Chronic alcoholism
  - C. Diuretic therapy
  - D. Diuretic phase of ATN
  - E. Post-obstructive diuresis
  - F. Hypercalciuric states
  - G. Primary or secondary hyperaldosteronism
  - H. Inappropriate antidiuretic hormone secretion
  - I. Idiopathic renal magnesium wasting
  - J. Gentamicin toxicity

a combination of decreased intake and increased gastrointestinal losses due to diarrhea or vomiting. Patients maintained for prolonged periods of time on intravenous fluids without magnesium may develop moderate hypomagnesemia.

Alcoholic patients develop hypomagnesemia, which probably results from several mechanisms. Ethanol ingestion has been shown to increase markedly urinary magnesium excretion. While this is a transitory phenomenon and presumably not an important one in the production of magnesium depletion, decreased intake due to abnormal dietary habits may be the major contributing factor to magnesium depletion in alcoholics.

A complete history, evidence of other manifestations of malnutrition (including low levels of plasma proteins, low cholesterol), presence of diarrhea or vomiting, recent bypass surgery, and the like help to differentiate individuals with decreased absorption of magnesium, due either to primary intestinal disease or decreased intake, from individuals who have increased magnesium excretion via the urine and develop hypomagnesemia on this basis.

III. Excessive Urinary Losses

Some patients with diabetic ketoacidosis may develop hypomagnesemia. While serum magnesium levels may be initially elevated during the period of ketoacidosis, they usually fall following insulin and fluid replacement. Increased urinary magnesium excretion has been described during the period of ketoacidosis. These urinary losses may continue during the initial period of treatment. It has been suggested that magnesium replacement is indicated in the treatment of patients with ketoacidosis.

Entities characterized by decreased salt and water absorption from the nephron and increased urinary volumes may also present with increased urinary losses of magnesium. Such entities include postobstructive diuresis, the diuretic phase of acute tubular necrosis, and the use of diuretic agents. Urinary magnesium excretion will be relatively high despite the presence of hypomagnesemia. This is somewhat different from the urinary levels of magnesium found in patients with malabsorption or decreased magnesium intake in whom the kidney can decrease magnesium excretion markedly. Determination of urinary magnesium levels, therefore, may be of help in the differential diagnosis of the cause of hypomagnesemia.

States characterized by hypercalciuria may also result in increased magnesium wasting via the kidney. This presumably relates, as discussed above, to the fact that calcium directly interferes with magnesium reabsorption by the nephron.

States characterized by volume expansion, such as inappropriate secretion of antidiuretic hormone or primary aldosteronism, may also present with increased losses of magnesium via the urine and hypomagnesemia. Renal magnesium wasting may be idiopathic in nature, and a hereditary basis for this renal defect in magnesium reabsorption has been suggested. This entity is presumably extremely rare and the diagnosis should only be made after other causes of renal magnesium wasting and hypomagnesemia have been excluded.

Clinical Problem

J. P., a 22-year-old white male, was admitted to the hospital because of severe diarrhea of 3 months' duration. The patient was in good health until 3 months prior to admission when he noticed an increase in the number of bowel movements from one up to three or four times daily. On certain occasions he noticed some mucus; however, he denied the presence of blood in the stools. Occasionally he had pain, colicky in nature and localized to the epigastrium with radiation to the left side of the abdomen. The patient stated that his appetite was good, and that his food intake had not decreased. However, he noticed a 25-pound weight loss over this 3-month period.

On physical examination he appeared well developed, poorly nourished, chronically ill, and in some acute distress. The physical examination was noncontributory, except for some epigastric tenderness and marked hyperreflexia. Trousseau and Chevosteck's signs were positive.

Laboratory studies showed the following: hemoglobin, 10.2 gm; hematocrit, 35%; WBC, 4200; sodium concentration, 138 mEq/liter; potassium, 3.2 mEq/liter; bicarbonate, 29 mEq/liter; chloride, 94 mEq/liter; BUN, 12 mg/dl; serum creatinine, 1.0 mg/dl; serum calcium concentration, 6.5 mg/dl; serum phosphorus, 3.1 mg/dl; and serum magnesium, 0.4 mg/dl; (normal 1.6–2.1 mg/dl). Chest roentgenograms and electrocardiograms were normal. Upper GI tract studies revealed an abnormal pattern in the small intestine. A small bowel biopsy was performed and was consistent with the diagnosis of nontropical sprue.

Because of profound hypocalcemia the patient received calcium intravenously, and most of the symptoms disappeared. Before calcium was administered, a blood sample for PTH was obtained. The next morning, the serum calcium concentration, which had been corrected by the intravenous administration of calcium, was again decreased (7.4 mg/dl). The patient was given 50 mEq of magnesium intravenously every 12 hours for 2 days and then continued on 50 mEq of magnesium per day. After 2 days of treatment the serum magnesium concentration increased to 1.3 mg/dl, and the serum calcium concentration returned to normal.

Questions

1. What is the most common cause of hypocalcemia in hospitalized patients?
2. Does the finding of a normal serum phosphorus concentration rule out the presence of hypoparathyroidism in this patient?
3. With a serum magnesium concentration of 0.4 mg/dl, does this patient have mild or severe magnesium depletion? Can you explain why this is important?

Discussion

This patient with diarrhea due to nontropical sprue presented with severe hypomagnesemia and hypocalcemia. The hypocalcemia was corrected transitorily by the intravenous administration of calcium. The day after intravenous calcium administration, the serum calcium concentration had again fallen to low levels. When magnesium was given, the hypocalcemia was promptly corrected. Measurement of PTH levels revealed a value of 9 μlEq/ml (normal range 2–10). However, in the presence of profound hypocalcemia, this concentration of PTH in blood is abnormal. If hypocalcemia is produced in a patient by the intravenous administration of EDTA, for example, the levels of PTH will usually rise three to five times above normal. In this particular patient, despite profound hypocalcemia, the concentration of PTH in blood was in the normal range, but the skeleton did not respond to this concentration of PTH by releasing calcium, and the patient had profound hypocalcemia. When magnesium was given the whole syndrome was reversed. A sample of blood for parathyroid hormone was obtained after the administration of magnesium. PTH levels in blood were increased threefold above the normal range.

This patient illustrates the multifactorial nature of the hypocalcemia that develops secondary to hypomagnesemia. In this patient, the profound magnesium depletion not only decreased the secretion of parathyroid hormone but also made the skeleton unresponsive to the normal amounts of circulating parathyroid hormone.

Hypermagnesemia

General Considerations

The most common cause of hypermagnesemia is renal insufficiency (Table 13-2). The kidney can excrete large magnesium loads; thus, even when magnesium influx is increased several times (by dietary means or in the form of laxatives or enemas), hypermagnesemia is seldom seen, unless a concomitant decrease in renal function is present. Mild hypermagnesemia is well tolerated; however, if serum magnesium levels increase to around 5–6 mg/dl, there may be a decrease in tendon reflexes, and some degree of mental obtundation. If the degree of hypermagnesemia increases, arrythmias and a fall in respiratory rate and blood pressure are frequently observed. If serum magnesium levels increase about 10 mg/dl, there is usually profound hypotension and severe mental depression. When magnesium levels increase further, to about 15 mg/dl, coma and death may occur.

In the past, large amounts of magnesium were used for the treatment of eclampsia, and some of these patients became comatose after correction of the hypertensive crisis. However, in those days, blood magnesium was measured in only a very few instances. In retrospect, knowing the large amounts of magnesium that these patients received, it is possible to ascribe some of the neurological symptoms that these women developed to profound hypermagnesemia. There are also reports in the literature in which profound hypermagnesemia was produced by the use of laxatives and enemas containing magnesium.

Hypermagnesemia is a late manifestation of renal insufficiency, and seldom does hypermagnesemia occur in patients with a GFR greater than 15 ml/min. Mild hypermagnesemia is seen in patients with GFR around 10 ml/min. However, more marked hypermagnesemia is seen usually in patients with GFR of less than 5 ml/min.

There is a remarkable adaptive change in the handling of magnesium per nephron in patients with renal failure. As mentioned above, hypermagnesemia is not seen until the GFR is 15 ml/min or less. This, in part, is due to an increased fractional excretion of magnesium, which can reach 30% to 60% of the filtered load in patients with profound renal insufficiency as compared to 5% in patients with GFRs of 120 ml/min. There is some evidence to indicate that the increased natriuresis per nephron occurring with chronic progressive renal disease may in part be responsible for this adaptation in magnesium excretion. However, recent evidence in experimental animals (dog) indicates that the increase in sodium excretion per remaining nephron is not responsible for the overall regulation of magnesium excretion in uremia. The increased excretion of magnesium per nephron observed in patients with far-advanced renal disease is probably not related to secondary hyperparathyroidism, since PTH administration has little effect on renal magnesium excretion. At present, the mechanisms responsible for the increased excretion of magnesium per

Table 13-2

Causes of Hypermagnesemia

I. Decreased renal excretion
   A. Acute renal failure
   B. Chronic renal disease
   C. Adrenocortical insufficiency
II. Increased entrance to ECF
   A. Laxatives containing magnesium
   B. Enemas containing magnesium
   C. Intravenous fluids containing magnesium
   D. Intramuscular administration of magnesium (eclampsia)

nephron in renal failure are not fully understood. Patients with chronic renal disease cannot further adapt to the ingestion of large amounts of magnesium when they are already excreting 30% to 60% of the filtered load. Therefore, if an increase in the ingestion of magnesium occurs, such as through the administration of laxatives or antacids (commonly used to bind phosphorus) containing magnesium, profound hypermagnesemia and death may occur.

Clinical Problem

S. H., a 35-year-old white male being maintained on chronic hemodialysis because of end-stage renal failure secondary to chronic pyelonephritis, was admitted to the hospital in coma. Apparently the patient was doing well and had been dialyzed uneventfully 3 days prior to admission. On physical examination the patient was semicomatose, but responded to pain. Blood pressure was 100/60, and respirations were 12 per minute. Funduscopic examination revealed a grade 2 hypertensive retinopathy. There was mild distention of neck veins at a 45° angle; the lungs were clear to auscultation and percussion. The heart revealed a grade 3/6 systolic murmur localized to the fifth intercostal space; the abdomen was soft and not distended. The liver was 2 cm below the right costal margin, the spleen and kidneys were not palpable, and there were no masses. There was 1+ pitting edema in both legs, and reflexes were absent.

Laboratory data revealed the following: hemoglobin, 7.5 gm/100 ml; hematocrit, 22%; BUN, 85 mg/dl; serum creatinine, 14 mg/dl; sodium concentration, 135 mEq/liter; potassium, 5.2 mEq/liter; bicarbonate, 18 mEq/liter; chloride, 104 mEq/liter; serum calcium, 8.9 mg/dl; phosphorus, 5.8 mg/dl; and magnesium, 13 mg/100 ml.

Because of profound hypermagnesemia the patient was dialyzed with a bath containing no magnesium for 12 consecutive hours. At the end of dialysis the serum magnesium concentration had decreased to 5 mg/100 ml. The patient became more alert and responsive, and the blood pressure increased to its usual levels of 160/90. Neurological examination improved; however, the hyporeflexia persisted. The patient received a second dialysis on his second hospital day, and the serum magnesium concentration corrected to normal levels.

Questions

1. What is the first therapeutic maneuver that should be undertaken in a comatose, uremic patient with a serum magnesium concentration of 13 mg/dl?
2. What is the most likely explanation for the hypermagnesemia in this patient?
3. Can all the clinical manifestations observed in this patient be explained by hypermagnesemia?

Discussion

It was difficult for the physicians who were taking care of this patient to understand how he developed extreme hypermagnesemia, since he had been doing well on hemodialysis for the past 4 years and had never had hypermagnesemia prior to this episode. After the severe hypermagnesemia was corrected by hemodialysis the patient was carefully interviewed by a physician looking for clues to explain the development of hypermagnesemia; apparently none were found. However, when a second physician interrogated the patient, it became apparent why he developed hypermagnesemia. The patient had been ingesting phosphate binders for the past 4 years in order to control his hyperphosphatemia. He ingested aluminum carbonate gel, 30 ml, three times a day (this binder does not contain magnesium). However, the patient ran out of medication and obtained another antacid from a different pharmacy. "This antacid the pharmacist recommended as being better than the previous one because it did not produce constipation." This antacid, which contains aluminum and magnesium, is usually prescribed in patients with peptic ulcer disease. In the absence of renal failure, it is an excellent drug. However, a patient with end-stage renal disease like the present one cannot excrete additional magnesium loads. This is particularly true for patients on dialysis in whom the GFR is less than 2 ml/min. The administration of antacids containing magnesium to uremic patients may produce severe hypermagnesemia and death in a relatively short period of time.

References

Anast, C. S., Winnacker, J. L., Forte, L. R., and Burns, T. W. "Impaired release of parathyroid hormone in magnesium deficiency." J. Clin. Endocrinol. Metab. *42:* 707, 1976.

Brady, J. P., and Williams, H. C. "Magnesium intoxication in a premature infant." Pediatrics 40: 100, 1967.

Chase, L. R., and Slatopolsky, E. "Secretion and metabolic efficacy of parathyroid hormone in patients with severe hypomagnesemia." J. Clin. Endocrinol. Metab. *38:* 363, 1974.

Chesly, L. C., and Tepper, I. "Some effects of magnesium loading upon renal excretion of magnesium and certain other electrolytes." J. Clin. Invest. *37:* 1362, 1958.

Coburn, J. W., Popovtzer, M. M., Massry, S. G., and Kleeman, C. R. "The physicochemical state and renal handling of divalent ions in chronic renal failure." Arch. Intern. Med. *124:* 302, 1969.

Hahn, T. J., Chase, L. R., and Avioli, L. V. "Effect of magnesium depletion on responsiveness to parathyroid hormone in parathyroidectomized rats." J. Clin. Invest. *51:* 886, 1972.

Hamburger, J. "Magnesium in acute renal failure." Clin. Chem. *3:* 333, 1957.

Heaton, F. W., and Parson, F. M. "The metabolic effect of high magnesium intake." Clin. Sci. *21:* 273, 1961.

Levi, J., Massry, S. G., Coburn, J. W., Llach, F., and Kleeman, C. R. "Hypocalcemia in magnesium-depleted dogs: Evidence for reduced responsiveness to parathyroid hormone and relative failure of parathyroid gland function." Metabolism *23:* 323, 1974.

MacManus, J., Heaton, F. W., and Lucas, P. W. "Decreased response to parathyroid hormone in magnesium deficiency." J. Endocrinol. *49:* 253, 1971.

Massry, S. G. "Pharmacology of magnesium." Ann. Rev. Pharmacol. Toxicol. *17:* 67, 1977.

Massry, S. G., Arieff, A. I., Coburn, J. W., Palmieri, G., and Kleeman, C. R. "Divalent ion metabolism in patients with acute renal failure: Studies on the mechanism of hypocalcemia." Kidney Int. *5:* 437, 1974.

Randall, R. E., Cohen, M. D., Spray, C. C., and Rossmeish, E. D. "Hypermagnesemia in renal failure. Etiology and toxic manifestations." Ann. Intern. Med. *61:* 73, 1964.

Steele, T. H., Wen, S. F., Evenson, M. A., and Rieselbach, R. E. "The contribution of the chronically diseased kidney to magnesium homeostasis in man." J. Lab. Clin. Med. *71:* 455, 1968.

Suh, S. M., Csima, A., and Fraser, D. "Pathogenesis of hypocalcemia in magnesium depletion." J. Clin. Invest. *50:* 2668, 1971.
Wacker, W. E. C., and Parisi, A. F. "Magnesium metabolism." N. Engl. J. Med. *278:* 658, 1968.
Walser, M. "Magnesium metabolism." Ergeb Physiol. Biol. Chem. Exp. Pharmakol. *59:* 185, 1967.

Chapter 14

Alterations of Serum Phosphate Concentration

General Considerations

Serum phosphorus concentrations are maintained within narrow limits ranging from 2.8 to 4.5 mg/dl in adults. Approximately 80% to 85% of the phosphorus is present in the skeleton. The rest is widely distributed throughout the body in the form of organic phosphate compounds. In the ECF, most of the phosphorus is present in the inorganic form. On an average diet 1 gm of phosphorus is ingested daily, of which approximately 70% is absorbed and the remainder is excreted in the stool.

Phosphorus absorption occurs mainly in the small intestine. Most of the inorganic phosphorus in serum (90% to 95%) is ultrafilterable at the level of the glomerulus. Approximately 7 gm of phosphorus is filtered daily by the kidney, of which 80% to 90% is reabsorbed by the renal tubules and the remainder excreted in the urine (about 700 mg on a 1 gm phosphorus diet). Micropuncture experiments have demonstrated that 60% to 70% of the filtered phosphorus is reabsorbed in the proximal tubule. However, there is also evidence that a significant amount is reabsorbed in the distal tubule.

Contradictory results have been obtained with regard to phosphorus secretion by the kidney. In certain animals, such as amphibians and birds, it has been clearly demonstrated that the kidney secretes phosphorus. However, the results obtained in mammals are controversial. Nevertheless, if phosphorus secretion occurs in mammals, this mechanism seems to play a minor role in the overall regulation of phosphate balance.

Regulation of Phosphorus Reabsorption

The reabsorption of phosphorus along the nephron is regulated by a series of factors, of which PTH is the most important. However, other factors, such as growth hormone, calcitonin, glucocorticoids, vitamin D metabolites, the degree of ECF volume expansion, the filtered load of phosphate, and the acid-base balance, also play a role in the regulation of PO_4 excretion.

Numerous studies have demonstrated the phosphaturic effect of PTH. PTH blocks the reabsorption of phosphorus both in the proximal and the distal tubule. The biological activity of PTH is mediated via stimulation of the adenylcyclase system and production of cyclic AMP. In the absence of PTH the maximal tubular reabsorptive capacity for phosphorus (TM_{PO_4}) is increased. Thus, patients with decreased or absent PTH characteristically have hyperphosphatemia. Extracellular fluid volume expansion is accompanied by a significant degree of phosphaturia, which may be shown to occur in the absence of PTH.

The effect of vitamin D and its metabolites on phosphate excretion by the kidney is still controversial. However, recent data suggest that vitamin D metabolites increase the reabsorption of phosphorus by the renal tubules. Thyrocalcitonin and growth hormone have opposite effects, the former being phosphaturic, while the latter increases phosphorus reabsorption.

Of interest is the fact that there is a diurnal variation in phosphorus excretion. Most of the studies indicate that excretion is minimal early in the morning until noon, gradually increasing in the afternoon, and reaching maximum values by evening. Although many factors are responsible for the regulation of phosphorus balance by the kidney in normal individuals, the amount of phosphorus in the diet plays a key role in the amount that ultimately will be excreted.

Hyperphosphatemia

General Considerations

Hyperphosphatemia (serum phosphate concentrations greater than 5 mg/dl in adults) is seen frequently in clinical medicine. By far the most common cause of hyperphosphatemia is a decrease in urinary phosphorus excretion secondary to renal failure. However, hyperphosphatemia can be the consequence of an increased intake of phosphorus or increased entrance of phosphate into the ECF from tissue breakdown. The causes of hyperphosphatemia are listed in Table 14-1.

Table 14-1

Causes of Hyperphosphatemia

I. Decreased renal excretion of phosphate
   A. Renal insufficiency
      1. Chronic
      2. Acute
   B. Hypoparathyroidism
   C. Pseudohypoparathyroidism
      1. Type I
      2. Type II
   D. Acromegaly
II. Increase in phosphate entrance to ECF
   A. Ingestion of PO_4 salts; intravenous administration of PO_4 salts
   B. Increased catabolism
   C. Neoplastic diseases
      1. Leukemia
      2. Lymphoma
   D. Pharmacologic administration of vitamin D metabolites
III. Miscellaneous
   A. Tumoral calcinosis
   B. Cortical hyperostosis
   C. Intermittent hyperphosphatemia
   D. Artifacts

Differential Diagnosis of Hyperphosphatemia

I. Decreased Renal Excretion of Phosphorus

A. Renal Insufficiency

Serum phosphate levels are maintained within normal limits until GFR values fall to 25–30 ml/min or below. Consequently, if the hyperphosphatemia is due to renal insufficiency, laboratory evidence of decreased GFR (increased serum creatinine and BUN values) will be evident.

The consequences of severe hyperphosphatemia in patients with chronic renal disease are multiple. There is evidence that phosphorus retention plays a key role in the development of secondary hyperparathyroidism. Experimental data in dogs have clearly demonstrated that if phosphorus ingestion is decreased during the development of renal insufficiency, secondary hyperparathyroidism can be prevented. Phosphorus retention may produce changes in ionized calcium with the consequent stimulation of the parathyroid gland. Also serum phosphorus levels may affect the metabolism of vitamin D. Vitamin D is first metabolized by the liver into 25-hydroxycholecalciferol and then by the kidney to its active metabolite, 1,25-dihydroxycholecalciferol. Thus, hyperphosphatemia may produce a fall in ionized calcium not only by precipitation of this ion but also by impairing the absorption of calcium from the intestine by decreasing the formation of 1,25-dihydroxycholecalciferol. A skeletal resistance to the action of PTH also may be a consequence of the decreased production of 1,25-dihydroxycholecalciferol.

In patients maintained on chronic hemodialysis the concentration of serum phosphorus, in general, correlates well with the severity of secondary hyperparathyroidism. It seems that those patients who do not adhere to therapeutic regimens and do not take phosphate binders develop severe and persistent hyperphosphatemia and profound secondary hyperparathyroidism.

Another consequence of the high levels of phosphorus in patients with far-advanced renal disease is the development of severe metastatic calcification. The precipitation of calcium is usually seen around the joints, mainly the hip, wrist, shoulder, and fingers. Vascular calcification sometimes produces ischemic changes, with necrosis and gangrene of the extremities. Precipitation of calcium in the skin may be responsible, in part, for the pruritus, a symptom that is usually seen in patients with far-advanced renal insufficiency.

In general, more drastic changes in serum phosphorus are seen in patients with acute renal failure in whom abrupt cessation of the GFR, profound oliguria, and increased tissue catabolism contribute to phosphate retention. Serum phosphorus in the range of 10–15 mg/100 ml is not unusual in patients with acute renal failure. The degree of hyperphosphatemia varies among patients and in part is related to the cause of the acute renal failure. Usually patients with severe trauma or even nontraumatic rhabdomyolysis may develop profound hyperphosphatemia. Characteristically these patients present low levels of serum calcium presumably due to precipitation in tissues as a consequence of severe hyperphosphatemia and lack of response of the skeleton to the action of parathyroid hormone.

B. Hypoparathyroidism

The most common cause of hypoparathyroidism results from injury of the parathyroid glands or their blood supply during thyroid, parathyroid, or radical neck surgery. Idiopathic hypoparathyroidism is a rare disease. The most striking symptom in patients with hypoparathyroidism is an increase in neuromuscular excitability resulting from a decrease in serum ionized calcium. Some patients may not have severe hypocalcemia and tetany, but increased neuromuscular excitability may be demonstrated by contraction of facial muscles in response to a stimulus over the facial nerve (Chvostek's sign) or by carpal spasm (Trousseau's sign) occurring 2 or 3 minutes after inflating a blood pressure cuff above systolic blood pressure around the arm. In other cases, psychiatric disturbances, paresthesias, numbness, muscle cramps, and dysphagia are also common symptoms.

As indicated before, in the absence of PTH there is an increase in tubular reabsorption of phosphorus by the kidney. Thus the excretion of phosphorus is greatly diminished until the serum phosphorus rises to 6–8 mg/100 ml; then the filtered load of phosphate is increased, and a new equilibrium is reestablished. In the absence of PTH, there is a decrease in osteoclastic activity with a consequent decrease in the mobilization of calcium from bone.

Patients with hypoparathyroidism are easily diagnosed by the presence of a low level of serum calcium, hyperphosphatemia, and undetectable levels of PTH. After several years of hypoparathyroidism other signs may become manifest, such as cataracts and bilateral symmetrical calcification of the basal ganglia on skull x-rays.

C. Pseudohypoparathyroidism

This is a rare condition characterized by end-organ resistance to the action of PTH. Characteristically, the kidney and the skeleton do not respond to the action of PTH. However, patients may have other congenital abnormalities on physical examination, such as short stature, round face, short metacarpal bones and phalanges, and some degree of mental retardation.

Biochemically, they are similiar to patients with hypoparathyroidism, having a low concentration of serum calcium and high serum phosphorus. However, there are two important points in the differential diagnosis. In the majority of patients with pseudohypoparathyroidism the levels of PTH in blood are elevated in contrast to patients with true hypoparathyroidism, in whom PTH is low or absent. Second, patients with pseudohypoparathyroidism are resistant to the administration of exogenous PTH. Characteristically, when exogenous PTH is given to patients with true hypoparathyroidism, they do respond by increasing the excretion of cyclic AMP and phosphate in the urine. However, patients with pseudohypoparathyroidism fail to increase the amount of cyclic AMP or phosphate in the urine. Recently, some patients with a normal response in cyclic AMP excretion in the urine but an absent phosphaturic response after PTH administration have been described. This type of pseudohypoparathyroidism has been named type II in contrast to the classical form which is known as type I pseudohypoparathyroidism.

D. Acromegaly

The hypersecretion of growth hormone may lead to the development of gigantism if the increased secretion occurs prior to the closure of the epiphyses or to acromegaly if excessive hormone secretion occurs after puberty. Acute administration of growth hormone to humans results in a decreased excretion of phosphate within 24 hours. It seems that the changes observed after the administration of growth hormone are not related to the changes in the GFR but to an increased reabsorption of phosphorus by the renal tubules. It is known that the concentration of serum phosphorus in children is higher than in adults, in the range of 5–8 mg/100 ml. It has been postulated that this may be due in part to increased circulating levels of growth hormone. This aspect, however, is still controversial.

II. Increased Entry of Phosphate to the Extracellular Fluid

A. Ingestion and Intravenous Administration of PO_4 Salts

In normal adults, an increase in dietary phosphorus rarely produces hyperphosphatemia; however, it may occur in patients ingesting laxatives containing phosphate salts. Several cases have been described, with patients developing profound hyperphosphatemia and hypocalcemia and some degree of renal insufficiency. In some patients, tetany was also present. Similar episodes of tetany following phosphate enemas have also been reported. In the newborn infant who is fed on cow's milk, hyperphosphatemia may develop and is considered to be an important factor in the genesis of neonatal tetany because the amount of phosphorus contained in cow's milk is much higher than that contained in human milk.

Intravenous phosphate administration has been used in the treatment of hypercalcemia of different etiologies. The administration of phosphate in the amount of 1–2 gm intravenously results in a prompt decrease in the concentration of serum calcium. Since the main mechanism by which phosphate infusion decreases serum calcium concentration is due to its precipitation in different organs and since better agents are now available to treat hypercalcemia, including saline expansion, diuretics, calcitonin, mitramycin, prostaglandin inhibitors, and the like, the author strongly believes that intravenous phosphate administration should be avoided in patients with hypercalcemia.

B. Increased Catabolism

Several conditions in which there is increased protein breakdown such as severe infections or muscle damage after intensive exercise are sometimes accompanied by hyperphosphatemia. Several mechanisms may play a role in these conditions, and hyperphosphatemia is not simply due to the exit of intracellular phosphate into the extracellular space. Hyperphosphatemia has been described in patients with ketoacidosis before treatment. Thus the combination of dehydration, acidosis, and tissue breakdown in different catabolic states is responsible for the development of hyperphosphatemia.

C. Neoplastic Diseases

Hyperphosphatemia has been described in patients with myeloproliferative disorders. Patients treated for lymphoblastic leukemia may develop hyperphosphatemia followed by a concomitant decrease in serum calcium concentration. The phosphate load originates primarily from the destruction of lymphoblasts, which have a greater amount of organic and inorganic phosphorus than mature lymphocytes.

D. Pharmacologic Administration of Vitamin D Metabolites

There is good evidence that vitamin D and its metabolites have a direct effect on phosphate transport across the gastrointestinal tract. Recently, potent metabolites of vitamin D, such as 25-hydroxycholecalciferol, 1,25-dihydroxycholecalciferol, and 1-α-hydroxycholecalciferol, have been used in the treatment of severe abnormalities of bone metabolism. It is possible that some of these metabolites may produce not only calcium but also phosphate mobilization from bone, increasing the entrance of these ions into the ECF. Physicians should be aware that these drugs potentially can produce hyperphosphatemia and ultimately should not be used in the presence of hypercalcemia because of the risk of metastatic calcification.

III. Miscellaneous

There is a series of rare clinical entities (tumoral calcinosis, cortical hyperostosis) that has been associated with hyperphosphatemia. In most of these conditions the mechanism for the development of hyperphosphatemia still remains unknown. The majority of these entities are characterized by hyperphosphatemia, heterotropic calcification around large joints, usually normal levels of PTH, and normal response to the administration of exogenous PTH.

Finally a common artifact that may increase the concentration of phosphate in serum is hemolysis. If the red cells are traumatized during centrifugation and hemolysis occurs, part of the intracellular phosphate will be present in the serum and will be measured as inorganic phosphorus, giving a falsely elevated value.

Clinical Problem

A 41-year-old truck driver was admitted to the hospital because of severe epigastric pain. The patient was in good health until 2 years prior to admission, when he was found to have a duodenal ulcer. Over the past 2 years because of epigastric discomfort the patient had been ingesting large amounts of calcium carbonate. On physical examination the patient was a well-developed, well nourished male in mild acute distress. Blood pressure was 125/75, pulse rate was 82 beats per minute and regular, respirations were 16 per minute, and temperature was 37.2° C. The entire physical examination was unremarkable, except for mild tenderness over the epigastrium. A rectal examination was normal, and stools for guaiac were negative.

On admission, laboratory data revealed the following: hemoglobin value, 14.2 gm; hematocrit, 43%; RBC, 4.8 million; WBC, 6000 with a normal differential; BUN level, 16 mg/100 ml; serum creatinine, 0.9 mg/100 ml; sodium concentration, 139 mEq/liter; chloride, 97 mEq/liter; potassium, 4.2 mEq/liter; carbon dioxide, 25 mEq/liter; serum phosphorus, 5.2 mg/100 ml (normal 2.8–4.5 mg/100 ml); and serum calcium, 11.1 mg/100 ml (normal 9–10.5 mg/l00 ml). Urinalysis, electrocardiogram, and chest x-ray were normal. Upper GI x-ray studies demonstrated a deformed duodenal bulb. The patient was fed a soft diet and received antispasmodic medications; after 2 days in the hospital his symptoms subsided. However, when the serum phosphorus and calcium determinations were repeated, they demonstrated the same abnormalities seen on admission.

Questions

1. What is the most logical explanation for the mild hyperphosphatemia and hypercalcemia observed in this patient?
2. What other laboratory studies should be obtained in the present case?

Discussion

The mild hypercalcemia observed in the patient may be related to the ingestion of the large amounts of calcium carbonate that the patient used for the treatment of abdominal pain. However, calcium carbonate binds phosphorus, so the patient should have had a normal or low level of serum phosphorus and not hyperphosphatemia. Thus, ingestion of calcium carbonate cannot explain both the hypercalcemia and the hyperphosphatemia.

Since the patient's renal function was normal and he did not ingest large amounts of phosphorus in the diet or receive phosphate salts intravenously, hypoparathyroidism may be the cause of the hyperphosphatemia. However, patients with hypoparathyroidism have low levels of serum calcium. Hypocalcemia in this patient may have been masked by the ingestion of large amounts of calcium carbonate in the diet. In order to rule out hypoparathyroidism, PTH levels were determined, and the concentrations were found to be two times above the normal range. Thus, the finding of an increased level of PTH in blood rules out the diagnosis of true hypoparathyroidism.

To further characterize the abnormalities in serum calcium and phosphorus levels, calcium carbonate was discontinued, and after a week serum calcium and phosphorus levels were again determined. At this time, the serum phosphorus level had increased to 6.2 mg/100 ml and the serum calcium level had decreased to 8.2 mg/100 ml. PTH determinations were repeated and found to be five times above the normal level. Thus, when the calcium carbonate was discontinued, the patient developed a picture characterized by hyperphosphatemia, hypocalcemia, and high levels of PTH. In view of these findings, the tubular reabsorption of phosphorus (TRP) was measured and found to be 85%, which is within the normal range. [In the presence of high levels of PTH, one would expect a low TRP (60% to 75%)]. Thus the diagnosis of pseudohypoparathyroidism was suspected. In order to confirm this diagnosis, PTH was injected intravenously to determine if the kidney was resistant to the action of PTH. Cyclic AMP and urinary phosphorus did not increase after the administration of PTH. The diagnosis made was pseudohypoparathyroidism type I, a condition in which the target organs, kidney and bone, are resistant to the action of parathyroid hormone.

Hypophosphatemia

General Considerations

This condition usually results from an increase in urinary phosphorus excretion or a decrease in the gastrointestinal absorption of phosphorus. However, hypophosphatemia also may be seen in a series of metabolic conditions, such as alterations in the metabolism of vitamin D, treatment of diabetic ketoacidosis, and treatment of prolonged malnutrition states.

Patients easily tolerate mild degrees of hypophosphatemia and are usually asymptomatic. However, if profound hypophosphatemia is present with serum phosphorus levels lower than 1.5 mg/100 ml, a series of hematological, neurological, and metabolic disorders may develop. In general the patients become anorectic, develop weakness, and mild bone pain may be present if the hypophosphatemia persists for several months. If the hypophosphatemia is severe, the amount of ATP in red cells and muscle is greatly diminished.

Severe phosphate depletion produces changes in erythrocyte metabolism that may predispose to hemolysis. Several investigators have demonstrated that the amount of 2,3-DPG in red cells is greatly reduced in the presence of profound hypophosphatemia. This compound plays an important role in promoting the release of oxygen from oxyhemoglobin. Other hematological disorders, such as phagocytic activity of leukocytes and platelet disorders, also have been described in the presence of severe hypophosphatemia. Patients with severe hypophosphatemia develop hypercalciuria. Since phosphate depletion promotes the conversion of 25-hydroxycholecalciferol to 1,25-dihydroxycholecalciferol, it is possible that during hypophosphatemia an increase in 1,25-dihydroxycholecalciferol augments calcium absorption from the gastrointestinal tract and calcium resorption from the skeleton, leading to an increase in calcium excretion by the kidney. Hypophosphatemia per se may also increase the absorption of calcium from the gastrointestinal tract. The mechanism is unknown. The mobilization of calcium from bone and the increased intestinal absorption of calcium will decrease the production of PTH. Decreased PTH levels may result in diminished calcium reabsorption by the kidney. All of the above factors may play a role in the development of hypercalciuria during hypophosphatemia. Phosphate depletion has a significant effect on bone, with the mineralization process being greatly impaired.

Differential Diagnosis Of Hypophosphatemia

Table 14-2 lists the causes of hypophosphatemia, which are discussed below.

I. Increased Renal Excretion of Phosphorus

A. Primary Hyperparathyroidism

Primary hyperparathyroidism is seen frequently in clinical medicine. In the majority of cases, a single adenoma is responsible for the increased production of PTH. However, there are cases in which two adenomas have been demonstrated. Chief-cell hyperplasia is less common in patients with primary hyperparathyroidism; however, it is by far the most common cause of secondary hyperparathyroidism. Elevated levels of immunoreactive PTH, hypercalcemia, hypophosphatemia, and a low reabsorption of phosphorus by the kidney are the hallmark of primary hyperparathyroidism.

Patients with primary hyperparathyroidism have a high incidence of gastric ulcer, renal stones, and psychiatric disorders. PTH activates the osteoclasts, which results in increased bone resorption and calcium mobilization. Some patients develop characteristic features in the x-rays, such as subperiosteal resorption of the phalanges, destruction of the clavicles, and profound demineralization. If the patients become hypercalcemic they may develop nausea, anorexia, loss of weight, polyuria, and polydipsia. If the hypercalcemia is severe, mental confusion could also be present, and in some cases there is a decrease in renal function. If the hypercalcemia is not corrected and persists for prolonged periods of time, the patient may develop nephrocalcinosis and impaired renal function. There are cases of primary hyperparathyroidism in which total serum calcium is within the normal range; however, if concomitant levels of ionized calcium and immunoreactive PTH are obtained, the diagnosis of primary hyperparathyroidism can be established in 95% of the cases. The treatment of this condition is surgery.

Table 14-2

Causes of Hypophosphatemia

I. Increased renal excretion of phosphorus
   A. Primary hyperparathyroidism
   B. Secondary hyperparathyroidism
   C. Renal tubular defects
   D. Diuretic phase of ATN
   E. Post-renal transplantation
   F. ECF volume expansion
II. Decrease in gastrointestinal phosphorus absorption
   A. Administration of PO_4 binders
   B. Malabsorption
   C. Starvation—malnutrition
III. Abnormalities in vitamin D metabolism
   A. Vitamin D-deficient rickets
   B. Vitamin D-resistant rickets
   C. Vitamin D-dependent rickets
IV. Miscellaneous
   A. Diabetes mellitus: during treatment for ketoacidosis
   B. Alcohol withdrawal
   C. Recovery phase of malnutrition
   D. Severe respiratory alkalosis

B. Secondary Hyperparathyroidism

The most frequent disease responsible for the development of secondary hyperparathyroidism is chronic renal disease. Hyperphosphatemia, rather than hypophosphatemia, occurs in chronic renal disease as a result of decreased phosphorus excretion via the kidney as GFR falls. However, certain conditions with decreased calcium absorption from the gastrointestinal tract, such as sprue, celiac disease, infiltration of small bowel, and the like, may produce secondary hyperparathyroidism and hypophosphatemia. In secondary hyperparathyroidism, serum calcium is usually low and is the factor that triggers the release of PTH. The levels of PTH may be very elevated, especially in patients with chronic renal disease, since the kidney plays an important role in the degradation of PTH. The levels of immunoreactive PTH may be 100 times normal in patients with chronic renal disease.

C. Renal Tubular Defects

There are many conditions in which the GFR may be normal, but different types of renal tubular defects result in decreased phosphorus reabsorption. In the classical syndrome described by Fanconi, the patients characteristically excrete not only increased amounts of phosphorus in the urine but also increased quantities of glucose, uric acid, and amino acids. There are other conditions in which only a renal tubular defect in phosphate transport is found. The cause of the hypophosphatemia in these conditions is relatively easy to ascertain, since in most of the patients the GFR is normal, and despite normal serum glucose, and low serum phosphorus and uric acid levels, the patient has glycosuria and increased urinary excretion of phosphorus, uric acid, and amino acids.

D. Diuretic Phase of Acute Tubular Necrosis

During the development of ATN, patients develop secondary hyperparathyroidism and phosphate retention. During the diuretic phase of ATN patients may excrete 4 or 5 liters of urine per day. In the presence of profound polyuria, persistent secondary hyperparathyroidism, and the frequent use of PO_4 binders the patients may develop severe hypophosphatemia. Usually the hypophosphatemia is only temporary and reverses back to normal in a very short period of time.

E. Post-Renal Transplantation

After renal transplantation, patients frequently develop profound hypophosphatemia. Since practically all the patients at the time of transplantation have severe secondary hyperparathyroidism, if the transplant is successful the GFR is greatly improved and the high levels of PTH in the blood will decrease the renal reabsorption of phosphorus, with the concomitant development of hypophosphatemia. However, some of these patients may also develop renal tubular defects, and there are patients in whom the hypophosphatemia persists for several years, even in the absence of secondary hyperparathyroidism. Thus the hypophosphatemia seen immediately after transplantation may result from a combination of factors: (1) ingestion of PO_4 binders; (2) secondary hyperparathyroidism; (3) improvement in renal function; and (4) tubular defects. When PO_4 binders are decreased or discontinued and hyperparathyroidism subsides, phosphorus levels return to normal in most patients. However, in some cases, hypophosphatemia does not subside, and this could be due to persistent hyperparathyroidism or to permanent tubular defects.

F. Extracellular Fluid Volume Expansion

Expansion of the extracellular space by the administration of solutions containing sodium will increase the excretion of phosphorus. An important mechanism by which ECF volume expansion produces phosphaturia is due to a dilution of ionized calcium and the release of PTH. However, studies in animals have demonstrated that even if the parathyroid glands are removed, volume expansion will decrease phosphorus reabsorption, and the phosphaturia will persist but be blunted. If this condition exists in clinical medicine, it is not of any importance and subsides when the expansion of the ECF is corrected.

II. Decrease in Gastrointestinal Phosphorus Absorption

A. Administration of PO_4 Binders

Phosphate binders, mainly aluminum salts (aluminum hydroxide, aluminum carbonate gel, and calcium carbonate), are drugs used in the treatment of hyperphosphatemia. However, when these drugs are given in excess, they may produce profound hypophosphatemia. These gels trap phosphorus in the small intestine and increase the amount of phosphorus in the stools. Thus, if the patients treated with phosphate binders are not followed closely, phosphate depletion may occur.

B. Malabsorption

Since most of the phosphorus is absorbed in the small intestine, gastrointestinal disorders, such as celiac disease, tropical and nontropical sprue, regional enteritis, and the like, may cause a decrease in the absorption of phosphorus. The degree of hypophosphatemia varies among patients, being extremely mild in some and severe in others. Recently, phosphorus malabsorption has been described in patients in whom bypass procedures for obesity have been performed. Gastrointestinal manifestations, diarrhea, abdominal pain, and a markedly decreased urinary excretion of phosphorus strongly suggest phosphorus malabsorption as the cause of the hypophosphatemia. Measurement of phosphorus in the stool, when the patients are ingesting a fixed phosphorus diet, will establish the diagnosis.

C. Starvation—Malnutrition

Most of the phosphorus ingested in the diet is present in proteins, especially milk, meat, cheese, eggs, and the like. In many parts of the world where protein consumption is poor, hypophosphatemia occurs. If malnutrition and hypophosphatemia occur in children, their overall growth is greatly diminished, and a series of metabolic disorders can be easily detected.

III. Abnormalities in Vitamin D Metabolism

Vitamin D and its metabolites play a key role in phosphate and calcium metabolism. Physiological amounts of vitamin D in the diet are necessary to maintain the normal mineralization process in bones as well as to increase the intestinal absorption of calcium and phosphorus. If vitamin D is deficient in the diet the amount of osteoid (uncalcified bone) tissue in the skeleton increases, and the normal mineralization front that is observed when bones are labeled with tetracycline is greatly diminished.

A. Vitamin D-Deficient Rickets

Vitamin D-deficient diets are responsible for a metabolic disorder known as rickets when it occurs in children and osteomalacia when it occurs in adults. Vitamin D deficiency in childhood causes severe deformities because of the rapid growth of bones. These deformities are characterized by soft lucent areas in the skull known as craniotabes and costochondral swelling or bending (known as rickettic rosary); the chest usually becomes flattened, and the sternum may be pushed forward to form the so-called pigeon chest. The volume of the thorax may be greatly reduced with impairment in respiratory function. Kyphosis is also frequently seen. There is a remarkable swelling of the joints, especially wrists and ankles, with characteristic anterior bowing of the legs. Fractures of the "green stalk" variety may also be present. In the adult form of the disease, the symptoms are not as striking, and usually are characterized by vague bone pain, weakness, radiolucent areas, and pseudofractures. The pseudofractures represent stress fractures in which the normal process of healing is impaired by the demineralization defect. Mild hypocalcemia may be present. However, hypophosphatemia is by far the most frequent biochemical alteration. This pathological process responds well to small pharmacologic doses of vitamin D. Unfortunately if the treatment is given after the deformities have already occurred, permanent deformities will be seen in these patients.

B. Vitamin D-Resistant Rickets or Familial Hypophosphatemic Rickets

This condition is an X-linked dominant disorder characterized by hypophosphatemia, reduced renal tubular reabsorption of phosphorus, decreased absorption of calcium and inorganic phosphate, and varying degrees of rickets or osteomalacia. The affected males are the homozygotes who exhibit a greater degree of hypophosphatemia and bone disease than the heterozygote females. Two key hypotheses have been postulated to explain this abnormality. The first one has proposed that there is a defect in the conversion of vitamin D to 25-hydroxy D_3. However, recently it has been demonstrated that the levels of 25 (OH) D_3 are normal in this condition. Furthermore, administration of 25 (OH) D_3 or 1,25 $(OH)_2$ D_3 does not correct the hypophosphatemia. The second hypothesis is that X-linked hypophosphatemic rickets results primarily from a defect in the reabsorption of inorganic phosphorus by the kidney and intestinal mucosa with subsequent malabsorption and renal phosphate wasting. There is some evidence that indicates that the decreased tubular reabsorption of phosphorus is not due primarily to an increase in PTH levels. It seems that a component of renal phosphate transport, which may be calcium-mediated, PTH-independent, may be abnormal and responsible for the increased phosphaturia.

C. Vitamin D-Dependent Rickets

This is a recessively inherited form of vitamin D refractory rickets. This condition is also characterized by hypophosphatemia, hypocalcemia, elevated levels of serum alkaline phosphatase, and sometimes generalized aminoaciduria and severe rickettic bone lesions. This condition usually responds to massive doses of vitamin D. Two main theories could explain the vitamin D-dependent state in this disease. One could be defective conversion of vitamin D into active metabolites and second, a defective ability of the target organs to respond to physiologic concentrations of vitamin D. Recently, it has been suggested that in this condition there is a genetic defect in the 25-hydroxycholecalciferol 1 hydroxylase D_3, the enzyme responsible for the production of 1,25 $(OH)_2$ D_3. When physiologic amounts of 1,25 $(OH)_2$ D_3 are given to patients with vitamin D-dependent rickets, serum phosphorus and calcium concentrations promptly return to normal. The pathogenesis of these genetic disorders should be interpreted with caution, since current research in the field of vitamin D is still providing new answers and modes of action for different metabolites of vitamin D. However, it is clear that several of these conditions could be easily reversed by modest pharmacologic doses of 1,25 $(OH)_2$ D_3, as in vitamin D-dependent rickets. On the other hand, it seems that a tubular defect may be the most logical explanation for vitamin D-resistant rickets.

IV. Miscellaneous

A. Diabetes Mellitus

When diabetes mellitus is poorly controlled and patients develop profound ketoacidosis, mild hyperphosphatemia and increased phosphorus excretion in the urine occur. However, when insulin is given and correction of the ketoacidosis occurs, serum phosphorus levels decrease rapidly and urinary phosphate excretion falls. A significant amount of phosphate enters the intracellular space, and some patients develop profound hypophosphatemia and profound weakness, presumably due to hypophosphatemia. Correction of the hypophosphatemia leads to the disappearance of these symptoms.

B. Alcohol Withdrawal

The pathogenesis of hypophosphatemia that is observed in some patients during alcohol withdrawal is not fully understood. The previous state of nutrition plays an important role in the development of hypophosphatemia. Many alcoholics develop borderline hypophosphatemia as a result of poor dietary intake or decreased phosphorus absorption. However, during treatment with glucose solutions, alcoholic patients may develop marked hypophosphatemia.

C. Recovery Phase of Malnutrition

Findings similar to those described above have been observed in patients with profound malnutrition who are receiving hyperalimentation without adequate phosphorus replacement. This condition is seen especially when the malnutrition is corrected by administration of large amounts of carbohydrates and low concentrations of proteins. It is critical that during dietary replacement in malnourished patients with high caloric diets substantial amounts of phosphorus be added to the diet to prevent the development of profound hypophosphatemia.

D. Severe Respiratory Alkalosis

Severe and prolonged respiratory alkalosis may be associated with profound hypophosphatemia. During respiratory alkalosis the amount of phosphorus excreted in the urine is greatly diminished. In contrast, patients receiving sodium bicarbonate intravenously may also develop hypophosphatemia, but in this condition there is an increase in urinary phosphorus excretion. It has been postulated that in respiratory alkalosis there is an increase in intracellular pH with activation of glycolysis and increased formation of phosphorylated carbohydrate compounds leading to a precipitous fall in serum phosphorus concentration. However, the hypophosphatemia produced by the administration of bicarbonate and the consequent development of metabolic alkalosis has been shown to be mainly secondary to a decrease in serum ionized calcium and release of parathyroid hormone.

Clinical Problem

H. W., a 54-year-old male, was admittd to the hospital because of weight loss, anorexia, nausea, vomiting, and mental confusion. The patient was apparently in good health until approximately 5 months prior to the present admission. He had had a hernia operation 10 years ago but otherwise was in good health and had never sought medical attention. On admission, he appeared chronically ill, dehydrated, and confused. He could not remember the name of the hospital nor the month of the year. On physical examination, his blood pressure was 130/85; pulse rate, 78 beats per minute and regular; respirations, 17 per minute; and temperature, 37.4° C. His physical examination was entirely within normal limits. Laboratory data revealed a normal hemoglobin value and hematocrit reading, normal electrolytes, a BUN of 25 mg/100 ml, and a serum creatinine of 1.3 mg/100 ml. Serum calcium concentration was 16 mg/100 ml; serum phosphorus, 1.5 mg/100 ml; and alkaline phosphatase, 98 units (upper limit of normal 85). His electrocardiogram was consistent with hypercalcemia but otherwise normal, chest x-ray was normal, and urinalysis was normal.

Questions

1. What is the most likely explanation for the symptoms and signs observed in this patient?
2. What other laboratory data should be obtained?

Discussion

Because of the hypercalcemia and hypophosphatemia without any other abnormalities in his electrolytes, chest x-ray, or urinalysis, primary hyperparathyroidism was suspected. Levels of immunoreactive PTH in blood were not determined. A surgeon, called in on consultation, advised that the patient undergo neck exploration and subtotal parathyroidectomy for the treatment of hypercalcemia. Prior to surgery, however, the patient received large amounts of saline and furosemide intravenously. With this regimen the serum calcium concentration was reduced to 12 mg/100 ml after 24 hours. Two days after admission to the hospital the patient had a neck exploration, and four normal parathyroid glands were found. However, one was removed, and histological examination revealed a normal architecture. Following surgery, there was no noticeable change in serum calcium or phosphorus levels. The patient was then transferred to Barnes Hospital for further studies. Laboratory findings were obtained at Barnes on admission and revealed a calcium concentration of 12.5 mg/100 ml and a phosphorus concentration of 1.8 mg/100 ml. Levels of PTH in blood were measured and found to be only slightly elevated.

This patient presents an interesting problem that biochemically is consistent with hyperparathyroidism. However, the radioimmunoassay for PTH revealed only a mild elevation in the blood levels of the hormone (14 μlEq/ml, normal is 10 μlEq/ml or less). If the patient had primary hyperparathyroidism, the PTH levels should be high, perhaps three to six times above normal. These findings, plus the history of normal histology of the parathyroid gland excised previously, rule out primary hyperparathyroidism. One wonders why the hypercalcemia did not suppress the release of PTH from the glands, in which case his blood PTH levels would be undetectable instead of slightly elevated. It is possible that we are dealing with a patient with an ectopic parathyroid-secreting tumor. Certain tumors may produce a peptide that biologically behaves like PTH increasing renal phosphorus excretion and bone resorption and thus leading to hypophosphatemia and hypercalcemia. However, this peptide may be immunologically different from the hormone secreted by the parathyroid glands; thus, when it is measured with the radioimmunoassay, the levels of PTH may be only slightly elevated because the PTH-like peptide is poorly recognized by the antibody used in this determination.

A complete workup was performed in the patient, including an IVP that revealed a mass in the right kidney. An arteriogram was performed and was consistent with the diagnosis of carcinoma of the right kidney. A right nephrectomy was performed without complications. Three days after surgery, the serum phosphorus and the serum calcium levels returned to normal. This patient illustrates the production of ectopic PTH-like material by a carcinoma of the kidney.

References

Agus, Z. S., Puschett, J. B., Seneskry, D., and Goldberg, M. "Mode of action of cyclic adenosine-3′,5′-monophosphate on renal tubular phosphate reabsorption in the dog." J. Clin. Invest. *50:* 617, 1971.

Amiel, C., Kuntziger, H., and Richet, G. "Micropuncture study of handling of phosphate by proximal and distal nephron in normal and parathyroidectomized rat. Evidence for distal reabsorption." Pflugers Arch. *317:* 93, 1970.

Beck, L. H., and Goldberg, M. "Mechanism of the blunted phosphaturia in saline-loaded thyroparathyroidectomized dogs." Kidney Int. *6:* 18, 1974.

Breuer, R. J., and LeBauer, J. "Caution in the use of phosphates in the treatment of severe hypercalcemia." J. Clin. Endocrin. *27:* 695, 1967.

Brickman, A. S., Coburn, J. W., and Norman, A. "Action of 1,25-dihydroxycholecalciferol, a potent kidney-produced metabolite of vitamin D_3 in uremic man." N. Engl. J. Med. *287:* 3, 1972.

Chase, L. R., Melson, G. L., and Auerbach, G. D. "Pseudohypoparathyroidism: Defective excretion of 3′,5′-AMP in response to parathyroid hormone." J. Clin. Invest. *48:* 1832, 1969.

Chen, T. C., Costillo, L., Korycka-Dahl, M., and DeLuca, H. "Role of vitamin D metabolites in phosphate transport of rat intestine." J. Nutr. *104:* 1056, 1974.

Corredor, D. G., Sabeh, G., Mendelsohn, L. D., Wasserman, R. E., Sunder, J. H., and Danowski, T. S. "Enhanced post glucose hypophosphatemia during starvation therapy of obesity." Metabolism *18:* 754, 1969.

Fuller, T. J., Carter, N. W., Barcenas, C., and Knochel, J. P. "Reversible changes of the muscle cell in experimental phosphorus deficiency." J. Clin. Invest. *57:* 1019, 1976.

Goldsmith, R. S., and Ingbar, S. H. "Inorganic phosphate treatment of hypercalcemia of diverse etiologies." N. Engl. J. Med. *274:* 1, 1966.

Gradowska, L., Caglar, S., Rutherford, W. E., Harter, H., and Slatopolosky, E. "On the mechanism of the phosphaturia of extracellular fluid volume expansion in the dog." Kidney Int. *3:* 230, 1973.

Kalbfleisch, J. M., Lindeman, R. D., Ginn, H. E., and Smith, W. O. "The effects of ethanol administration on urinary excretion of magnesium and other electrolytes in alcoholic and normal subjects." J. Clin. Invest. *42:* 1471, 1963.

Knochel, J. P. "The pathophysiology and clinical characteristics of severe hypophosphatemia." Arch. Intern. Med. *137*: 203, 1977.

Kowarski, S., and Schachter, D. "Effects of vitamin D on phosphate transport and incorporation into mucosal constituents of rat intestinal mucosa." J. Biol. Chem. *244:* 211, 1969.

Lotz, M., Zisman, E., and Bartter, F. C. "Evidence for a phosphorus depletion syndrome in man." N. Engl. J. Med. *278:* 409, 1968.

Mercado, A., Slatopolsky, E., and Klahr, S. "On the mechanisms responsible for the phosphaturia of bicarbonate administration." J. Clin. Invest. *56:* 1386, 1975.

Oppe, T. E., and Redstone, D. "Calcium and phosphorus levels in healthy newborn infants given various types of milk." Lancet *1:* 1045, 1968.

Popovtzer, M. M., Robinette, J. B., DeLuca, H. F., and Holick, M. F. "The acute effect of 25-hydroxycholecalciferol on renal handling of phosphorus." J. Clin. Invest. *53:* 913, 1974.

Puschett, J. B., Beck, W. S., Jr., Jelonek, S., and Fernandez, P. C. "Study of the renal tubular interactions of thyrocalcitonin, cyclic adenosine-3′,5′-monophosphate, 25-hydroxycholecalciferol, and calcium ion." J. Clin. Invest. *53:* 756, 1974.

Rodriquez, H. J., Villarreal, H., Jr., Klahr, S., and Slatopolsky, E. "Pseudohypoparathyroidism Type II. Restoration of normal renal responsiveness to parathyroid hormone by calcium administration." J. Clin. Endocrinol. Metab. *39:* 693, 1974.

Slatopolsky, E., Caglar, S., Pennell, J. P., Taggart, D. D., Canterbury, J. M., Reiss, E., and Bricker, N. "On the pathogenesis of hyperparathyroidism in chronic experimental renal insufficiency in the dog." J. Clin. Invest. *50:* 492, 1971.

Territo, M. C., and Tanaka, K. R. "Hypophosphatemia in chronic alcoholism." Arch. Intern. Med. *134:* 445, 1974.

Travis, S. F., Sugerman, H. J., Ruberg, R. L., Dudrick, S. J., Delivoria-Papadopoulos, M., Miller, L. D., and Oski, F. A. "Alterations of red cell glycolytic intermediates and oxygen transport as a consequence of hypophosphatemia in patients receiving intravenous hyperalimentation." N. Engl. J. Med. *285:* 763, 1971.

Yawata, Y., Hebbel, R. P., Silvis, S., Howe, R., and Jacob, H. "Blood cell abnormalities complicating the hypophosphatemia of hyperalimentation: Erythrocytes and platelet ATP deficiency associated with hemolytic anemia and bleeding in hyperalimented dogs." J. Lab. Clin. Med. *84:* 643, 1974.

Zusman, J., Brown, D., and Nesbit, M. "Hyperphosphatemia, hyperphosphaturia, and hypocalcemia in acute lymphoblastic leukemia." N. Engl. J. Med. *289:* 1336, 1973.

Chapter 15

Alterations of Serum Potassium Concentration

General Considerations

Potassium is an essential cation located predominantly in the intracellular space. Total body potassium is roughly 3600 mEq, with the ECF space containing only 65–70 mEq. Muscle mass contains approximately 3000 mEq of potassium; the liver, 200 mEq; and red cells, 300 mEq. Approximately 100 mEq of potassium is ingested in the average American diet per day. Under normal circumstances, 90% of this amount is excreted by the kidney (80–90 mEq/day), and the stools will contain 10% (8–15 mEq/day). Because potassium is located primarily in the intracellular space (98%), it is difficult to fully monitor any changes in body stores of this cation.

The intracellular location of potassium is critical in the maintenance of an electrical potential difference between the extracellular and intracellular spaces. This electrical gradient is maintained by the active movement of potassium into and sodium out of the cell by a coupled pump referred to as the sodium-potassium pump. While the intracellular concentration of potassium is approximately 150 mEq/liter, the amount that is freely exchangeable is considerably less than that, probably in the range of 40–50 mEq/liter. Maintenance of the intracellular concentrations of potassium and sodium is dependent upon the presence of adequate amounts of adenosine triphosphate (ATP) and on the activity of an ATPase in the cell membrane, with selective affinity for sodium or potassium, which hydrolyzes ATP and is referred to as the sodium-potassium dependent ATPase pump.

Conducting tissues are polarized, with the cell being negative on the inside and positively charged on the outside. This activity across the membrane is referred to as the potential difference (PD) and is quantitatively described by the Nernst equation [$PD = -61(\log Ki/Ko)$]. Ki refers to the intracellular potassium concentration, while Ko refers to the extracellular potassium concentration. The normal potential difference in resting tissue is approximately –80 to –90 mv. This is an index of the irritability of contractile tissue, and during muscle contraction or nerve conduction, potassium moves out of the cell and sodium moves into the cell. The force of contraction or the rate of conduction of nerve impulses is directly proportional to the generation of the electrical potential, which is dependent upon the intracellular and extracellular potassium concentrations. Variations in the ratio between intracellular and extracellular potassium will critically affect muscle and nervous activity.

Since the maintenance of the intracellular potassium concentration is presumably dependent upon the sodium-potassium ATPase pump, anything that affects the activity of this pump will affect this ratio. Some factors known to affect this pump include concentrations of magnesium, sodium, and potassium. For instance, high extracellular potassium concentrations will tend to depress the sodium-potassium pump. Certain drugs may directly inhibit the activity of the pump, including the cardiac glycosides and also diuretics such as ethacrynic acid and furosemide.

Regulation of Body Potassium

Potassium is handled primarily by the kidney. Although sweat may contain potassium concentrations of 10–15 mEq/liter and the concentration is responsive to aldosterone, the amount of potassium lost per day via this route is usually negligible. Stool losses of potassium average about 10 mEq/day, and, except under conditions in which there is an excessive loss of diarrheal fluid, are not a major mechanism for potassium loss. Thus the kidney becomes the critical regulating organ.

Potassium is freely filtered at the glomerulus. The proximal tubule reabsorbs approximately 60% to 70% of the filtered load of potassium. The majority of the reabsorption is passive following the bulk reabsorption of salt and water in this portion of the nephron. Recent evidence would suggest that a certain portion of the potassium is actively reabsorbed. The thin segments of Henle's loop do not contribute greatly to potassium reabsorption. The only change that does occur is probably a result of the concentration gradients generated in the medullary interstitium. The thick ascending limb, on the other hand, may account for the reabsorption of 10% to 15% of the filtered load of potassium. Reabsorption in this segment is presumed to be passive following electrical gradients generated by the active reabsorption of chloride.

Final regulation of urinary potassium excretion occurs in the distal tubule and collecting duct. Figure 15-1 is a schematic representation of a distal tubular cell and depicts the postulated pathways of potassium secretion. The distal tubular cell, for the purposes of discussion, is illustrated as having two pumps at the peritubular side.

Pump 1 is considered to be a coupled sodium-potassium pump and, as outlined above, is referred to as the sodium-potassium ATPase pump. Its primary activity is presumably related to the maintenance of intracellular cation composition, extruding sodium from the cell interior to the peritubular capillary, and taking up potassium into the cell from the peritubular capillary. The activity of this pump may be affected by different agents, such as aldosterone, insulin, diuretic agents, and digitalis, and will determine, along with other

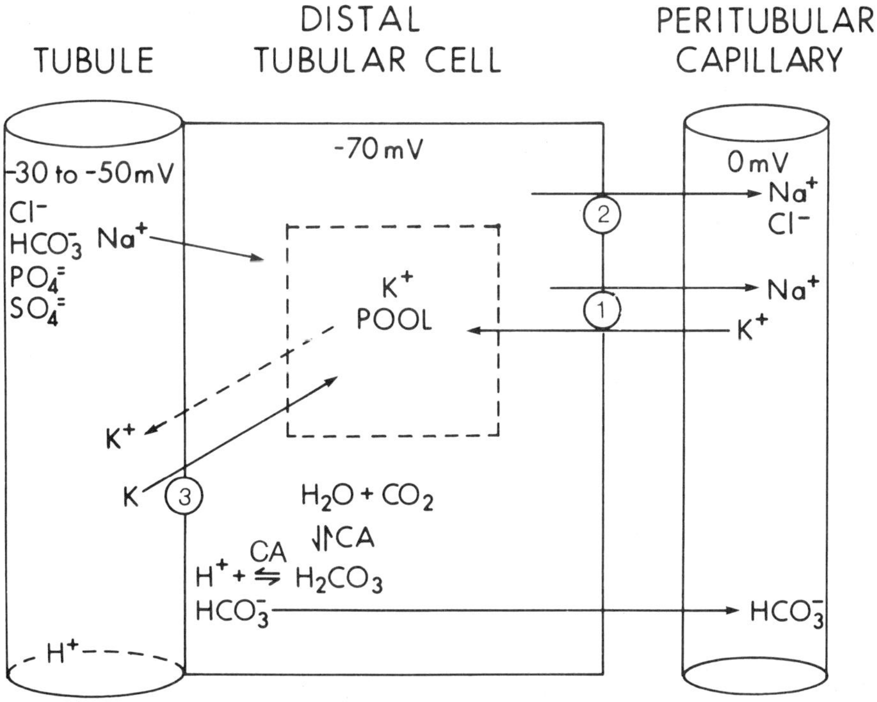

Fig. 15-1.

Postulated pathways of potassium secretion in distal tubular cells of the kidney.

factors to be discussed later, the size of the intracellular potassium pool, which in turn will determine the amount of potassium secreted into the final urine. Thus the activity of the sodium-potassium ATPase pump is critical to potassium homeostasis.

Pump 2 is considered to be an electrogenic sodium pump, presumably responsible for sodium chloride reabsorption. As sodium is actively reabsorbed from the tubular lumen, a potential difference (lumen negative) develops. The magnitude of the potential difference depends primarily on sodium reabsorption but also on the relative concentrations of chloride, bicarbonate, phosphate, and sulfate present in the distal tubule and on the rate of potassium and hydrogen secretion into the tubular lumen. This negativity of the tubular lumen will allow for the passive movement of potassium from the distal tubular cell interior down its electrochemical gradient into the tubular lumen. Increased sodium reabsorption or a rise in impermeant anions will increase the lumen negativity and favor potassium or hydrogen secretion into the tubular fluid.

The final regulation of potassium excretion presumably depends on a pump (pump 3) capable of reabsorbing potassium from the tubular lumen back into the cell interior. The important parameters affecting potassium secretion by the distal tubule will depend upon factors affecting the three pumps and the concentration of potassium and hydrogen within the distal tubular cell.

When potassium intake is increased, secretion of potassium in the distal nephron increases proportionately to maintain homeostasis. On the other hand, under conditions of extremely low potassium intake, reabsorption of this cation may continue along the distal nephron to prevent excessive losses of potassium. However, even with potassium depletion the urinary excretion of potassium seldom falls below 10 mEq/day. Thus, continuing potassium losses may occur despite hypokalemia.

Reabsorption of potassium has not been fully defined for the collecting duct. It is obvious, however, that this portion of the nephron plays a major role in potassium homeostasis. From the available literature, it is concluded that net addition of potassium to the collecting duct occurs and may be responsive to aldosterone. Furthermore, significant reabsorption of potassium occurs along this segment of the nephron. Reabsorption of potassium in the collecting duct appears to be tightly coupled to sodium excretion. The difficulty in interpreting the contributions of the collecting duct and the distal tubule to potassium homeostasis relates partially to species differences.

The data presented above are predominantly those obtained from micropuncture, microperfusion, or isolated nephron segment studies. There are some difficulties in interpreting the data now available, since two nephron populations exist. Micropuncture and microperfusion studies have examined the role of proximal and distal tubules of superficial cortical nephrons. The exact function of the deeper juxtamedullary nephrons in potassium handling has not been fully delineated. Excretion of potassium in the final urine obviously reflects the functional capabilities of both nephron populations.

Factors Responsible for the Renal Regulation of Potassium Excretion

Excretion of potassium by the kidney is dependent upon many factors, including acid-base status, anion excretion, urine flow rate, and potassium intake.

Acid-Base Status

Acid-base balance is critical in potassium homeostasis. The secretion of distal tubular potassium is affected by the rate of hydrogen secretion. During acidosis, intracellular potassium concentrations will fall and hydrogen ion concentrations will rise in response to an intracellular shift of this ion. Since sodium reabsorption continues, creating a negative tubular lumen, it will obligate the secretion of hydrogen, and relatively less potassium will be excreted in the urine during acidosis despite hyperkalemia. On the other hand, under conditions of alkalosis, hydrogen will move out of the cell and potassium will therefore move into the cell, producing a relatively increased intracellular pool of potassium. This will allow for more potassium and less hydrogen loss in the urine, despite a decreased plasma potassium concentration.

Nonreabsorbable Anions

Potassium secretion into the distal tubular lumen is predominantly a passive phenomenon, with the potassium ion moving down an electrochemical gradient generated by the reabsorption of sodium and the greater concentration of potassium in the cell interior as compared to the tubular lumen. As the positively charged sodium is actively reabsorbed, negatively charged anions (poorly reabsorbed) are left behind. This will result in an increase in the lumen negativity and favor the movement of the positively charged potassium ions. If there are increased amounts of nonreabsorbable or poorly reabsorbable anions present within the lumen of the distal tubule, the negative electrical gradient will increase, allowing for more potassium loss. Therefore, under conditions in which excessive amounts of bicarbonate, sulfate, phosphate, or the like are delivered to the distal tubule, increased amounts of potassium are excreted in the urine.

Urine Flow Rate

Fluid flow rate in the distal tubule is critical to the excretion of potassium. Under conditions of rapid fluid movement, with excessive urinary losses of salt and water, potassium losses with increase. On the other hand, under conditions of dehydration with slow urine flows, less sodium and potassium are lost. The mechanism for this altered excretion of potassium will increased distal tubular flow is not entirely clear but may relate to either the amount of sodium reabsorbed or maintenance of a high chemical gradient for potassium along the distal tubule due to the rapid removal and low concentrations of tubular lumen potassium. While potassium homeostasis is dependent upon urine flow rates, it is not necessarily dependent upon the GFR, except when the latter is extremely reduced. Potassium balance will be maintained despite significant reductions in the GFR, with the amount of excreted potassium actually exceeding the filtered load (filtered load = GRF × plasma concentration of potassium).

Intracellular Potassium Concentrations

As is obvious from the above discussion, potassium secretion in the distal nephron is dependent primarily upon the intracellular potassium concentration and on the electrical gradient generated by sodium reabsorption. Any factor that affects the intracellular potassium concentration will, of necessity, affect potassium secretion. For instance, when increased amounts of potassium are ingested, regulatory factors come into play and intracellular potassium concentrations will rise, thus allowing for increased losses. The regulatory factors that may affect intracellular potassium during ingestion of large amounts of this ion include both aldosterone, which is directly stimulated by the potassium concentration, and insulin, which may play a critical role in the acute shift of potassium from extracellular to intracellular compartments. Both hormones tend to increase intracellular potassium concentration, presumably by stimulating sodium-potassium ATPase pump mechanisms (pump 1, Fig. 15-1). While acute compensation after excessive amounts of administered potassium may be due to several factors, aldosterone plays one of the major roles in regulating potassium excretion by the distal nephron and the collecting duct. Aldosterone will increase sodium transport across cell membranes and increase potassium uptake by cells. Thus the net effect of excessive amounts of aldosterone is to augment sodium reabsorption, increase intracellular potassium concentrations, and therefore promote potassium losses, leading to a volume expanded state associated with hypokalemia. Similar, although less marked, changes are produced by corticosterone, as might be seen in patients with Cushing's syndrome.

Hypokalemia

General Considerations

Hypokalemia is usually defined as a plasma potassium concentration of less than 3.5 mEq/liter. Hypokalemia may be relative or absolute. Relative hypokalemia is present when changes in acid-base balance cause potassium shifts into the cells, so that total body potassium may, in fact, be normal, but plasma concentrations are depressed. Absolute hypokalemia, on the other hand, reflects a fall in both intracellular and extracellular potassium concentrations.

One of the frequent laboratory findings seen concomitantly with hypokalemia is metabolic alkalosis. A brief discussion of its etiology is included here. Figure 15-2 depicts the sequence of events leading to hypokalemic alkalosis. As potassium is lost from the ECF space, potassium shifts from the ICF to the ECF space, producing a decrease in intracellular potassium concentration. In order to maintain electroneutrality, both sodium and hydrogen ions will move into the intracellular space. This process occurs essentially in all tissues and produces two results. First, the movement of hydrogen from the ECF to the ICF will leave an unbuffered base in the ECF, causing mild alkalosis. Second, sodium ions will also move into the intracellular space, causing movement of water from ECF to ICF and contraction of the ECF, further increasing the apparent alkalosis.

The main effects of hypokalemia, however, occur at the level of the kidney. A process similar to that seen in other body tissues occurs in the renal tubular cells, leading to a decrease in intracellular potassium. Since sodium reabsorption continues to maintain ECF volume as hydrogen moves into tubular cells and intracellular potassium decreases, hydrogen ion rather than potassium will be lost in the urine. As will be described in Chapter 16, the hydrogen generated within the distal tubular cells comes from carbonic acid. For every hydrogen produced, one bicarbonate is generated. The hydrogen secreted into the urine is trapped by ammonia or phosphate and is lost. The bicarbonate thus generated moves into the ECF, producing the observed alkalosis. Correction of this alkalosis obviously requires the replacement of potassium, and, on occasion, chloride, body stores of which may also be depleted.

Clinical Features and Systemic Effects of Hypokalemia

The organ systems most significantly affected by hypokalemia include skeletal muscle, heart, kidneys, and the gastrointestinal tract. Potassium directly affects the irritability of all contractile tissues, since the resting membrane potential is a direct function of the natural logarithm of the ratio of the concentration of potassium within the cell to potassium outside the cell. In conditions in which extracellular potassium concentrations fall acutely, there may be increased irritability. On the other hand, when chronic, prolonged loss of potassium occurs, both intracellular and extracellular potassium concentrations fall and irritability may not be significantly affected. Although tetany has been described in acute potassium losses, the most frequent physical finding in patients with profound hypokalemia is one of muscle weakness leading to paralysis. Most patients presenting with plasma potassium levels of 2.5 mEq/liter or less will complain of moderate muscle weakness. As the plasma levels of potassium fall below 1.5 mEq/liter, a condition of areflexic paralysis may

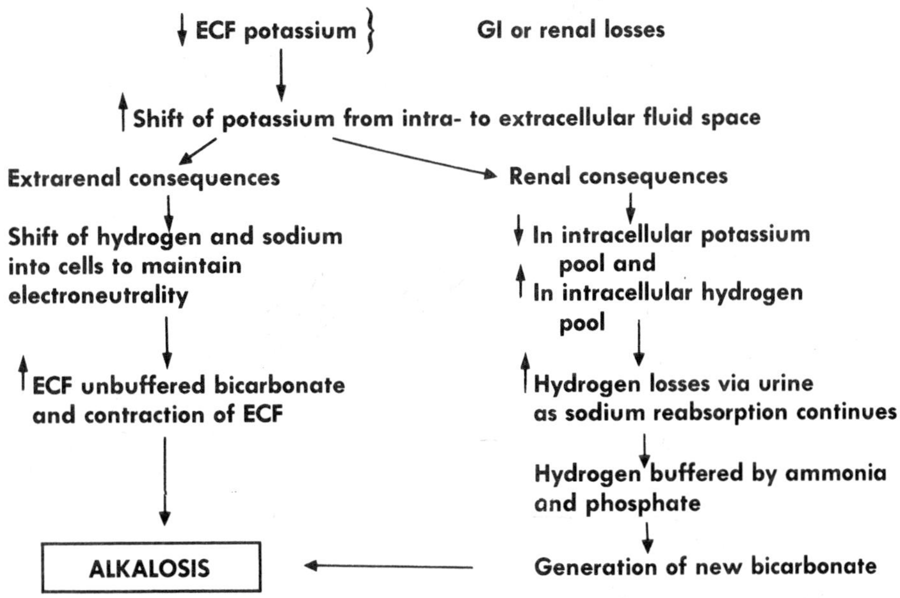

Fig. 15-2.

Generation of metabolic alkalosis as a complication of hypokalemia.

occur. At this point, respiratory depression may be an immediate threat to survival. While the rate at which hypokalemia develops will have the major effect on muscle activity (e.g., more rapid potassium loss will lead to a more severe weakness), extreme potassium depletion under any circumstance will lead to profound weakness and paralysis. Myoglobinuria may be a consequence of severe, acute hypokalemia.

Potassium significantly affects cardiac function. Changes in cardiac function will depend upon whether there is (1) a change in only the extracellular potassium; (2) a small change in the intracellular potassium; or (3) a large change in the intracellular potassium. Acute, purely extracellular potassium loss is rare and is infrequently seen in clinical circumstances. However, it may occur during brisk diuresis or with other excessive urinary losses of potassium. These acute potassium losses may cause hyperpolarization, since intracellular potassium may remain normal as extracellular potassium falls. This situation will lead to premature ventricular contractions, frequent ectopic tachycardias, and widening of the QRS complex. With small changes in intracellular potassium concentration, cardiac output begins to fall, since the force of myocardial contractility is dependent upon the intracellular potassium concentration. While this may not be clinically evident, significant changes in the electrocardiogram may be present, including early depression of the ST segment with a decreased amplitude of the T wave. U waves may also be present, as well as first-degree A-V block. In patients who have severe depletion of intracardiac potassium concentration, accentuation of the above electrocardiographic changes are seen, with total flattening of the ST segment, absence of the T wave, prominent U waves, significant widening of the QRS complex, and second- or even third-degree A-V block. Furthermore, as the intracellular potassium concentration falls, contractility progressively decreases, leading to marked ventricular irregularity and profound heart failure. These extremely large losses of potassium are associated with abnormalities in structure as well as function, causing swelling of the myocardial cell with intrinsic damage of the myocardial fiber as concentrations of potassium fall below 2 mEq/liter in plasma.

Under most circumstances, mild changes in plasma potassium are well tolerated and generate little cardiovascular change. It must be remembered, however, that patients receiving digitalis are extremely prone to the cardiac complications of hypokalemia and may present with significant cardiac irregularity, acute digitalis intoxication, and fatal arrhythmias, with only modest losses in total body potassium.

Potassium depletion also affects the gastrointestinal tract by decreasing gastric and small intestinal motility and, at times, may lead to a paralytic ileus.

Severe prolonged potassium depletion also produces characteristic structural and functional disturbances in the kidney, but usually several months are required for significant renal impairment to occur. Histological changes in the kidney include multiple vacuoles in the proximal tubular epithelium. In profound hypokalemia, there is inability to concentrate the urine, even after prolonged water restriction. On the other hand, diluting capabilities are well maintained. Mechanisms associated with inability to concentrate the urine may relate to an inability to maintain normal medullary hypertonicity or to an impaired response to antidiuretic hormone. Patients will complain of polyuria, polydipsia, and nocturia. There is also an increased incidence of pyelonephritis in these individuals.

The previous paragraphs have outlined the major clinical manifestations associated with mild to severe hypokalemia. When reviewing the section on differential diagnosis for causes of hypokalemia, pertinent historical and physical findings will be obvious. In general, however, the patient with significant hypokalemia will present with complaints of weakness, constipation, polyuria, and polydipsia. Patients may also present with complaints of tingling or localized neurological defects associated with moderate hypokalemia. Symptoms of congestive heart failure, palpitations, or tachycardia will also be manifest if severe hypokalemia is present.

On physical examination, the patients will usually appear fatigued and lethargic. Blood pressures will most often be normal or slightly depressed, relating to the degree of depression of cardiac output. Hypertension may be present if the cause of hypokalemia is hyperaldosteronism, Cushing's syndrome, or if the patient has been treated with diuretics for hypertension. Pulses will be variable, depending upon the presence of arrhythmias, tachycardias, or A-V block. Patients with hypertension, depending upon cause, may present with grade II to IV retinopathy according to the Kirkendall-Armstrong classification. Chest examination will reveal clear lung fields in the absence of congestive heart failure, although hyporespiration may be present if the potassium depletion is severe. Cardiac examination may reveal increased cardiac size if severe potassium depletion or significant hypertension is present. An atrial or ventricular diastolic gallop may be present. Significant arrhythmias, either atrial or ventricular, may be present with or without the presence of ectopic tachycardias. Abdominal examination is usually negative in the absence of specific gastrointestinal complaints, although hypoactivity of bowel sounds or paralytic ileus may be present if the potassium depletion is severe. Peripheral examination will reveal evidence of diffuse muscle weakness with strength decreased symmetrically under most circumstances. Significant muscle pain may be present in patients who have severe acute potassium depletion associated with myoglobinuria. Otherwise, palpation of the muscles is usually negative. There also may be edema of the lower extremities associated with evidence of congestive heart failure. Neurological examination will typically reveal hyporeflexia and, as the degree of hypokalemia becomes more severe, areflexia and paralysis. When paralysis is present, evidence of seizure or severe mental obtundation may also be present.

Differential Diagnosis of Hypokalemia

Table 15-1 lists the causes of hypokalemia, which are discussed below.

I. Gastrointestinal Causes

A. Decreased Potassium Intake

Although it is rare, hypokalemia may occur because of markedly decreased potassium intake. For significant hypokalemia and potassium depletion to occur, however, depressed intake must take place over a prolonged period of time, since only 10–15 mEq/day are lost obligatorily in the urine. It would be very difficult to decrease potassium intake to this level except in extreme starvation or in patients with anorexia nervosa. Since potassium content is high in meats, in fruits such as bananas and tomatoes, and in vegetables such as spinach and potatoes, complete abstinence from these foods would be required to produce hypokalemia.

B. Loss of Hydrochloric Acid

A more common cause of potassium depletion is persistent vomiting from conditions such as pyloric stenosis or persistent gastroenteritis or from gastric suction without adequate replacement of potassium. The usual concentration of potassium in gastric contents is approximately 15 mEq/liter, which would not explain the degree of hypokalemia seen in these patients. A more important consequence of either vomiting or gastric aspiration, however, is the loss of fixed acid. Hydrogen ion secreted by the stomach is produced by the hydration of carbon dioxide to carbonic acid, a reaction catalyzed by the enzyme carbonic anhydrase. For every hydrogen secreted into the gastric lumen, one bicarbonate is produced and reabsorbed into the plasma. Thus, in patients with accelerated hydrogen loss from gastric contents, excessive amounts of unbuffered bicarbonate will enter the plasma, producing systemic alkalosis. As hydrogen moves from the intracellular to the extracellular space to buffer the bicarbonate, potassium moves into the intracellular space, increasing the intracellular potassium concentration. This shift, as discussed before, will significantly augment urinary potassium excretion. Furthermore, since volume depletion also occurs, aldosterone secretion will increase, further accelerating urinary potassium losses. Thus, in patients with vomiting or gastric aspiration, a hyperkaliuric state persists despite hypokalemia. The renal losses of potassium can be marked, depending upon the amount of hydrogen lost by gastric aspiration.

C. Defective Potassium Absorption

Any condition associated with rapid gastrointestinal transit may be associated with defective absorption of potassium and other constituents. By diverting gastric or duodenal contents or pancreatic secretions directly into the colon or by bypassing large segments of ileum, absorption is significantly impaired, leading rapidly to volume depletion and hypokalemia. Entities characterized by rapid intestinal transit time or malabsorption, such as the Zollinger-Ellison syndrome, sprue or other forms of steatorrhea, or the postgastrectomy syndrome, will lead to excessive losses of potassium. Potassium depletion in these instances usually involves a prolonged illness. Inflammatory bowel disease, because of rapid transit and reduced absorption, may also lead to a hypokalemic state.

Table 15-1

Causes of Hypokalemia

- I. Gastrointestinal causes
  - A. Decreased potassium intake
    - 1. Starvation
    - 2. Anorexia nervosa
  - B. Loss of hydrochloric acid
    - 1. Vomiting from pyloric stenosis or gastroenteritis
    - 2. Gastric aspiration without adequate replacement
  - C. Defective potassium absorption
    - 1. Fistulas
      - a. Biliary
      - b. Pancreatic
      - c. Gastrocolic
    - 2. Zollinger-Ellison syndrome
    - 3. Malabsorption
    - 4. Postgastrectomy dumping syndrome
    - 5. Inflammatory bowel disease
      - a. Regional enteritis
      - b. Ulcerative colitis
  - D. Increased intestinal secretion of potassium
    - 1. Diarrhea, usually infectious
    - 2. Villous adenomas
  - E. Induced lesions
    - 1. Laxative abuse
    - 2. Repeated enemas
    - 3. Use of exchange resins
- II. Renal causes
  - A. Diuretic therapy
    - 1. Mercurial diuretics
    - 2. Furosemide and ethacrynic acid
    - 3. Thiazide diuretics
    - 4. Carbonic anhydrase inhibitors
  - B. Renal tubular or parenchymal diseases
    - 1. Renal tubular acidosis
      - a. Proximal type
      - b. Distal type
    - 2. Fanconi syndrome
    - 3. Chronic pyelonephritis
  - C. Adrenal steroids
    - 1. Primary hyperaldosteronism
      - a. Adrenal adenomas
      - b. Adrenal hyperplasia
      - c. 17-α-hydroxylase or 11-β-hydroxylase deficiencies
      - d. Dexamethasone or glucocorticosteroid suppressible hyperaldosteronism
    - 2. Secondary hyperaldosteronism
      - a. Associated with decreased "effective plasma volume"
        - i. Cirrhosis
        - ii. Congestive heart failure
        - iii. Hypoalbuminemia
      - b. Bartter's syndrome
      - c. Associated with malignant hypertension
    - 3. Cushing's syndrome
      - a. Excessive ACTH production from the anterior pituitary gland
      - b. Exogenous ACTH production (malignancy)
      - c. Exogenous cortisol production (malignancy)
    - 4. Adrenal steroid therapy
    - 5. Licorice ingestion

Table 15-1—continued

III. Miscellaneous causes related to intracellular shifts of potassium
   A. Systemic alkalosis either respiratory or metabolic
   B. Infusion of large amounts of glucose
   C. Familial hypokalemic paralysis

D. Increased Intestinal Secretion of Potassium

Patients who have severe diarrhea, usually induced by infectious agents, whether viral or bacterial, may lose excessive amounts of potassium in the range of 30–50 mEq/liter of stool. Villous adenomas may be associated with excessive potassium secretion and may quite rapidly lead to potassium depletion. They may be present in the rectum or along the entire colon.

E. Laxatives and Exchange Resins

One of the common causes of hypokalemia is the excessive use of laxatives or repeated enemas, which produce rapid transit and defective absorption of potassium and chronic potassium wasting. A careful history is required to exclude these possibilities. Finally, the excessive use of exchange resins such as Kayexalate (a sodium for potassium exchange resin) may lead to potassium losses via the stool and hypokalemia.

In summary, then, a frequent site of potassium loss is the gastrointestinal tract. Potassium depletion may occur secondary to excessive hydrogen loss as a result of vomiting (in this instance, potassium is mainly lost via the kidney) or secretory mechanisms within the bowel leading to excessive potassium loss in the stool, such as occurs in infectious diarrhea or villous adenomas. Conditions associated with defective absorption, as seen in certain fistulas, malabsorption syndromes, or other conditions associated with rapid transit, may lead to potassium depletion. Except for vomiting or gastric aspiration, in which urinary potassium concentrations will be high, the urinary potassium concentration in patients with excessive gastrointestinal losses of potassium is low, thus alerting the physician to the possibility of a gastrointestinal cause for hypokalemia.

II. Renal Causes

A. Diuretic Therapy

Probably the single most important cause for the renal loss of potassium is diuretic therapy. Although the mechanisms of action of diuretics are not the same, most diuretics are associated with potassium wasting. These include the mercurial diuretics, ethacrynic acid, furosemide, the thiazide diuretics and their derivatives, and carbonic anhydrase inhibitors. Diuretics may lead to potassium wasting because of excessive distal delivery of sodium and chloride, in which case augmented distal sodium reabsorption occurs associated with an increased electronegativity of the tubular lumen, causing increased potassium losses. Increased flow of fluid in the distal nephron also contributes to excessive potassium secretion. Carbonic anhydrase inhibitors result also in increased bicarbonate concentrations in the distal nephron, which in turn increases the electronegativity of the tubular lumen, promoting potassium wastage. It must also be remembered that patients receiving diuretics, because of volume depletion, may also have excessive levels of plasma aldosterone, which contributes to the secretion and excretion of potassium in the urine. Whatever the mechanism, potassium losses through the use of diuretics may lead to severe hypokalemia. It may become necessary to augment the potassium intake or to use potassium-sparing diuretics such as triamterene or spironolactone in patients receiving diuretics to protect against the development of hypokalemia.

B. Renal Tubular Disease

Specific renal tubular diseases are also associated with hypokalemia. Renal tubular acidosis (RTA) of the proximal variety, with or without Fanconi syndrome, is often associated with hypokalemia. In conditions in which bicarbonate reabsorption is defective, as in proximal RTA, increased distal delivery of a poorly reabsorbable anion occurs, resulting in an increase in the electronegativity of the tubular lumen and potassium losses by the distal nephron. In distal RTA, individuals are unable to maintain a hydrogen gradient between the tubular lumen and the cell either because of decreased hydrogen ion secretion or because excessive amounts of secreted hydrogen may "leak back" from tubular lumen into cells. Since sodium reabsorption continues, potassium may be lost to maintain electroneutrality. A similar circumstance may also occur in chronic pyelonephritis, where interstitial and distal tubular disease may affect the ability of the individual to generate adequate hydrogen gradients to maintain acid-base balance. Under these circumstances, potassium wasting may occur.

C. Adrenal Steroids

Adrenal steroids are known to promote urinary potassium losses. The most potent kaliuretic hormone, of course, is aldosterone. Causes of primary hyperaldosteronism (see Chapter 6 on hypertension) include (1) hyperaldosteronism with adenoma or hyperplasia of the zona glomerulosa; (2) 11-β-hydroxylase or 17-α-hydroxylase deficiency; and (3) syndromes associated with excessive secretion of aldosterone-like compounds from the adrenal gland. In these disease states, there is increased sodium for potassium exchange in the distal nephron leading to volume expansion, hypertension, and potassium losses.

Conditions of secondary hyperaldosteronism also lead to hypokalemia. These include any condition in which there is a decreased plasma volume. As described elsewhere, patients who have severe hypoalbuminemia, nephrotic syndrome, cirrhosis, or congestive heart failure will have increased aldosterone secretion in response to a decreased "effective" plasma volume. Patients with malignant hypertension may also develop secondary hyperaldosteronism as a consequence of renal ischemia, causing increased renin production and angiotensin II generation.

The unique clinical entity referred to as Bartter's syndrome is also a form of secondary hyperaldosteronism. It appears that this syndrome is due to an increased release of prostaglandins from the renal medulla leading to renal vasodilatation and increased sodium losses thus producing a state of chronic volume depletion. Volume depletion and/or augmented prostaglandin production are associated with increased renin release by the kidney, which then causes secondary hyperaldosteronism. The patient will therefore present with a clinical picture compatible with hyperaldosteronism but without hypertension.

Cushing's syndrome is also associated with hypokalemia because of the mild kaliuretic effect of the glucocorticoid hormones. Usually the degree of hypokalemia and the hypertension are less severe. Of course, the use of exogenous steroids must be excluded in any patient who presents with hypokalemia. Since glycyrrhizic acid, a by-product of licorice metabolism, has aldosterone-like activity, excessive ingestion of licorice could produce a syndrome indistinguishable from hyperaldosteronism.

III. Miscellaneous Causes

A. Systemic Alkalosis (Respiratory or Metabolic)

The translocation of potassium between intracellular and extracellular fluid compartments is dependent not only upon the potassium intake but also upon acid-base status. As the concentration of bicarbonate increases in the ECF space, hydrogen will shift from the ICF space as a buffering mechanism. This shift is associated with a potassium and sodium shift from ECF compartment to the ICF space. Thus, modest hypokalemia will occur without a net loss of total body potassium. The milk-alkali syndrome is an example of this condition.

Respiratory alkalosis is associated with a fall in plasma pCO_2 (carbonic acid), depressing the denominator of the Henderson-Hasselbalch equation and raising the plasma pH. The reader is referred to the chapter on respiratory alkalosis for a complete differential diagnosis. Thus, despite a depressed plasma bicarbonate induced by renal compensation, hypokalemia may occur in response to a shift of hydrogen as outlined above.

B. Infusion of Large Amounts of Glucose

During the infusion of glucose, both potassium and phosphate are transported from the extracellular to the intracellular fluid compartment. Modest hypokalemia and hypophosphatemia may occur. The patients receiving prolonged infusions of glucose are most frequently malnourished and may also be receiving amino acids or lipid as an energy source in hyperalimentation. Significant hypokalemia may develop in these patients and potassium supplementation will be necessary.

C. Familial Hypokalemic Paralysis

Familial hypokalemic paralysis is a rare, dominant, inherited condition associated with a fall in plasma potassium reflecting intracellular shifts of the cation and coincident weakness. Symptoms usually begin in adolescence, are primarily nocturnal, are severe, and last for one or more days. Attacks may be precipitated by vigorous exercise, during sleep, or by ingesting a large amount of carbohydrate, suggesting a defect in carbohydrate transport or metabolism. Weakness usually begins in the legs and ascends to the arms, usually sparing the cranial nerves. Respiratory paralysis is rare. The attacks are variable and not necessarily related to the fall in plasma potassium. Weakness of the proximal muscle groups usually persists between the attacks. Electrocardiographic abnormalities may be seen with severe reductions in plasma potassium. Pathologically the muscles contain numerous vacuoles that are derived from the sarcoplasmic reticulum. Treatment with oral potassium chloride will reverse most attacks. Acetazolamide therapy may be an effective form of prophylaxis.

Laboratory Considerations in Patients with Hypokalemia

After a careful history and physical examination, certain laboratory data should be obtained in patients with suspected hypokalemia. Urinalysis should be performed with special reference to specific gravity, the presence of glucose or protein in the urine, and any formed elements on microscopic examination. A complete blood count, including WBC, hematocrit, and differential count, is indicated. Serum sodium, potassium, chloride, CO_2, BUN, and creatinine determinations are necessary to document the severity of the hypokalemia and alkalosis and the possibility of associated renal involvement. A chest x-ray to elucidate cardiac size and evidence of congestive heart failure and an electrocardiogram to demonstrate the possible changes of hypokalemia as outlined earlier should be obtained immediately. Depending upon the patient's primary presenting complaint (i.e., nausea, vomiting, or diarrhea), a KUB roentgenogram is indicated, as well as a stool guaiac.

Patients with primary gastrointestinal causes of hypokalemia will frequently have mild to moderate dehydration. Measurement of the urinary electrolytes will reveal an increased urinary potassium and a depressed urine sodium in patients with protracted vomiting. Urine potassium values will often be in the range of 50–60 mEq/liter, despite plasma levels of potassium in the range of 2–3 mEq/liter, while urinary sodium values may be as low as 2–10 mEq/liter. Of course, in patients presenting with evidence of protracted vomiting, specific upper gastrointestinal roentgenograms, as well as surgical consultation, should be obtained if indicated.

Patients presenting with evidence of diarrhea or malabsorption will require stool analysis for electrolytes, occult blood, and fat content. In these circumstances, the patient's urine will reveal very low levels of potassium (5–10 mEq/liter), reflecting the systemic hypokalemia, and depressed urinary sodiums if the patient has evidence of volume depletion. Of course the workup of diarrhea, malabsorption, and the like requires specific x-ray studies, including an upper gastrointestinal roentgenogram, small bowel follow-through, and a barium enema. Proctoscopy should be performed on all such patients.

For patients with renal potassium wasting, a careful history will often elucidate treatment with diuretics, which should be discontinued until the potassium stores are replenished. Whatever the cause, in renal potassium wasting, urinary potassium levels will be higher than would be expected for the degree of hypokalemia and may range anywhere from 20–50 mEq/liter. A depressed plasma bicarbonate, a low plasma pH, and a urinary pH in the range of 5 should suggest proximal renal tubular acidosis. Distal RTA may generate similar laboratory values, but the urinary pH is rarely lower than 6.0. If the Fanconi syndrome is suspected, measurements of amino acids, glucose, and phosphate should be obtained to ascertain the amount excreted in the urine. In any patient with renal potassium wasting, an IVP with a postvoiding film for residual is necessary to determine renal size, evidence of pyelonephritis, obstructive uropathy, or the like. Urine cultures are indicated if pyelonephritis is suspected. If there is no obvious cause for gastrointestinal losses or primary renal losses of potassium and the patient presents with evidence of hypertension, alkalosis, and hypokalemia, then hyperaldosteronism, or Cushing's syndrome if the pertinent historical and physical findings are present, should be suspected. Patients who have hyperaldosteronism will have increased urinary potassium levels associated with a low plasma potassium and moderate alkalosis, as described in Chapter 6 on hypertension. If the hypokalemia does not respond to potassium supplementation, or if continuing excessive potassium losses occur despite attempts at correction of the plasma potassium levels, then the patient should be admitted for evaluation of hyperaldosteronism. Pertinent laboratory data should be obtained as outlined in Chapter 6 on hypertension.

Clinical Problem

W. M., a 53-year-old white female, was admitted to the hospital with complaints of chronic constipation, colicky upper abdominal pain, and nausea of 3 months' duration. She was in good health until 7 years prior to this admission when she was admitted elsewhere with the diagnosis of "uremic poisoning." She was found to have lower urinary tract obstruction secondary to urethral trauma incurred during the birth of her first child. She was treated by bladder catheterization and then urethral dilatation, with resolution of the symptoms. Plasma creatinine or BUN levels from that admission were not available. She was placed on Lasix, 40 mg, and Diazide, 1 tablet daily, which she had continued to take since that time without potassium supplementation.

The patient did well until 1 year prior to admission when she saw her physician because of weakness, easy fatigability, and depression. A diagnosis of depression was made, and she was treated with diazepam and amitriptyline hydrochloride. However, her symptoms progressed, and were associated with intermittent cramping abdominal pain which was treated with Donnatal for the 6 months prior to admission. Three months prior to admission the patient complained of severe, crampy, midabdominal pain and constipation unrelieved by laxatives. Upper and lower gastrointestinal roentgenograms and an intravenous pyelogram were normal. The patient was then referred for further evaluation.

The patient denied vomiting, melena, hematemesis, nocturia, polyuria, frequency, urgency, or history of urinary tract infection. She had been dilated on three occasions over the past 7 years to correct urethral stricture.

Her past medical history was negative except for a total abdominal hysterectomy at the age of 26 for uterine carcinoma. She takes no other medications except for those noted above.

She is married, has two children and lives with her husband. She drinks only socially and does not smoke. Her family history was noncontributory.

The patient has noted dizziness on standing for the past 12 months. No syncopal episodes have occurred. She denied shortness of breath, cough, hemoptysis, or chest pain. Occasional edema of the feet has been noted over the past 7 years.

On physical examination the patient presented as a healthy woman appearing her stated age. She was cheerful, alert, and pleasant. Blood pressure in the right and left arms was 120/70 mm Hg supine and 100/60 mm Hg standing. The pulse rate was 84 beats per minute and regular when supine, increasing to 92 when standing. Respirations were 14 per minute, and she was afebrile. Her skin turgor was normal and her mucous membranes moist.

Results of examination of her head, eyes, ears, nose, and throat were normal. Her chest was clear, and no cardiomegaly, murmurs, or gallop rhythms were noted. There was mild midepigastric and periumbilical tenderness to palpation without masses being felt. The liver, kidneys, and spleen were not enlarged. Auscultation revealed hypoactive bowel sounds. Rectal examination was normal, with a negative stool guaiac. Pelvic examination showed a closed vaginal vault without abnormalities. There was no peripheral edema, and the pulses were normal. The neurological examination was negative except for a slight hyporeflexia of the knee and ankle jerks. No evidence of upper extremity weakness was noted, but significant proximal lower extremity weakness was present.

Questions

1. Could this patient's entire symptom complex be explained by electrolyte abnormalities?
2. What plasma and urinary electrolyte determinations are most critical in this patient?
3. What roentgenograms are indicated at this time?

Discussion

The patient was admitted for evaluation of gastrointestinal complaints. As part of the initial screening evaluation, several tests were obtained. The plasma chemistries revealed: sodium concentration, 138 mEq/liter; potassium, 1.7 mEq/liter; bicarbonate, 46 mEq/liter; chloride, 77 mEq/liter; BUN level, 46 mg/dl; serum creatinine, 1.9 mg/dl; and fasting blood glucose, 89 mg/dl. Arterial blood gases were: pH, 7.55; pCO_2, 46; PO_2, 88. Urinalysis was normal, with a specific gravity of 1.008 and a pH of 5.0, and was negative for glucose, protein, or formed elements. Chest roentgenogram was normal without evidence of pulmonary disease or cardiomegaly. The electrocardiogram revealed the following abnormalities: (1) slight increase in P wave amplitude; (2) prolongation of the QT interval (.52); (3) evidence of U waves in precordial and limb leads. The electrocardiogram in Figure 15-3 illustrates these points.

It is obvious from the above data that the patient has severe metabolic alkalosis and hypokalemia. It is likely that the patient's symptoms are related to the hypokalemia induced by diuretic therapy. The changes in plasma creatinine and BUN levels may reflect intrinsic renal disease or ECF volume contraction induced by the diuretics. At this point, 24-hour urine chemistries were obtained and the results were as follows: volume, 1.8 liters; sodium, 12 mEq/liter; and potassium, 50 mEq/liter, with a creatinine clearance of 86 ml/min corrected for 1.73 m^2.

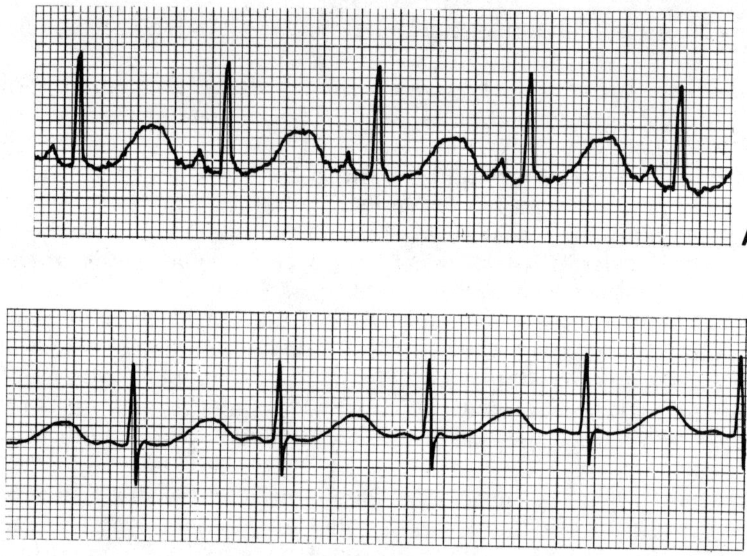

Fig. 15-3.

While severe metabolic alkalosis may accompany hyperaldosteronism, this diagnosis seems unlikely, since hypertension is not present. Also there are no clinical signs compatible with the development of secondary hyperaldosteronism, although Bartter's syndrome cannot be excluded at this time. Finally, in view of an extremely high urinary potassium with a low plasma potassium, a renal loss of potassium secondary to diuretic therapy is most likely, since the patient has had no vomiting.

The diuretic therapy was discontinued and oral potassium supplementation begun. Over the next 7 days the plasma potassium rose to 2.8 mEq/liter, with a plasma chloride level of 88 mEq/liter; bicarbonate, 36 mEq/liter; BUN, 30 mg/dl; and creatinine, 1.0 mg/dl. Repeat creatinine clearance at this time was 96 ml/min corrected for 1.73 m^2. Repeat gastrointestinal x-rays and IVP were not performed, since recent examinations were normal.

The patient was followed carefully in the clinic after discharge. Within 2 months plasma potassium levels were 4.4 mEq/liter; CO_2, 26 mEq/liter; creatinine, .8 mg/dl; and BUN, 16 mg/dl. Creatinine clearance at that time was 118 ml/min corrected for 1.73 m^2.

The patient did not become hypertensive, and after discontinuation of potassium supplementation, her plasma chemistries have been normal on repeated determinations. She has noted marked improvement in her strength, no further abdominal pain or constipation, and her electrocardiogram has returned to normal.

Hyperkalemia

General Considerations

Hyperkalemia is defined as a plasma potassium level greater than 5.0 mEq/liter. It is a relatively uncommon clinical entity but has potentially lethal consequences. Hyperkalemia may be relative or absolute. Relative hyperkalemia occurs when there are shifts of tissue potassium stores to the ECF space without an increase in total body potassium concentration. Absolute hyperkalemia occurs when there is an increase in both intracellular and extracellular potassium concentrations.

Clinical Manifestations of Hyperkalemia

Hyperkalemia occurs less frequently than hypokalemia, but its consequences are much more severe. The electrical excitability of any tissue depends on the difference between the resting membrane potential (Em) and the threshold potential (Et). (Excitability = Em – Et.) The membrane potential is primarily determined by the log of the ratio of intracellular (Ki) to extracellular (Ko) potassium [Em = -61.5 log(Ki/Ko)]. If the extracellular potassium is suddenly increased with little or no change in the intracellular potassium concentrations, the membrane potential will be significantly decreased approaching threshold potential, thus reducing excitability toward zero. The patient will therefore manifest depolarization block and paralysis. On the other hand, with chronic potassium excess, both intracellular and extracellular potassium concentrations rise, and membranes are only partially depolarized leading to hyperexcitability. The excitability can be affected by several maneuvers, including translocation of the potassium from the extracellular to intracellular space and removal of the excess potassium or depression of the threshold potential by the administration of calcium.

It is obvious from the above discussion that patients presenting with hyperkalemia will have symptoms involving primarily the cardiovascular and neuromuscular systems. Cardiac contractility is not affected by hyperkalemia, but significant arrhythmias may occur as a result of conduction changes. Electrocardiographic changes usually occur, with plasma potassium levels over 7 mEq/liter. Initially, tall, peaked, tented T waves are seen with a normal QT interval. Usually with modest increases in plasma potassium, decreased amplitude of the P waves occurs with a prolonged P-R interval. As hyperkalemia progresses, atrial asystole is seen with widening of the QRS complex leading to a sine wave. Finally, plasma potassium concentrations greater than 10 mEq/liter lead to ventricular standstill. The effects of hyperkalemia on cardiac function may be seen with smaller increases in plasma potassium if there is associated hyponatremia, hypocalcemia or acidosis.

Figures 15-4 to 15-6 illustrate the electrocardiographic (ECG) changes in several patients presenting with severe hyperkalemia. Figure 15-4 illustrates the ECG changes in a patient with a plasma potassium level of 8.4 mEq/liter. There is decreased amplitude of the P wave as well as tall peaked T waves.

Figure 15-5 illustrates the ECG changes in a patient presenting with a plasma potassium level of 11.4 mEq/liter. There is absence of the P wave, indicating atrial asystole. The QRS is widened and blends with the T wave, leading to a sine wave formation. The tracing is most typical of ventricular flutter.

Figure 15-6 demonstrates the ECG changes in the same patient illustrated in Figure 15-5 after the intravenous administration of 10 mg of calcium gluconate. Here, the widening of the QRS complex has been reversed. The rhythm is probably an irregular nodal tachycardia. Note that there are no P waves in this tracing, and the tall, tented T waves are not present. Patients with hyperkalemia will therefore present primarily with cardiac arrhythmias leading to ventricular fibrillation and death.

Although the major effects of hyperkalemia are on cardiac function, neuromuscular changes are also seen. Changes in muscle strength or nerve conduction velocities are usually not evident with plasma potassium levels below 8 mEq/liter. Above this level, weakness occurs, usually beginning in the lower extremities and ascending to the upper extremities. Respiratory depression may occur, but the cranial nerves and central nervous system are rarely affected, even with plasma potassium levels above 9 mEq/liter.

Plasma potassium levels above 8 mEq/liter are rarely observed, even in acute renal failure. Several mechanisms protect the patient from rapid elevations in plasma potassium. Figure 15-7 illustrates the proposed mechanism for chronic and acute potassium adaptation. When plasma potassium concentrations are chronically elevated, aldosterone levels rise. Recent evidence would suggest that muscle stores of potassium are actually lowered by elevated plasma aldosterone levels. If an acute potassium load then occurs, increased muscle uptake of potassium takes place, thus protecting the individual from fatal hyperkalemia. Furthermore, aldosterone stimulates distal tubular and collecting duct peritubu-

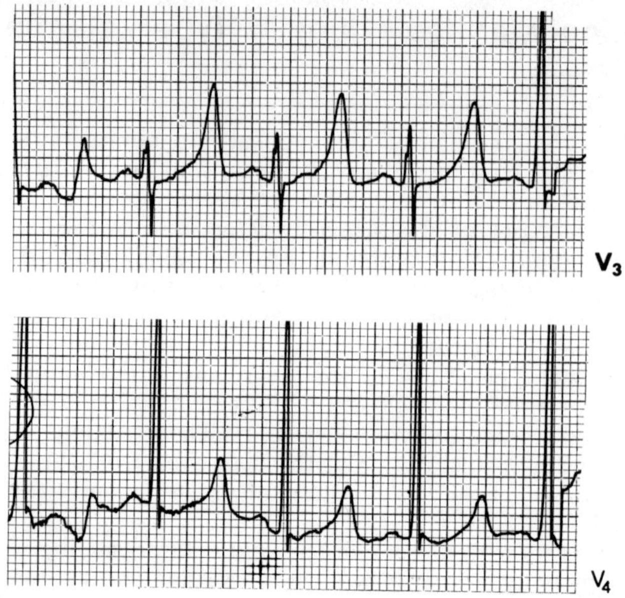

Fig. 15-4.

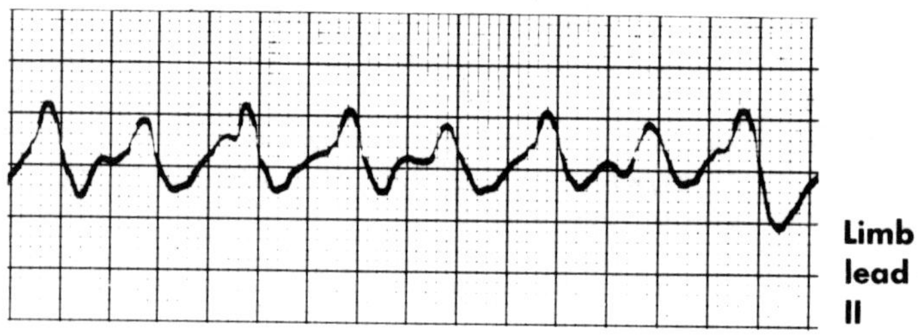

Fig. 15-5.

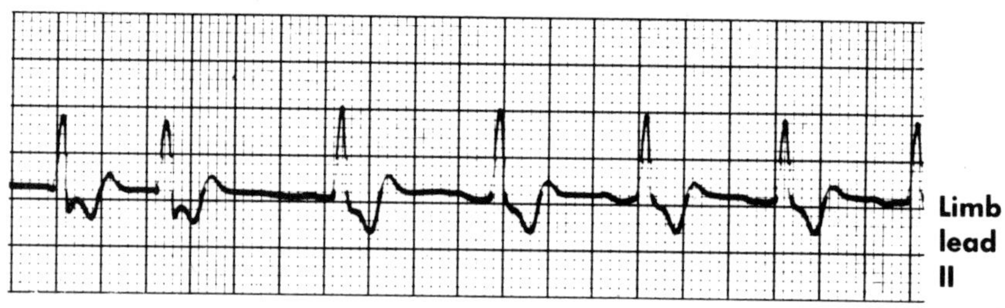

Fig. 15-6.

lar potassium uptake, which augments potassium excretion by the kidney. Insulin also appears to play a major role in acute potassium adaptation. When an acute rise in plasma potassium levels occurs, an increased insulin release follows, which rapidly accelerates

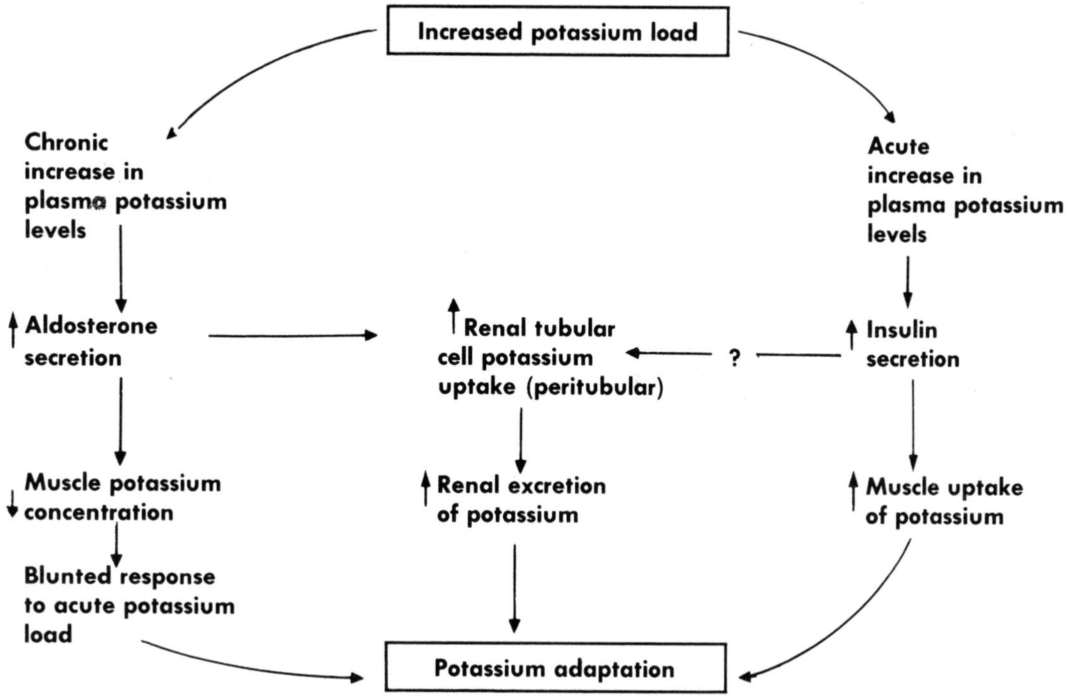

Fig. 15-7.

Proposed mechanism for chronic and acute potassium adaptation.

muscle potassium uptake either directly in response to glucose uptake or via stimulation of the sodium-potassium ATPase enzyme system. Although the chronic effects of increased plasma insulin levels on renal potassium handling are not known, it is possible that augmented renal contraluminal uptake of the cation occurs, followed by increased urine excretion.

Both of these control mechanisms are of critical importance in protecting the individual from fatal hyperkalemia. While they probably are of more critical importance in patients with acute or chronic renal failure, they also play a role in potassium adaptation in normal individuals.

Differential Diagnosis of Hyperkalemia

The most frequent causes of hyperkalemia are listed in Table 15-2 and discussed below.

I. Acute and Chronic Renal Failure

Renal failure accounts for the majority of patients who present with hyperkalemia. Acute renal failure from any cause (acute tubular necrosis, acute glomerulonephritis,

Table 15-2

Causes of Hyperkalemia

I. Acute or severe chronic renal failure
   A. Continued potassium intake
   B. Accelerated catabolism
   C. Acidosis
   D. Administration of potassium-containing solutions
   E. Gastrointestinal bleeding
   F. Hemolysis
II. Translocation of potassium from the intracellular to the extracellular fluid space
   A. Acidosis
   B. Severe catabolism
   C. Rhabdomyolysis
   D. Familial hyperkalemic periodic paralysis
III. Mineralocorticoid deficiency states
   A. Addison's disease
   B. Hyporeninemic hypoaldosteronism
IV. Administration of aldosterone antagonists or potassium-sparing diuretics
   A. Spironolactone
   B. Triamterene
V. Miscellaneous causes
   A. "Pseudohyperkalemia" of myeloproliferative disorders
      1. Hyperkalemia associated with thrombocytosis
      2. Hyperkalemia associated with granulocytosis
   B. Hemolysis at the time of blood sampling
   C. Intravenous administration of potassium

trauma, or vascular compromise) will frequently lead to hyperkalemia. For a complete discussion on the causes of acute renal failure, the reader is referred to Chapters 7 and 8. Since the kidney is the major organ responsible for potassium homeostasis, a marked and sudden loss of renal function will lead to hyperkalemia if intake is not curtailed. Furthermore, patients with renal failure are frequently acidotic, causing a shift of potassium from the intracellular to the extracellular fluid space. Also, accelerated catabolism frequently accompanies acute renal failure, and with tissue breakdown, there is release of intracellular potassium. Other potential sources of potassium, such as blood in the gastrointestinal tract, necrotic tissue, hemolysis, or administration of blood, are poorly tolerated by patients with renal insufficiency and will accelerate the rate of rise of plasma potassium levels.

While hyperkalemia is a frequent complication of acute renal failure, it is usually not seen with chronic renal failure unless excessive potassium is administered. Patients with chronic renal failure maintain potassium homeostasis even with severe reductions in the GFR. The amount of potassium excreted by these patients may actually exceed the filtered load (filtered load = GFR × plasma concentration of potassium), demonstrating that net secretion has occurred. However, when the GFR is below 2 or 3 ml/min the excretory capacity of the residual nephrons for potassium is frequently exceeded, despite dietary restriction, and hyperkalemia occurs. A more frequent cause of hyperkalemia, however, is the administration of potassium salts. Hypokalemia may be seen in patients with chronic renal disease but correction of the deficit should be undertaken slowly and carefully. Intravenous potassium is rarely needed, and supplementation should be given orally if possible. Hyperkalemia may be produced by the administration of outdated blood, gastrointestinal bleeding, severe catabolism, or hemolysis if the GFR is severely reduced.

II. Translocation of Potassium from the Intracellular to the Extracellular Fluid Space

The sudden shift of potassium from the ICF to the ECF space may cause hyperkalemia. Patients with normal renal function may develop transient hyperkalemia with the rapid onset of acidosis, such as lactic acidosis or ketoacidosis, which is rapidly reversed by correction of the acidosis. With excessive release of tissue stores of potassium such as may occur with severe catabolism or rhabdomyolysis, the renal excretory capacity for potassium may be exceeded, causing transient hyperkalemia. Accelerated catabolism is rarely a cause of fatal hyperkalemia, but modest elevations of the plasma potassium concentration may be seen. Elevations of plasma potassium levels may occasionally be seen with rhabdomyolysis and may be severe if acute renal failure due to myoglobinuria supervenes. The most common causes for rhabdomyolysis are crush or thermal injuries. Thermal injuries may occur after prolonged exposure to extreme cold, with heat stroke, or with malignant hyperthermia after general anesthesia. Rhabdomyolysis also occurs after vigorous exercise in unconditioned individuals, with arterial embolism, and in alcoholics.

Familial hyperkalemic periodic paralysis is a rare cause of hyperkalemia. The syndrome usually occurs during potassium ingestion and presumably reflects a shift of potassium from muscle cells to the ECF space. The disease is manifested in early childhood and is typified by mild, short-lived, intermittent episodes of muscle weakness. The weakness usually occurs after vigorous exercise and affects the lower extremities first, progressing to the upper extremities. The cranial nerves are rarely involved. Proximal muscle weakness usually persists between attacks. The plasma potassium level may rise to 7 mEq/liter, causing electrocardiographic abnormalities, cardiac arrhythmias, and, on occasion, ventricular tachycardia. The exact cause of the syndrome is unknown. The disease is most effectively treated by the administration of glucose and insulin or calcium salts. Acetazolamide has also been effective in preventing recurrent attacks.

III. Mineralocorticoid Deficiency States

Since aldosterone is a major regulatory hormone of potassium homeostasis, its absence may lead to hyperkalemia. While isolated aldosterone deficiency is exceedingly rare, *primary adrenal insufficiency (Addison's disease)* may be associated with severe depression of plasma aldosterone levels. Adrenal insufficiency associated with panhypopituitarism is not associated with hyperkalemia, since aldosterone secretion rates remain normal. Addison's disease occurs in 1 patient out of 100,000 population. The disease is not manifested unless 85% of the gland is destroyed. The most common causes of adrenal insufficiency include tuberculosis, fungal infections and idiopathic atrophy of the gland. Rarely, amyloidosis or metastatic replacement of the gland by tumor may lead to adrenal failure. The patients are hyperpigmented as a result of excessive melanocyte-stimulating hormone (MSH) production, since cortisol production is severely curtailed, eliminating negative feedback. Appetite is decreased, hypoglycemia may occur during stress, and hypotension may be life-threatening. Since aldosterone levels are greatly reduced, renal sodium wasting with hyponatremia develops associated with hypovolemia, reduced cardiac output and reduction in cardiac size. The associated hypotension leads to increased catabolism and release of tissue potassium stores. The increased load of potassium, as well as the reduced renal blood flow and deficiency of aldosterone, leads to the hyperkalemic state.

The disease is usually insidious with few early symptoms. As levels of aldosterone and cortisol decrease, weakness, weight loss, hypotension, anorexia, nausea, and vomiting supervene. Hyperpigmentation occurs late in the disease course, being more prominent at body folds, scars, and exposed areas. The disease culminates in Addisonian crisis, with profound shock usually occurring during episodes of stress such as surgery or trauma. Immediate therapy with intravenous sodium chloride and glucocorticoids is necessary.

The recently described syndrome of *hyporeninemic hypoaldosteronism* causes hyperkalemia and acidosis. The syndrome is usually associated with mild reductions in renal function, and the hyperkalemia is rarely fatal, although plasma potassium levels of 7.0 mEq/liter have been described. The disease is usually seen in patients with diabetes mellitus or interstitial nephritis. The presumed mechanism relates to defective release of renin from the juxtaglomerular cells, probably induced by the underlying renal disease. Since aldosterone release from the adrenal cortex is primarily dependent upon angiotensin II levels, modest hypoaldosteronism occurs. Potassium directly stimulates aldosterone release, which may explain why severe hyperkalemia, profound sodium wasting, and hypovolemia are not usually seen in these patients. The patients most frequently have reductions in GFR of 30% to 50% of predicted values, with modest elevations of plasma potassium levels (5.0–6.5 mEq/liter) and a mild acidosis, which is more severe than one would expect for the degree of renal impairment. The patients respond to a 9-α-fluorohydrocortisone with a return of potassium levels to normal and correction of the acidosis.

IV. Administration of Aldosterone Antagonists or Potassium-sparing Diuretics

Spironolactone is a specific pharmacologic antagonist of aldosterone that produces its effects by competitive binding to aldosterone-receptor sites in the distal convoluted tubule. By binding to these sites, spironolactone blocks the effects of aldosterone. Moderate natriuresis occurs associated with retention of potassium. When used as a diuretic, spironolactone rarely produces hyperkalemia. However, if potassium supplementation or diets rich in potassium are used concomitantly, fatal hyperkalemia may occur. Furthermore, hyperkalemia may also occur if the drug is used in patients with moderate reductions in renal function.

Triamterene is also a potassium-sparing diuretic. It is not an aldosterone antagonist, and recent evidence would suggest that its site of action is the collecting duct. Its mode of action is to inhibit sodium exchange for either potassium or hydrogen. Under most circumstances, triamterene will not cause hyperkalemia, but if renal impairment exists or if potassium supplements or a diet rich in potassium are used concomitantly, elevations in plasma potassium may be seen. Patients with diabetes mellitus are especially prone to the development of hyperkalemia with the use of this drug.

V. Miscellaneous Causes

Chronic granulocytic leukemia is characterized by abnormal proliferation of immature granulocytes in the bone marrow as well as the spleen and liver. The disease occurs in patients over the age of 40. The complaints include fatigue, weakness, and fullness in the abdomen. On examination, both the spleen and liver are enlarged. A leukocytosis with a WBC over 50,000 and variable degrees of anemia and thrombocytosis are found. A small percentage of these patients may present with modest hyperkalemia (plasma potassium level, 5.0–6.5 mEq/liter), despite normal renal function. The exact mechanism for the hyperkalemia is unclear but may reflect potassium release from platelets during coagulation. In patients with markedly elevated white blood cell counts, release of potassium from these cells may also cause hyperkalemia. The condition is referred to as "pseudohyperkalemia," since the potassium release usually occurs at the time of blood sampling. Pseudohyperkalemia also occurs whenever blood samples are hemolyzed when they are drawn.

Under most circumstances the renal capacity to excrete potassium cannot be exceeded. However, when very large boluses of potassium are injected intravenously, renal excretion may be exceeded by the rate of administration of the cation, and fatal hyperkalemia may occur. Certain patients tolerate potassium administration less well, especially aged, debilitated, dehydrated patients and those with preexisting renal disease. Potassium should rarely be administered intravenously; when given by this route, concentrations of potassium should never exceed 40–60 mEq/liter of administered fluid.

Laboratory Considerations

All patients with suspected hyperkalemia require immediate evaluation. A complete blood count, including a platelet count, serum electrolytes (sodium, potassium, chloride, bicarbonate), BUN, creatinine, calcium, and arterial pH, pCO_2 and PO_2 levels, should be immediately obtained. An electrocardiogram is required to document the severity of the hyperkalemia. The type of immediate therapy will be dictated by the ECG changes. If only peaked T waves are present, insulin, glucose, and bicarbonate given intravenously will suffice. If widening of the QRS as well as T wave changes are present, calcium should be administered, immediately followed by the above recommended procedure.

Most patients with hyperkalemia have depressed renal function and 24-hour urines for creatinine, sodium, and potassium levels are necessary. Urine cultures are also indicated. Long-term correction of hyperkalemia in these patients will depend upon the severity of the reduction in the GFR (hemodialysis, Kayexalate, etc.).

If the patients present with normal renal function, the presence of lactic acidosis or ketoacidosis can be suspected from the electrolytes and the presence of a large anion gap (see Chapter 16 on metabolic acidosis). Measurement of plasma and urine myoglobin is indicated if rhabdomyolysis is suspected. Of course, hemolysis at the time of blood sampling must be excluded. Myeloproliferative disorders will be obvious from the complete blood count. Stool guaiacs should be obtained to rule out gastrointestinal bleeding.

Addison's disease can be suspected from the history and physical examination. Plasma cortisol levels must be obtained. Urinary potassium levels will be lower than expected for the degree of hyperkalemia, and an increased urine sodium with polyuria may be present.

Hyporeninemic hypoaldosteronism is rare but can be suspected if the patient is a diabetic or has interstitial nephritis, with a modest reduction in the GFR, low urine potassium levels, elevated plasma potassium levels, and acidosis more severe than one would expect for the degree of renal impairment. Increased intake or the use of potassium-sparing diuretics must be excluded in these patients.

Familial hyperkalemic periodic paralysis is very rare and is diagnosed only by exclusion. The history and physical examination are most helpful. During acute attacks, elevated plasma potassium levels with normal or low urinary potassium values are seen. Acidosis is not present. Renal function is normal, and Addison's disease is excluded by normal plasma cortisol levels.

Special reference to blood pH and potassium levels has to be made. If the patient is acidotic the plasma potassium levels probably reflect a release from the ICF space. Total body potassium levels are usually not elevated in this situation, and therapy with bicarbonate is rapidly effective and well tolerated by most patients, assuming that the ECF volume is not markedly expanded. On the other hand, if the blood pH is normal and the plasma potassium level is elevated, the total body potassium level is increased. Bicarbonate is ineffective in this situation and glucose and insulin are only transiently beneficial. Potassium must be removed from the body either by exchange resins (Kayexalate) or by dialysis. Also, if hyperkalemia occurs in the face of a normal pH, development of acidosis will cause rapid increases in the plasma potassium with potentially fatal consequences.

Clinical Problem

G. H. was a 47-year-old white female with chronic pyelonephritis documented by biopsy. She was followed as an outpatient in the Renal Clinic. She had been stable with a creatinine clearance of 5 ml/min, BUN 50 mg/dl, negative urine cultures, hematocrit 30%, calcium 9.0 mg/dl, phosphorus 4.5 mg/dl, and a normal electrocardiogram and chest film. She had been maintained on a diet containing 50 gm protein, 600 mg phosphorus, 50 mEq potassium, and 5 gm sodium chloride. The patient was seen monthly in the clinic until 3 months prior to admission when she discontinued her visits. On the day of admission, the patient presented to the emergency room complaining of shortness of breath and weakness. She admitted to dietary indiscretion with excessive salt intake over the past 2 months associated with increasing pedal edema and shortness of breath. For the 7 days prior to admission the patient noted a significant increase in dyspnea associated with two-pillow orthopnea and occasional paroxysmal nocturnal dyspnea, necessitating her visit to the emergency room. She denied chest pain or hemoptysis, fever, or chills but had a chronic cough presumably secondary to cigarette smoking.

The patient also admitted to increasing weakness and fatigue for the 7 days prior to admission. She noted the weakness primarily in the lower extremities, manifested by difficulty arising from a sitting position and unsteady gait. The symptoms usually became more severe as the day progressed.

She denied frequency, urgency, or dysuria but admitted to nocturia three times per night. Her appetite had remained good without nausea or vomiting, abdominal pain, diarrhea, or melena.

The patient's medications prior to her discontinuation were: furosemide, 80 mg P.O. each morning; methyldopa, 250 mg P.O. q.i.d.; aluminum hydroxide capsules, one q.i.d.; ferrous sulfate, 300 mg P.O. t.i.d.; Os-Cal, 250 mg P.O. q.i.d.; and multivitamins, one tablet each morning.

The patient admitted to chronic cigarette abuse, smoking 40 cigarettes per day for 25 years. She had documented chronic obstructive lung disease with a morning cough productive of one-half cup of clear sputum. The remainder of the system review was negative with the exception of mild hypertension well controlled by medication.

Her past medical history revealed a hysterectomy for uterine fibroids 5 years prior to admission and Billroth II procedure for duodenal ulcer 3 years previously. Family history was noncontributory. The patient had discontinued clinic visits and all medication because of financial problems induced by her husband's loss of employment.

Upon physical examination the patient presented as an acutely ill female, somewhat lethargic but arousable, with both tachypnea and hyperpnea. Blood pressure was 160/100, right arm, supine; pulse rate, 128 beats per minute and regular; respirations, 39 per minute; temperature, 37.2° rectally. Funduscopic examination revealed a grade I hypertensive retinopathy (Kirkendall-Armstrong classification). Carotid pulses were 2+ without bruits. The jugular veins were distended to the angle of the jaw at 45° and filled from below. The chest had an increased anteroposterior diameter; there was use of accessory muscles during respiration. Chest was tympanitic to percussion, with dullness at both bases. Auscultation revealed diffuse rales bilaterally, with inspiratory and expiratory wheezes both anteriorly and posteriorly. The point of maximal cardiac impulse could not be felt. There was moderate cardiomegaly to percussion. Both an atrial and ventricular diastolic gallop were present. There was a grade II/VI systolic murmur along the left sternal border radiating into the axilla. The abdomen was soft, nontender; there was no palpable spleen or kidneys. The liver edge was palpable 8 cm below the right costal margin and was tender. Total liver span was 12 cm. Slight edema of the abdominal wall was present. On rectal examination there were no masses; stool guaiac was 2+ positive. Extremities showed 3+ edema to the thigh bilaterally; pulses were 2+. Range of motion was normal. On neurological examination, the patient was lethargic but arousable and oriented to time, person and place. Cranial nerves were intact. A slight decrease in pinprick sensation was noted in both lower extremities. Upper extremity reflexes were 2+ and symmetrical with good strength. Reflexes were 1–2+ in the lower extremities with significant diffuse weakness primarily of extension and flexion at the knee. Babinski's reflexes were not present.

Questions

1. What laboratory determinations are most critical at this time?
2. Does this patient's chronic lung disease play any role in her recent symptoms?

3. How could congestive heart failure compound this patient's problems?

Discussion

The patient presented to the emergency room in pulmonary edema. The chest x-ray revealed severe cardiomegaly with pulmonary edema and bilateral pleural effusions. The electrocardiogram revealed sine wave formation (see Fig. 15-5) compatible with severe hyperkalemia. Serum electrolytes, BUN, creatinine, glucose, and complete blood count were drawn. Arterial blood gases and pH were also obtained. Calcium (10 ml of calcium gluconate) was given slowly through the intravenous route, with conversion of the electrocardiogram to an irregular nodal rhythm (see Fig. 15-6). Thereafter the patient was placed on a monitor. Plasmaphoresis was begun immediately via a central venous catheter followed by the administration of 100 ml of 10% glucose and 10 units of regular insulin. Sodium bicarbonate was also administered (88 mEq) via a peripheral vein. The patient received nasal O_2 at a rate of 5 liters/min and 120 mg furosemide was given intravenously. The bladder was catheterized and 200 ml of straw-colored urine obtained. The urine protein was 1+; glucose negative; SG, 1007. The microscopic examination was unremarkable except for 5 to 8 WBCs per high-power field. The serum electrolyte levels were as follows: sodium, 132 mEq/liter; potassium, 11.4 mEq/liter; chloride, 121 mEq/liter; CO_2, 10 mEq/liter; BUN, 156 mg/dl; creatinine, 16 mg/dl; and glucose, 108 mg/dl. The arterial pH was 7.0; pCO_2, 38; PO_2, 46. The hematocrit was 23%, with a WBC of 6200 and a normal differential count.

The patient had chronic metabolic acidosis secondary to her renal failure. Excessive ingestion of fruits, as well as gastrointestinal bleeding, significantly increased potassium entry into the ECF. Respiratory compensation for her metabolic acidosis, despite her chronic lung disease, played a major role in maintenance of acid-base balance prior to the development of her congestive heart failure. With the onset of pulmonary edema and an elevation in the plasma pCO_2 (and hence carbonic acid), the arterial pH began to fall, leading to a severe metabolic acidosis. This relatively acute exacerbation and increased potassium intake led to the severe hyperkalemia.

Because of the presence of severe congestive heart failure, with hyperkalemia and acidosis in addition to her chronic renal failure, conservative management with calcium, bicarbonate, and glucose was not possible. The patient did not respond to the original dose of furosemide and a repeat dose of 400 mg intravenously produced little result. The patient was therefore acutely hemodialyzed with rapid resolution of her pulmonary edema, correction of the acidosis, and return of her electrocardiogram to normal. During the first 2 hours of the procedure, however, calcium gluconate (10 ml) had to be administered on two occasions via a peripheral vein because of conversion of the electrocardiogram to a sine wave configuration.

The patient has been maintained on intermittent hemodialysis since that time with no further episodes of congestive heart failure or significant hyperkalemia. Upper gastrointestinal x-rays revealed a marginal ulcer that was treated conservatively with complete resolution.

References

Adler, S. "An extrarenal action of aldosterone on mammalian skeletal muscle." Am. J. Physiol. *218:* 616, 1970.

Alexander, E. A., and Levinsky, N. G. "An extrarenal mechanism of potassium adaptation." J. Clin. Invest. *47:* 740, 1968.

Bennett, C. M., Clapp, J. R., and Berliner, R. W. "Micropuncture study of the proximal and distal tubule in the dog." Am. J. Physiol. *213:* 1254, 1967.

Conn, J. W. et al. "Licorice-induced pseudohyperaldosteronism." JAMA *205:* 492, 1968.

Fowler, N., Giebisch, G., and Whittenbury, G. "Distal tubular tracer microinjection study of renal tubular potassium transport." Am. J. Physiol. *229:* 1227, 1975.

Grantham, J. J. "Renal transport and excretion of potassium." *In:* The Kidney, B. M. Brenner and F. C. Rector (eds.). W. B. Saunders, Philadelphia, p. 299, 1976.

Grantham, J. J., Burg, M. B., and Orloff, J. "The nature of transtubular Na and K transport in isolated rabbit renal collecting tubules." J. Clin. Invest. *49:* 1815, 1970.

Gross, J. B., and Kokko, J. P. "Effects of aldosterone and potassium-sparing diuretics on electrical potential differences across the distal nephron." J. Clin. Invest. *59:* 82, 1977.

Hiatt, N., Yamakawa, T., and Davidson, M. B. "Necessity of insulin in transfer of excess infused potassium to intracellular fluid." Metabolism *23:* 43, 1974.

Huth, E. J., and Squires, R. D. "The relation of the cardiovascular phenomenon to metabolic changes in a patient with chronic hypokalemia." Circulation *14:* 60, 1956.

Malnic, G. M. de Millo Aires, and Giebisch, G. "Potassium transport across renal distal tubules during acid-base disturbances." Am. J. Physiol. *221:* 1192, 1971.

Malnic, G., Klose, R. M., and Giebisch, G. "Micropuncture study of renal potassium excretion in the rat." Am. J. Physiol. *206:* 674, 1964.

Malnic, G., Klose, R. M., and Giebisch, G. "Micropuncture study of distal tubular potassium and sodium transport in rat nephron." Am. J. Physiol. *211:* 529, 1966.

Reineck, H. J., Osgood, R. W., Ferris, T. F., and Stein, J. H. "Potassium transport in the distal tubule and collecting duct of the rat." Am. J. Physiol. *229:* 1403, 1975.

Relman, A., and Schwartz, W. B. "The kidney in potassium depletion." Am. J. Med. *24:* 764, 1958.

Santensanio, F., Faloona, G. R., Knochel, J. P., and Unger, R. H. "Evidence for a role of endogenous insulin and glucagon in the regulation of potassium homeostasis." J. Lab. Clin. Med. *81:* 809, 1973.

Schultze, R. G. "Recent advances in the physiology and pathophysiology of potassium excretion." Arch. Intern. Med. *131:* 885, 1973.

Schultze, R. G., Taggart, D. D., Shapiro, H., Pinnell, J. P., Caglar, S., and Bricker, N. S. "On the adaptation in potassium excretion associated with nephron reduction." J. Clin. Invest. *50:* 1061, 1971.

Verberckmoes, R. et al. "Bartter's syndrome with hyperplasia of renomedullary cells: Successful treatment with indomethacin." Kidney Int. *9:* 302, 1976.

Weidmann, P. et al. "Syndrome of hyporeninemic hypoaldosteronism and hyperkalemia in renal disease." J. Clin. Endocrinol. Metab. *36:* 965, 1973.

Weiner, M. W., and Epstein, F. H. "Signs and symptoms of electrolyte disorders." *In:* Clinical Disorders of Fluid and Electrolyte Metabolism, M. H. Maxwell and C. R. Kleeman (eds.). McGraw-Hill, New York, p. 635, 1972.

Wright, F. S., Strieder, N., Fowler, N. D., and Giebisch, G. "Potassium secretion by distal tubule after potassium adaptation." Am. J. Physiol. *221:* 437, 1971.

Chapter 16

Alterations of Acid-Base Balance

General Considerations

Clinical abnormalities of acid-base balance occur frequently in medical practice. These abnormalities relate either to an increase or a decrease in the number of hydrogen ions entering or leaving the ECF or to an extracorporeal gain or loss of base. Sustained acid-base abnormalities most often result from disease of one of the two major organs concerned with acid-base regulation, the lung and the kidney. The clinical and particularly the laboratory manifestations of acid-base disturbances are determined by the interplay between two opposing forces: (1) the pathophysiological factors that operate to lower or raise hydrogen activity (or pH) of body fluids, and (2) the defense mechanisms attempting to restore pH toward normal.

A rational approach to the diagnosis and management of acid-base abnormalities requires an understanding of the physiologic processes concerned with hydrogen ion regulation. Conceptual clarity in the area of acid-base has been abetted by the widespread utilization of the Bronsted-Lowry concept of acids and bases. In this view, simply stated, an acid is a proton (H^+) donor and a base is a proton (H^+) acceptor. Buffers minimize changes in hydrogen ion (H^+) by converting strong (completely ionized) acids and bases into weaker (less completely dissociated) bases and acids, respectively. In humans and other mammals the bicarbonate-carbonic acid pair is the major physiologically active buffer system of the ECF. The efficacy of this system results chiefly from the precise regulation of the buffer pair in body fluids by the kidney and the lungs. The pH of plasma is given by the ratio of bicarbonate to carbonic acid (dissolved carbon dioxide) as formulated in the Henderson-Hasselbalch equation:

$$pH = pK + \log \frac{HCO_3^-}{H_2CO_3 \text{ or } \alpha \text{ x } pCO_2}$$

where α, the solubility constant for CO_2, has a value of .03 at 37° C. In a normal individual the above expression will have the following numerical values:

$$7.4 = 6.1 + \log \frac{26 \text{ mEq/liter}}{1.3 \text{ mEq/liter}} .$$

The denominator of the Henderson-Hasselbalch equation, the plasma carbon dioxide tension (pCO_2), is maintained within very narrow limits by the excretion of carbon dioxide by the lungs. While pH changes may be minimized through changes in extracellular fluid pCO_2, the integrity of plasma pH depends upon the availability of bicarbonate ions in the ECF. The kidneys are concerned with the stabilization of the numerator of the Henderson-Hasselbalch equation, the concentration of bicarbonate ions in plasma.

Each day in the normal individual, on a protein intake of approximately 1–2 gm/kg body weight, the processes of metabolism result in the addition of approximately 60 mEq of nonvolatile acid to body fluids. This same amount of bicarbonate ions in the ECF is consumed to buffer this surplus acid. Restoration of serum bicarbonate consumed in buffering either metabolically produced or exogenous hydrogen ions occurs both by virtually complete reabsorption of filtered bicarbonate ("reclamation") and by the regeneration of bicarbonate ions formed in conjunction with the production and excretion of titratable acid and ammonium (de novo synthesis of bicarbonate). These processes require the transfer of hydrogen ions into the tubular lumen of the nephron. The hydrogen ions are generated in the tubular cells by the hydration of carbon dioxide under the catalytic influence of the enzyme, carbonic anhydrase. When excesses of extracellular bicarbonate occur, these are corrected by the renal excretion of a larger than normal fraction of filtered bicarbonate.

Because the carbonic acid-bicarbonate pair constitutes the principal buffer system of the ECF, measurement of its components provides a meaningful and convenient expression of the acid-base status of the organism. The pathophysiologic forces that tend to alter pH are of two general types: metabolic and respiratory. Metabolic acid-base disturbances are due to processes that alter body fluid pH primarily by changing the concentration of the numerator of the Henderson-Hasselbalch equation, that is, the concentration of plasma bicarbonate. Respiratory acid-base disturbances result from primary changes in the respiratory component or denominator of the equation, which is measured as pCO_2.

A series of overlapping defense mechanisms tend to maintain ECF fluid pH within narrow limits. The defense mechanisms consist of at least three well-defined systems: (1) The presence of extracellular and intracellular buffers, which provide an almost instantaneous and first line of defense against changes in pH. (2) Compensation, a process much slower in its onset of action than buffering but somewhat more effective in returning pH toward normal. The respiratory system constitutes the compensatory defense in metabolic disorders, while the kidney assumes this role in respiratory disorders. (3) Correction, a process that restores the acid-base abnormality and its measurable parameters to normal. This process occurs only when the disease causing the primary disorder is cured or so modified that the lungs can correct the respiratory component and the kidneys can completely correct the metabolic component of the acid-base equation.

Laboratory Considerations

In evaluating the acid-base status of a patient, it is necessary to determine any two of the three values (pH, pCO_2, HCO_3^-) in the Henderson-Hasselbalch equation; the third value may then be easily calculated or read directly from a nomogram. The initial screening procedure traditionally employed in the evaluation of the acid-base status of a patient is the examination of the "carbon dioxide (CO_2) content" of plasma or serum. This measurement reflects the total number of mols of CO_2 liberated from both bicarbonate and carbonic acid, and because of the relatively small amount of carbonic acid (1.3 millimol at a pCO_2 of approximately 40 mm Hg), the value for the CO_2 content approximates the bicarbonate concentration of the ECF. Normal values for CO_2 content are 26–28 millimol/liter and can be measured in venous blood. A low CO_2 content is found in metabolic acidosis, where the bicarbonate concentration has been diminished by buffering an increased load of hydrogen ions. But the CO_2 content is also diminished in respiratory alkalosis, where the kidneys have excreted bicarbonate in compensation for a primary reduction in the pCO_2 of body fluids due to hyperventilation. An increase in the CO_2 content is found in metabolic alkalosis, where bicarbonate concentrations are increased proportionately more than the pCO_2. The CO_2 values are also increased, however, in respiratory acidosis, where the kidneys have synthesized more than the normal amount of bicarbonate in response to a primary retention of CO_2 by the lungs. Although the clinical setting frequently will aid in evaluating a deviation from normal in the CO_2 content, the latter determination alone rarely is sufficient to allow for precise analysis of an acid-base disturbance. Thus the appropriate interpretation of an acid-base abnormality and the subsequent design of therapy must begin with the measurement of the blood pH.

Sampling of blood anaerobically from an artery is not a difficult procedure, and determination of pH using any of a number of commercially available pH meters is simpler than many of the other commonly performed laboratory procedures. On the same sample of anaerobic arterial blood, only one other analysis need be performed to obtain all the requisite data necessary to evaluate an acid-base abnormality. The additional parameter measured can be either the pCO_2, using a pCO_2 electrode, or the CO_2 content, measured manometrically. With any two of the three values for pH, pCO_2 [which can be converted readily to H_2CO_3, pCO_2 in millimeters of mercury multiplied by the solubility coefficient, $\alpha(.0301) = H_2CO_3$ in millimols per liter], and CO_2 content, the third value can be derived using a standard nomogram. It should be remembered that pH and pCO_2 values ideally should be determined in arterial or arterialized capillary blood. Venous blood pH is usually about .03 units lower than arterial pH, and considerably more variations occur with the venous pCO_2.

The acid-base status of a patient also may be evaluated using the Astrup technique, which involves measurement of the initial pH of an anaerobic blood sample and the pH of the same sample equilibrated with two different known concentrations of carbon dioxide. From these determinations, it is possible to calculate the so-called base excess or base deficit with the use of a nomogram. This approach and that of the whole blood buffer base previously described by Singer and Hastings, however, do not, in the author's judgment, provide a more accurate description of acid-base relationships than the traditional measurements of pH, pCO_2, and CO_2 content. Indeed, these extra units introduce certain conceptual complexities into an area that already is surrounded by an inordinate amount of unnecessary confusion.

Normal Regulation of Acid-Base Balance

Approximately 40–60 mEq of hydrogen ions are produced daily from metabolism on a diet containing 1–2 gm of protein per kilogram of body weight. These protons must be buffered within body fluids and ultimately eliminated if a progressive rise in hydrogen ion concentration is to be averted. In addition to the production of hydrogen ions from metabolism, large quantities of carbon dioxide (approximately 13,000–15,000 mEq/day) are evolved from the complete combustion of carbohydrates and fats. While carbon dioxide, per se, is a gas and does not contain hydrogen ion in its molecular structure, operationally in body fluids, it is an acid. Thus, CO_2 is in equilibrium with its hydrated form $H_2O{\cdot}CO_2$ or H_2CO_3, and the latter, carbonic acid, is the principal weak acid of the ECF. A portion of the molecules of H_2CO_3 dissociate at the pH of body fluids, and hydrogen ions are released into solution ($H_2CO_3 \rightleftarrows HCO_3 + H^+$). The regulatory system, therefore, must not only effect excretion of metabolic hydrogen ion but it must also be equipped to trap the large quantities of CO_2 produced in the tissues; convey the CO_2 to the excretory organ, the lung, without altering the pH of the conducting medium, the blood; and then excrete the CO_2 into the external environment, again without allowing a serious change in the number of freely dissociated hydrogen ions in body fluids.

An understanding of the acid-base regulatory system may be facilitated by tracing the path of a hydrogen ion that enters body fluids in the course of normal metabolic processes. The sequence to be described is depicted in Figure 16-1. Hydrogen ion entering body fluids is shown to combine with the bicarbonate ion in the ECF. Bicarbonate is a relatively strong base, and the collision between the hydrogen ion and the bicarbonate ion results in the trapping of the former by the latter and the formation of a new compound, carbonic acid. The hydrogen ion thus disappears from the solution and so does an equimolar concentration of bicarbonate. As already indicated, carbonic acid, although weak, is still an acid, and some of the newly formed H_2CO_3 molecules will dissociate, releasing part of the trapped hydrogen ion back into solution. Thus, at the end of the day, were the bicarbonate buffering mechanism the only defense against the intrusion of hydrogen ions, there would be a decrease in bicarbonate ion concentration in the ECF, an increase in hydrogen ion activity, and an associated shift in pH in an acid direction.

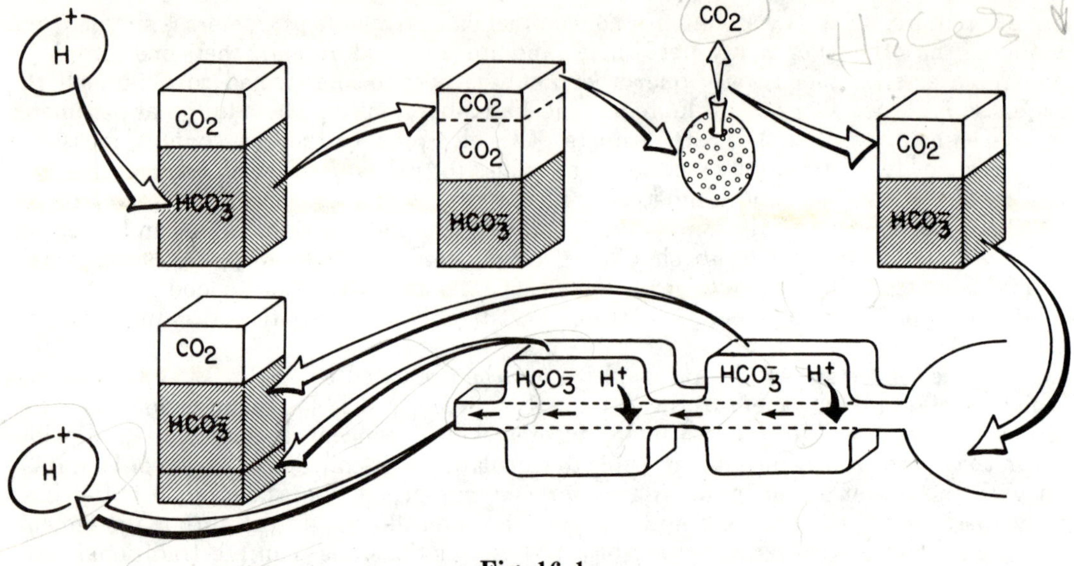

Fig. 16-1.

Overall scheme of the acid-base regulatory system (see text for description). (Reproduced by permission from Modern Treatment *5:* 635, 1968.)

This sequence, however, does not constitute the complete regulatory system. The second phase of the control system also is depicted in Figure 16-1. As the bicarbonate ion concentration diminishes and the carbonic acid concentration increases, the CO_2 gas tension (pCO_2) will rise because H_2CO_3 is in equilibrium with CO_2. Either the increase in pCO_2 or the increase in hydrogen ion concentration or both will stimulate the respiratory center, resulting in an increase in the depth and rate of respiration, and an increase in the pulmonary excretion of CO_2 will restore the pCO_2 to its original (normal) level of 40 mm Hg. This will help to correct the deviation in the pH of ECF induced by the initial accession of hydrogen ions, for as CO_2 is excreted, carbonic acid (H_2CO_3) concentrations diminish and the concentration of hydrogen ions in the ECF diminishes. The respiratory contribution will restore the pH toward its initial value. It will not, however, completely correct the alteration, for the bicarbonate consumed in the initial buffering of the hydrogen ions must still be replenished. It is the kidney that accomplishes this process.

The initial biological responsibility of the kidney is to conserve all the bicarbonate filtered in that the loss of bicarbonate into the urine would simply increase the propensity for the development of acidosis. The second responsibility of the kidney is to synthesize new bicarbonate in an amount equal to that utilized in the initial buffering of the metabolic hydrogen ions. These two functions are accomplished by the tubular epithelial cells through a singular mechanism. Hydrogen ions within the tubular epithelial cells (formed by the hydration of CO_2 and the subsequent dissociation of intracellular H_2CO_3 yielding protons and bicarbonate) are secreted into the tubular lumen. The excretion of the H^+ from an epithelial cell leaves a bicarbonate ion behind, and it is this bicarbonate that will enter the ECF. Whether the bicarbonate ion leaving an epithelial cell serves as a "reabsorbed" ion replacing one in the tubular fluid or a newly synthesized ion (replacing a bicarbonate ion in the ECF previously consumed in buffering) depends upon the presence or absence of bicarbonate in the tubular fluid. In the proximal tubule, where bicarbonate is still present in the tubular fluid, the secreted hydrogen ions combine with the bicarbonate, forming H_2CO_3. This H_2CO_3 is rapidly dehydrated, forming CO_2 and water; CO_2 diffuses back across the cell, and the water enters the water pool in the tubular fluid. Until all the bicarbonate in the tubular fluid is consumed, the epithelial cell bicarbonate that returns to the ECF serves only to replace that filtered. Once the tubular fluid is free of bicarbonate ions, however, each hydrogen ion that is secreted into the tubular lumen leads to a new bicarbonate ion entering the ECF. The hydrogen ions secreted into bicarbonate-free tubular fluid are buffered by ammonia and phosphate, both of which will remove protons from solution, bind them within their molecular structures and then release only a small percentage of the total number bound. Hence, the capacity of the kidney to excrete hydrogen ions and thus to engage in the de novo synthesis of bicarbonate ions is increased greatly by the presence of these two buffers. It follows that the amount of buffers available for excretion will determine the capacity of the tubular cells to restore bicarbonate to body fluids. These steps are shown schematically in Figure 16-1. All the filtered bicarbonate is converted to CO_2 and water by hydrogen ion secretion, but an equimolar quantity of bicarbonate enters the ECF from the tubular epithelial cells, thereby preventing the loss of base into the urine. In the more distal portions of the nephron the synthesis of new bicarbonate ions balances exactly the number of bicarbonate consumed in the initial buffering of metabolic ions in the ECF. Finally, because both the hydrogen ions and the bicarbonate ions arise in equimolar concentrations from the same parent carbonic acid molecules, there is a one-to-one equality between the number of hydrogen ion excreted as NH_4 and titratable acid (titratable acid refers to the hydrogen ion buffered by phosphate) and the number of new bicarbonate ions delivered to the ECF. Under steady-state conditions the rate of hydrogen ion excretion in the urine exactly balances the rate of metabolic production of hydrogen, and the net rate of synthesis of new bicarbonate exactly balances the bicarbonate used in the buffering of the metabolic hydrogen ions.

The trapping and excretion of the large quantities of CO_2 formed in metabolism is accomplished by the red blood cells. The CO_2 combines reversibly with hemoglobin; trapping occurs at the level of tissues where the CO_2 is evolved, and release occurs in the lungs where the CO_2 is excreted. So efficient is this system of CO_2 trapping and transport that the pH of CO_2 rich venous blood is only about .03 units lower than that of arterial blood.

When the integrated regulatory system becomes damaged or when its regulatory capacity is exceeded, abnormalities in the pH of body fluid evolve. This will be the subject of the remainder of this section.

Metabolic Acidosis

General Considerations

Metabolic acidosis results when the rate of addition of hydrogen ions to the ECF exceeds the rate of excretion of hydrogen ions or when base is lost from the body in excess of the rate of replenishment. The hallmark of metabolic acidosis is a decrease in blood pH characterized by a primary decrease in plasma bicarbonate concentration. The bicarbonate concentration can be decreased in three ways: (1) by the addition to body fluids of a readily dissociated (strong acid) that is buffered by bicarbonate; (2) by the loss of bicarbonate from body fluids via the gastrointestinal tract or the kidneys; and (3) by the rapid dilution of the ECF space.

The sequence of events that transpires with an increased rate of hydrogen ion addition to body fluids is exactly the same qualitatively as that referred to in Figure 16-1 for normal metabolism. The only difference is that the load is greater and the compensation is incomplete. The added hydrogen ions are buffered by bicarbonate ions, resulting in the conversion of bicarbonate to carbonic acid. This diminishes the bicarbonate ion concentration and increases the carbonic acid concentration. Some of the newly formed H_2CO_3 molecules will dissociate, and the H^+ will reenter the solution. Thus, an increase in hydrogen ion activity of the ECF will occur. The increase in pCO_2 or the decrease in pH will stimulate the respiratory center, and pCO_2 levels generally will be reduced to below normal in consequence of the augmented rate of pulmonary excretion of carbon dioxide. But the arterial pH, nevertheless, remains on the acid side of normal, for the pulmonary compensation is less than complete. A key factor in controlling the fall in hydrogen ion activity and ultimately in restoring pH to normal is the rate of reconstitution of bicarbonate ions. The kidney, by regenerating bicarbonate and simultaneously excreting an increased number of protons, will effect definitive restoration of pH to normal. Obviously, the administration of bicarbonate and the interruption of the events leading to the enhanced rate of delivery of hydrogen ions into the ECF will decrease the time required for the definitive correction of metabolic acidosis.

The loss of base leads to an increase in the dissociation of hydrogen ions from carbonic acid according to the Henderson-Hasselbalch equation. In addition, reduction in base concentration will diminish the buffering capacity of the ECF to further addition of hydrogen ions. It has been postulated that the decrease in pH (increase in hydrogen ion activity) as a result of metabolic acidosis stimulates peripheral carotid and aortic chemoreceptors to increase ventilation initially. However, the steady-state increase in ventilatory response seems to be dependent primarily on the change in pH in the interstitium of the central nervous system. The lag in the maximal decrease in arterial pCO_2 leads to a more severe acidosis during the acute phase, but as the arterial pCO_2 falls to a steady-state level, the pH rises toward normal. It must be emphasized that respiratory compensation for chronic metabolic acidosis (which takes between 12 and 24 hours) is never complete. Therefore, the pH never returns to preexisting normal values, although with very mild acidosis, pH may decrease only to the lower limits of the normal range. By determining the response in many patients, a predictable relationship between the fall in plasma bicarbonate and the fall in arterial pCO_2 has been established. In general, to estimate the degree of appropriateness of the respiratory compensation to metabolic acidosis, it has been suggested that for every decrement in plasma bicarbonate of 1 millimol/liter, the arterial pCO_2 should fall by 1–1.5 mm Hg. If lesser or greater changes in arterial pCO_2 are observed, a mixed acid-base disturbance involving a primary respiratory disorder should be suspected.

Clinical Features and Systemic Effects of Metabolic Acidosis

The clinical manifestations of metabolic acidosis are dependent, in part, on the signs and symptoms of the primary disorder responsible for the production of the acidosis. However, depending on its severity, acidosis per se may directly produce signs and symptoms. With severe metabolic acidosis, left ventricular function is depressed and peripheral vascular resistance falls. This effect may result in a decrease in blood pressure, pulmonary edema, arrythmias (particularly ventricular fibrillation), and tissue hypoxia. The respiratory compensatory effort may be manifested by an increase in the depth and rate of respiration sometimes referred to as Kussmaul respiration, which is especially prominent when plasma bicarbonate levels have decreased to 15 mEq/liter or less. Central nervous system manifestations may occur, including changes in mentation, confusion, and sometimes convulsive disorders. With profound metabolic acidosis, hypotension may be unresponsive to the use of pressor agents, and restoration of normal pressor response may be obtained only after correction of the acid-base abnormality. Chronic acidosis may lead to osteopenia and osteoporosis as a result of the buffering of hydrogen ions by calcium carbonate in bone. This may contribute to bone disease, particularly in conditions such as chronic renal failure and renal tubular acidosis.

Laboratory Findings in Metabolic Acidosis

The primary laboratory finding of metabolic acidosis is a decrease in plasma pH. There is a decrease in plasma bicarbonate concentrations and, as a compensatory mechanism, a tendency to a decrease in arterial pCO_2. Laboratory data will reveal a decrease in total CO_2 content and an increased or normal anion gap (discussed later); plasma potassium concentrations may be normal or increased (even in the face of some total body potassium deficits) as a result of the shift of intracellular potassium into the ECF compartment as the cellular hydrogen ion activity increases. Urine pH may be acid or alkaline, depending on the nature of the disturbance, and in general the kidney increases its excretion of acid mainly by a rise in urinary ammonium. Titratable acid increases somewhat, but since the quantity of titratable buffers in the urine (mainly phosphate) change little, the increase in titratable acid is relatively fixed.

Differential Diagnosis of Metabolic Acidosis

From the point of view of the laboratory, metabolic acidosis is best classified as hyperchloremic or normal anion gap metabolic acidosis and metabolic acidosis characterized by an increased anion gap.

Anion Gap

When anions other than chloride replace the bicarbonate consumed in the buffering of hydrogen ions in the ECF during metabolic acidosis, routine laboratory studies may fail to show the nature of these anions. The anion gap consists of the unmeasured anions. The magnitude of the gap is estimated by subtracting the sum of chloride plus bicarbonate concentrations from the sodium concentration in the plasma or serum. Normally a difference of 8 to 12 mEq/liter exists (made up predominantly by the plasma proteins, phosphate, and sulfate). If hydrogen ions have been added to the ECF with another anion such as lactate, beta-hydroxybutyrate or acetoacetate, a widening of the gap will be observed. By defining the nature of the anion replacing the bicarbonate, the nature of the offending metabolic acid and generally the approach to therapy will be revealed (Fig. 16-2).

The differential diagnosis of metabolic acidosis may be approached by dividing the causes of this disorder into two groups: metabolic acidosis occurring with normal anion gap (hyperchloremic acidosis) and metabolic acidosis in which the anion gap is increased. The conditions in which metabolic acidosis occurs with a normal anion gap are usually due to external losses of bicarbonate via the gastrointestinal tract or the kidneys. The only exception to this relates to dilution of the extracellular space by chloride-containing solutions or the addition to body fluids of hydrochloric acid or derivatives such as arginine hydrochloride or ammonium chloride which, in the final analysis during metabolic processes, will yield hydrochloric acid. Table 16-1 lists the potential causes of metabolic acidosis.

I. Normal Anion Gap (Hyperchloremic Acidosis)

A. Renal Loss of Bicarbonate

1. Use of Carbonic Anhydrase Inhibitors

These drugs inhibit the enzyme responsible for the hydration of carbon dioxide. This process is important in the secretion of H^+ and consequently in the reabsorption of bicarbonate by the renal tubule. One of the pharmacologic effects of such inhibitors is an increased bicarbonate excretion in the urine. The drug most commonly used among the inhibitors of carbonic anhydrase is acetazolamide (Diamox), which is used in cases of glaucoma to decrease intraocular pressure and also as a diuretic. An adequate history may reveal whether or not the patient is using such drugs.

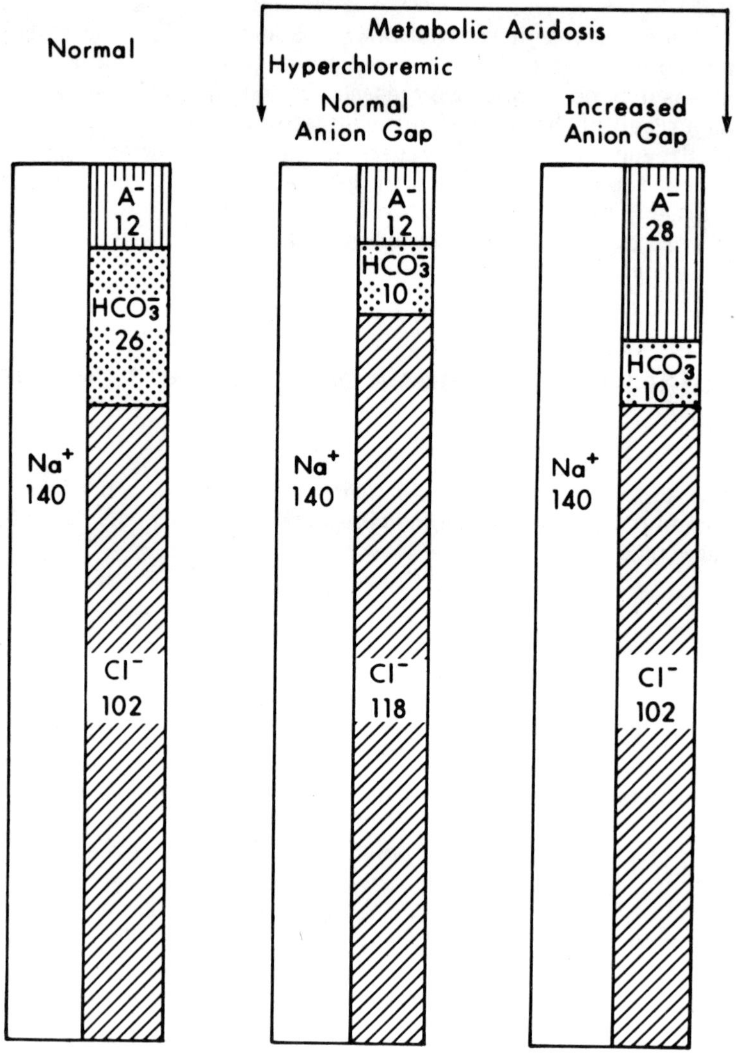

Fig. 16-2.

Anion gap under conditions of normal acid-base balance and during metabolic acidosis. Values are given in milliequivalents per liter.

2. Renal Tubular Acidosis

Renal tubular acidosis (RTA) is a metabolic hyperchloremic acidosis that occurs in patients with a nonazotemic renal acidification defect. Actually, all patients with renal disease and acidosis have an underlying inability of the renal tubules to secrete hydrogen ions (and reabsorb bicarbonate), and this is the cause of their acidosis. These disorders have in common the inability of the renal tubules to secrete sufficient hydrogen to allow the body to remain in acid-base balance.

There are two major types of RTA with several admixtures and hybrids; the two recognized forms are the proximal and the distal. The *distal variety,* also referred to as *classic RTA,* is characterized by an inability of the distal nephron to establish or maintain a hydrogen ion gradient such as the normal nephron can produce. The normal kidney can produce an acid urine pH of 4.7, which represents a urine-to-plasma concentration ratio for hydrogen ions of approximately 800:1. By contrast, patients with classic RTA cannot excrete a urine more acidic usually than pH 6 irrespective of the severity of their systemic

Table 16-1

Causes of Metabolic Acidosis

I. Normal anion gap (hyperchloremic acidosis)
  A. Renal loss of bicarbonate
    1. Use of carbonic anhydrase inhibitors
    2. Renal tubular acidosis—proximal and distal
  B. Gastrointestinal loss of bicarbonate
    1. Diarrhea
    2. Fistulas or drainage of the small bowel or pancreas
    3. Ureteral sigmoidostomy or ileal loop conduit
    4. Use of anion-exchange resins
  C. Other causes
    1. Dilutional acidosis
    2. Addition of HCl, NH_4Cl, arginine, or lysine hydrochloride
    3. Hyperalimentation
II. Metabolic acidosis with increased anion gap
  A. Increased acid production (noncarbonic acid)
    1. Increased β-hydroxybutyric and acetoacetic acid production
      a. Insulin deficiency (diabetic ketoacidosis)
      b. Starvation or fasting
      c. Ethanol intoxication
      d. Hypoglycemia with ketosis and low alanine levels in plasma
    2. Increased lactic acid production
      a. Tissue hypoxia (circulatory insufficiency, etc.)
      b. Muscular exercise
      c. Administration of phenformin, particularly in diabetics
      d. Ethanol ingestion
      e. Systemic diseases (leukemia, diabetes mellitus, cirrhosis, pancreatitis)
      f. Type I glycogen storage disease
      g. Fructose-1,6-diphosphatase deficiency
    3. Conditions in which the nature of the organic acid responsible for the acidosis has not been clearly established
      a. Methanol intoxication
      b. Ethylene glycol intoxication
      c. Paraldehyde intoxication
      d. Salicylate intoxication
      e. Methylmalonic aciduria
      f. Propionyl Co A carboxylase deficiency
    4. Increased sulfuric acid
      a. Methionine administration
  B. Decreased acid excretion
    1. Acute renal failure
    2. Chronic renal failure

acidosis. The lower limit of urine pH of 6 in turn limits the amount of hydrogen that can be excreted as ammonium. Since the amount of buffers in the urine is limited, the pH of 6 also limits the excretion of titratable acid. (It should be remembered that the pK of phosphate, the main buffer responsible for the excretion of titratable acid, is 6.8. Hence, a portion of the phosphate will not be titrated at urine pH's of 6 or above.) The inability to excrete hydrogen ions at a rate comparable to their rate of formation and, consequently, the failure to regenerate the bicarbonate consumed daily results in the development of systemic acidosis. If urinary buffer is increased (e.g., by infusion of intravenous phosphate), more hydrogen ions can be excreted within the limitations of urine pH. This indicates that the defect in distal RTA relates to an inability to generate an adequate hydrogen ion gradient between urine and plasma rather than to the quantity of hydrogen ion that may be excreted.

Although the rate of ammonium excretion in patients with distal RTA is high for the relatively alkaline urine, it is insufficient to provide the cation necessary for the excretion of fixed anions such as sulfate, phosphate, and the like in the urine. Hence, these anions obligate the urinary excretion of cations such as sodium, potassium, and calcium. This results in depletion of these cations with reduction of the ECF volume, potassium depletion, and rickets or osteomalacia. The increased calcium and phosphate excreted into the alkaline urine often causes kidney stones or nephrocalcinosis. Since proximal reabsorption of most of the filtered bicarbonate is intact in distal RTA, the amount of sodium bicarbonate required to correct the hyperchloremic acidosis is relatively modest. Furthermore, this modest amount of sodium bicarbonate prevents the potassium depletion and the demineralization of bone.

Distal or classic RTA is seen in (1) sporadic, congenital, primary form; (2) certain hypergammaglobulinemic states; (3) nephrocalcinosis, which may result from a number of genetic and metabolic disorders including hyperthyroidism, hyperparathyroidism, hereditary fructose intolerance, etc.; (4) nephrotoxicity due to drugs in the distal nephron: amphotericin B, vitamin D intoxication, toluene inhalation; (5) medullary sponge kidney; (6) renal transplantation; (7) possibly pyelonephritis; and (8) collagen disorders (lupus erythematosus) and Sjogren's syndrome.

The other variety, *proximal RTA,* may be characterized by a large excretion of bicarbonate in the urine. A disorder in bicarbonate reabsorption located in the proximal tubule delivers increased amounts of bicarbonate into the distal nephron that surpass the capacity of this segment for bicarbonate reabsorption. An alkaline urine is excreted, and a hyperchloremic systemic acidosis develops. When plasma bicarbonate falls to very low levels, the distal reabsorptive mechanisms may be able to reabsorb the small amount of bicarbonate that is delivered past the proximal tubule. The urine may then again become maximally acidified to pH 4.7 and thus indicate the intact state of the distal tubular hydrogen ion secretory mechanism.

The proximal nature of the reabsorptive defect for bicarbonate is sometimes also suggested by the presence of concomitant defects in proximal reabsorptive activity such as aminoaciduria, glycosuria, and phosphaturia. The hallmark of proximal RTA therefore is normal acidification in the presence of normal renal function when plasma bicarbonate concentrations are low and excretion of alkaline urine as plasma bicarbonate is raised by the administration of exogenous bicarbonate.

In proximal RTA, attempts to restore serum bicarbonate to normal levels by administering sodium bicarbonate are generally unsuccessful. The higher the plasma bicarbonate, the larger the quantity of bicarbonate that escapes proximal reabsorption and is excreted in the urine. The loss of sodium in the alkaline urine results in contraction of the ECF volume, which in turn enhances aldosterone secretion. In the presence of increased aldosterone, large quantities of sodium delivered to the distal tubule enhance potassium secretion into the urine, and potassium depletion ensues. Demineralization of the skeleton occurs owing to phosphate loss, systemic acidosis, and secondary hyperparathyroidism, so that the situation, in this respect, resembles classic distal RTA. The inability to correct the hyperchloremic acidosis completely except with large amounts of sodium bicarbonate, the failure of such therapy to prevent the potassium loss, the ability to reduce urinary pH at low levels of plasma bicarbonate, and the frequent association with other proximal tubular reabsorptive defects all distinguish the proximal from the distal type of RTA.

Proximal or bicarbonate wasting renal tubular acidosis is associated with multiple proximal tubular defects, such as Fanconi syndrome as a result of genetically transmitted systemic diseases (e.g., cystinosis, Wilson's disease, hereditary fructose intolerance, and Lowe's syndrome) or intoxication by heavy metals (cadmium poisoning) or drugs (outdated tetracyclines). It also may be seen in disorders of increased protein excretion, such as the nephrotic syndrome and multiple myeloma, and in vitamin D deficiency. In the absence of other defects of proximal tubular function as a primary form, proximal RTA may be seen as presumably sporadic or inherited, drug induced (e.g., sulfonamides), and during acute phases of rejection in renal transplantation.

B. Gastrointestinal Loss of Bicarbonate

1. Diarrhea

Diarrhea may be characterized by excretion of fluid containing bicarbonate in excess of the concentration present in plasma. With severe diarrhea, stool may contain concentrations of bicarbonate between 30 and 50 mEq/liter. Large quantities of potassium may also be lost, and metabolic acidosis with hypokalemia may be seen.

2. Fistulas or Drainage of the Small Bowel or Pancreas

Secretions of the small bowel, pancreatic juice, and biliary tract are rich in bicarbonate. Losses to the exterior from such fluids may lead to marked hyperchloremic acidosis. The bile may contain as much as 60 mEq/liter of bicarbonate, while the pancreatic secretion, which in many instances exceeds 2 liters/day, may contain bicarbonate concentrations as high as 120 mEq/liter.

3. Ureteral Sigmoidostomy or Ileal Loop Conduit

Patients who have undergone complete cystectomies, especially for malignancy of the bladder, are subjected to the construction of artificial bladders either in the form of ureteral sigmoidostomies or ileal loop conduits. While the first procedure has been almost completely abandoned, many patients who underwent this procedure one or two decades ago frequently developed hyperchloremic acidosis. The mechanism probably involves retention in the sigmoid of urine with reabsorption of water and chloride and secretion of bicarbonate. This leads, of course, to a decrease in bicarbonate concentration in body fluids and an increase in chloride. With ileal bladders, hyperchloremic acidosis is uncommon. However, in certain instances when the ileal segment is extremely long or an antiperistaltic loop has been constructed or when the stoma of the ileal loop is obstructed, metabolic acidosis may occur. Under these conditions, prolonged exposure of the urine to the ileal mucosa will occur with exchange of chloride for bicarbonate, resulting in loss of bicarbonate from body fluids.

4. Use of Anion-Exchange Resins

Gastrointestinal losses of bicarbonate may also occur during the use of certain anion-exchange resins. Cholestyramine, a resin used to treat bile acid retention, has some affinity for bicarbonate and may exchange chloride for bicarbonate. The use of this resin in patients with a certain degree of renal functional impairment has been reported to result in the development of hyperchloremic metabolic acidosis due to increased loss of bicarbonate via the stool and inability of the kidney to generate new bicarbonate to replace those losses.

C. Other Causes of Normal Anion Gap (Hyperchloremic) Metabolic Acidosis

1. Dilutional Acidosis

Dilutional acidosis is occasionally seen as a mild hyperchloremic acidosis resulting from expansion of the ECF volume with chloride-containing solutions. This is a mild and rapidly corrected abnormality, and the decreases in plasma bicarbonate are modest.

2. Addition of Hydrochloric Acid, Ammonium Chloride, Argine Hydrochloride, or Lysine Hydrochloride

Administration of hydrochloric acid or other substances, such as ammonium chloride, lysine hydrochloride, or arginine hydrochloride, that may yield hydrochloric acid as the final product may result in the development of hyperchloremic acidosis. The administration of hydrochloric acid, a substance that dissociates almost completely and is buffered by bicarbonate, leads to an increase in the plasma concentration of chloride and a decrease in the plasma concentration of bicarbonate.

3. Hyperalimentation Acidosis

Amino acid infusates that contain inorganic cations in significant excess of organic anions may cause a metabolic acidosis with hyperchloremia. Metabolism of these amino acid cations to tissue protein releases hydrogen, which is buffered by bicarbonate. The accompanying anion in the infusates is usually chloride, which accounts for the hyperchloremia. If the cationic amino acids are balanced by organic anions, metabolic acidosis may be avoided because metabolism of organic anions consumes hydrogen.

II. Metabolic Acidosis Associated with an Increased Anion Gap

A. Increased Acid Production

1. Increased β-hydroxybutyric and Acetoacetic Acid Production

In these conditions the increased rate of acid production takes place intracellularly. In consequence of the relative or absolute state of insulin deficiency, the amount of glucose entering the cells is diminished, and there is an increased rate of breakdown of fat. When the production of fatty acids, exceeds the rate at which they can be metabolized, two relatively strong fatty acids β-hydroxybutyric acid and acetoacetic acid, begin to accumulate in the ICF. Because these acids are almost completely dissociated at the pH of body fluids, 1 mol of either of the fatty acids will liberate virtually 1 mol of hydrogen ions; the pH of the intracellular water thus will fall progressively, and hydrogen ions will begin to enter the ECF. The newly acquired extracellular hydrogen ions will be buffered by bicarbonate, decreasing the concentration of bicarbonate in the ECF. The anion residue from the dissociated acid (ketoacid) will also enter the ECF and will replace the bicarbonate that is consumed in equimolar concentrations. This results in a metabolic acidosis with an increased anion gap. The increment in anion gap should approximate the decrement in bicarbonate. The hallmark is the accumulation of ketone bodies in the ECF. A previous history, a family history of diabetes, and the presence of hyperglycemia, glycosuria, and the like will help in establishing the diagnosis of diabetes mellitus. Other conditions such as starvation or fasting, ethanol intoxication, and hypoglycemia with hypoalaninemia may also result in accumulation of ketone bodies in the ECF and in metabolic acidosis with an increase in the anion gap. A pertinent history and particularly the laboratory data may be of help in establishing the diagnosis.

2. Increased Lactic Acid Production

The metabolic production of hydrogen ions also occurs intracellularly in consequence of an increase in the rate of production of lactic acid. Lactic acid is the end product of glycolysis, and in anaerobic metabolism 1 mol of glucose will give rise to 2 mol of lactate. Normally, in aerobic metabolism the rate of lactate synthesis from the reduction of pyruvate is a carefully regulated process. An increase in the production of lactic acid has been recorded in a variety of conditions, at least some of which have hypoxia as a common denominator. Lactic acidosis may also be seen during extreme muscular exercise; with the administration of DBI (phenformin), an oral hypoglycemic agent that has some capacity to uncouple oxidation from phosphorylation; in leukemics and patients with diabetes mellitus; in glycogen storage disease; and in hereditary fructose-1,6-diphosphatase deficiency. Cirrhosis and pancreatitis also have been associated with lactic acidosis. A metabolic acidosis with an increased anion gap is present, and when lactate and pyruvate ratios are determined, a marked increase in lactic acid and in the ratio of lactate to pyruvate is observed.

The concept of excess lactate or an increase in the ratio of lactate to pyruvate has been used to indicate the two ways in which lactate levels can be elevated. If pyruvate is elevated, lactate will increase but the ratio may remain unchanged. If anaerobic glycolysis is accelerated (by hypoxia, for example) and sufficient NAD is not available to reconvert lactate to pyruvate, lactate will increase out of proportion to pyruvate and an increased ratio of lactate to pyruvate will result. In general, it is this latter circumstance that is associated with metabolic acidosis with an increased anion gap.

3. Conditions in Which the Nature of the Organic Acid Responsible for the Acidosis Has Not Been Clearly Established

a. Methyl Alcohol Ingestion. The accidental or suicidal ingestion of methyl alcohol may lead to severe metabolic acidosis. An unexplained increase in plasma osmolality may be a clue as to previous ingestion of alcohol. Profound acidosis and retinitis, which can lead to blindness, develop after a latent period averaging 12 to 18 hours. This delay in onset of clinical disorders is related to the slow oxidation of methyl alcohol by alcohol dehydrogenase to formic acid, which then forms formaldehyde. The interference by formic acid with oxidative metabolism leads to the accumulation of organic acids, particularly lactate, which accounts for the acidosis.

b. Ethylene Glycol Ingestion. Ingestion of ethylene glycol can lead to CNS disturbances, cardiovascular collapse, respiratory failure, severe metabolic acidosis, and acute renal failure. The initial metabolic degradation involves alcohol dehydrogenase with formation of glyoxalic acid, an intermediate that is further metabolized to oxalic acid and formic acid. The acidosis results from the accumulation of organic acids, particularly lactate, that are formed as oxidative metabolism is interfered with by formic acid. Oxalate accumulation is believed to be the major factor in the acute renal failure that develops. Oxalate crystals in the urine may be evident, and an accumulation of oxalate crystals may be seen in renal tubules on biopsy.

c. Paraldehyde Poisoning. Chronic ingestion of paraldehyde may cause moderate to severe metabolic acidosis. The acids responsible for the increase in anion gap have not been identified. This disturbance is seen both with outdated or decomposed paraldehyde and with fresh paraldehyde. Occasionally, a false-positive test for blood ketones may be obtained under these conditions and may confuse the clinical picture. A history of paraldehyde intake is important in establishing the diagnosis.

d. Salicylate Poisoning. Accidental, therapeutic, or suicidal ingestion of large amounts of salicylate compounds or derivatives may lead to serious metabolic acidosis. Blood levels of salicylate greater than 30 mg% are considered to be in the toxic range. Salicylates may produce initial stimulation of the respiratory center, which leads to hyperventilation, a decrease in arterial pCO_2, and marked excretion of bicarbonate in the urine. This is a picture of compensated respiratory alkalosis. However, as salicylate is metabolized and dissociates in body fluids, a metabolic acidosis ensues. Plasma bicarbonate decreases and the anion gap increases. The acids responsible for this increase in anion gap include salicylic acid and intermediates in biochemical pathways that are inhibited by salicylate. If the respiratory component of salicylate intoxication is prevented and bicarbonate stores are not depleted initially by a compensatory renal mechanism, the severity of the metabolic acidosis is ameliorated, at least in experimental animals. Salicylism should be suspected in patients with a history of aspirin ingestion, nausea, vomiting, the finding of unexplained hyperventilation, prolonged prothrombin time, a low serum uric acid, and a positive urine ferric chloride test. The diagnosis, of course, can be confirmed by determining the blood levels of salicylate.

e. Methylmalonic Aciduria. Since 1967, about 20 children with known vitamin B_{12} deficiency with prominent abnormalities in methylmalonate metabolism have been studied.

The clinical findings of these children are similar, but their response to vitamin B_{12} administration has allowed their separation into two distinct categories: those who respond to vitamin B_{12} administration with reduction in methylmalonate excretion and those whose methylmalonic aciduria is unaffected by vitamin B_{12} supplementation. Life-threatening metabolic ketoacidosis has been the clinical hallmark in all these children. Several children had the onset of their disease within the first month of life. Arterial pH values of 6.91–7.1 have been documented in several, associated with serum bicarbonate concentrations of 5 mEq/liter or less. The acidosis was responsible for failure to thrive or developmental retardation in at least 11 of these children when they were first seen. Persistent growth failure or CNS retardation has not been observed in any of the children who have survived their episodic ketoacidosis.

f. Propionyl Co A Carboxylase Deficiency. In 1961, Childs et al. described a male infant with episodic metabolic ketoacidosis, protein intolerance, and remarkably elevated plasma glycine concentration. More than a dozen children with closely similar clinical and biochemical findings have since been described. Many of these children were found subsequently to have methylmalonic aciduria. The observation that in at least four patients no methylmalonic acid was detected in the urine indicated that methylmalonic aciduria and ketonic hyperglycinemia were not identical diseases. Recently, data have been presented that demonstrate that these children have a primary defect in propionyl Co A carboxylase, the enzyme that catalyzes the conversion of propionyl Co A to D-methylmalonyl Co A. The clinical course is characterized by recurrent attacks of ketoacidosis, precipitated by infections or protein ingestion, and by developmental retardation, electroencephalographic abnormalities, and osteoporosis.

4. Increased Sulfuric Acid

a. Methionine Administration. Administration of 13.9 gm of DL-methionine to normal subjects for 5 to 6 days has been shown to produce a small reduction in serum CO_2 content associated with acidification of the urine and increased excretion of ammonium. The changes in acid excretion have been shown to be related to the observed reductions in serum CO_2 content and to the calculated acid retention.

B. Decreased Acid Excretion

1. Acute or Chronic Renal Failure

In the acidosis of renal failure, the rate of production of hydrogen in the body may not be excessive, but the decreased renal function, especially the marked decrease in the GFR, prevents excretion of the anions of the strong acids generated during metabolism, and sulfate, phosphate, and organic anions accumulate at the expense of a lower plasma bicarbonate concentration. In every case, however, it is the retained hydrogen ion, not the retained anion, that is responsible for the systemic acidosis. With acute renal failure and almost total cessation of the GFR, the daily acid load resulting from diet and metabolism is handled only by buffering. A marked fall in plasma bicarbonate may occur rather rapidly. In the presence of fever, infection, trauma, and an increased catabolic state, the accession of hydrogen ions from tissues may markedly increase, and the acidosis may become extremely severe.

In patients with chronic renal disease, two major types of metabolic acidosis are seen. The most common type is a metabolic acidosis characterized by an increased anion gap with accumulation of strong acids, such as phosphate, sulfate, and organic anions. There is, as renal mass decreases, a compensatory increase in the rate of acid excretion per nephron, especially in the form of ammonium. This allows for maintenance of balance, although with decreased plasma bicarbonate concentrations for prolonged periods of time. As the number of nephrons is reduced below a critical level, acid balance can no longer be maintained, and metabolic acidosis results. As renal function decreases, the ability to excrete titratable acid remains almost intact, but the total amount of ammonium excreted per day decreases. It should be remembered that under normal conditions, about two thirds of the acid excreted by the kidney is excreted in the form of ammonium and one third in the form of titratable acid (approximately 40 mEq/day in the form of ammonium and 20 mEq/day in the form of titratable acid). With chronic renal disease, titratable acid excretion is preserved until late in the disease course. However, ammonium excretion decreases progressively, and an inversion in the ratio of excretion of ammonium to titratable acid occurs. It should also be remembered that once the GFR has fallen to low levels, plasma bicarbonate, under steady-state conditions, very seldom falls below 15 mEq/liter in patients with chronic renal disease. However, these patients are still in positive H+ balance, and the lack of a continuous fall in plasma bicarbonate relates to the buffering of bone salts, particularly calcium carbonate by hydrogen ions. This will prevent progressive metabolic acidosis but will result in loss of minerals from bone and osteopenia.

Another pattern observed in chronic renal disease in certain patients is that of hyperchloremic acidosis. This type of acidosis is seen particularly in patients with interstitial disease, polycystic kidney disease, and pathological entities that compromise mainly the medullary structures of the kidney. Evidence of renal insufficiency with retention of nitrogen products, elevation of serum creatinine and BUN levels, tendency toward hyperkalemia, development of anemia, and the like are all hallmarks of chronic renal insufficiency. Their presence will help to ascribe the metabolic acidosis to renal disease.

Clinical Problem

A 41-year-old white housewife was first seen at Barnes Hospital in 1966 for evaluation of long-standing nephrocalcinosis and nephrolithiasis. At age 16, she first suffered from back pain, chills, and fever, and a diagnosis of kidney stones was made. In 1958, a left ureterolithotomy was performed. An intravenous pyelography performed at that time showed no nephrocalcinosis. She was asymptomatic until 1963. At that time, after the birth of the last of her four children, she began again to pass stones with great frequency. In 1964, she complained of fatigue, weakness, dyspnea, and intermittent gross hematuria. Intravenous pyelography at that time revealed extensive bilateral nephrolithiasis and nephrocalcinosis. The BUN, serum calcium, and serum phosphorus levels were all then within normal limits. In 1966, she was admitted for the first time to Barnes Hospital, and intravenous pyelograms revealed nephrocalcinosis. A bone survey was negative. Physical examination was essentially within normal limits except for scars from previous surgery.

Biochemical analysis revealed the following: total carbon dioxide, 17.5 mEq/liter; chloride, 114 mEq/liter; sodium, 142 mEq/liter; and potassium, 3.5 mEq/liter. Calcium, 10 mg%; PO_4, 2.3 mg%; and BUN, 15 mg%. Examination of the urine revealed a pH of 6.9, 1+ proteinuria and zero to three red blood cells as well as many white blood cells per high-power field. A urine culture was obtained and subsequently reported as negative. The blood pH was 7.32. The creatinine clearance was 85 ml/min. After ammonium chloride loading for 2 days, serum content of carbon dioxide decreased to 14 mEq/liter, but her urine pH, tested on two occasions, was never lower than 6.5. The patient was then discharged on a regimen of 50 mEq of sodium bicarbonate and potassium citrate per day.

During the 6 months following discharge the patient continued to pass stones despite an increase in alkaline therapy to 130 mEq of cation per day. Analysis of several stones passed during this period revealed that they were mainly composed of calcium carbonate and calcium phosphate. During 1967 the patient continued to pass numerous stones, and early in the spring of 1968, two large stones remained impacted in the right ureter. Another ureterolithotomy was then performed. In the summer of 1968, following an increase in alkaline therapy, there was an elevation of plasma bicarbonate to almost normal values, with levels oscillating between 22 and 24 mEq/liter. There was some suggestive evidence on IVP of decreased nephrocalcinosis. By December of 1969 the degree of nephrocalcinosis was definitely decreased on the right side.

Questions

1. What do you consider to be the most likely entity responsible for the metabolic acidosis?
2. Can you name three or more causes of renal nephrocalcinosis?
3. What is the Fanconi syndrome?

Discussion

The association of persistently alkaline or slightly acid urine with hyperchloremic acidosis in a patient with normal renal function, recurring kidney stones, and nephrocalcinosis leaves little doubt about the diagnosis of the syndrome of renal tubular acidosis in this case. The inability to maximally acidify the urine decreases the daily excretion of both ammonia and titratable acid. Hence, patients such as the one reported here develop positive hydrogen ion balance as a result of their inability to excrete the daily hydrogen load originating from diet and metabolism. This retained hydrogen will be buffered by bicarbonate in plasma, and a decrease in the total carbon dioxide content of plasma will be observed. A progressive fall in plasma bicarbonate presumably does not occur, because the persistent positive hydrogen ion balance will lead to titration of bone with buffering by the calcium carbonate present in bone. This presumably leads to the development of hypercalciuria with increased stone formation and nephrocalcinosis.

As mentioned previously, primary renal tubular acidosis in adults may be discovered in four ways: (1) the presenting symptom may be a periodic paralysis similar to familial periodic paralysis except that there is a chronic persistent hypokalemia between the attacks of paralysis; (2) there may be bone pain and a characteristic waddling gait found on investigation to be due to rickets or osteomalacia; (3) the patient, as in this case, may present with typical renal colic due to the passage of renal stones; and (4) the conditions may be discovered entirely by accident if the abdomen is x-rayed for other unrelated conditions. In the fully developed disease, as in this case, the diagnosis is made by the finding of chronic acidosis with an abnormally low plasma bicarbonate and arterial pH associated with an alkaline, neutral, or only slightly acid urine.

It should be remembered that about 50% of cases of renal tubular acidosis show bilateral nephrocalcinosis, the calcification being located in the medullary portion of the kidney. Renal tubular acidosis is the third most common cause of bilateral nephrocalcinosis, being exceeded in number of cases only by primary hyperparathyroidism and chronic pyelonephritis. At least 14 families with multiple cases have been reported, suggesting that renal tubular acidosis is caused by a dominant hereditary factor with incomplete penetrance. The disease has also been reported following the administration of certain drugs such as amphotericin B and outdated tetracycline. The functional defect of renal tubular acidosis may also be found in conditions causing severe hyperglobulinemia. Multiple myelomatosis may cause a condition resembling the Fanconi syndrome, but other types of hyperglobulinemia may produce a pure renal tubular acidosis without aminoaciduria or other disorders of proximal tubular reabsorption.

Renal tubular acidosis, as mentioned before, has been associated with cryoglobulinemia, hyperglobulinemic purpura, and the juvenile type of cirrhosis of the liver. In the case reported here, none of the entities mentioned was present, and this reported case is believed to be a case of familial renal tubular acidosis. At least another member of the family has subsequently been identified to have renal tubular acidosis.

Renal tubular acidosis, as in this case, usually responds well to therapy with sodium citrate or other alkalinizing salts. An appropriate mixture of sodium citrate and sodium bicarbonate, as employed in the present case, as well as potassium citrate in an effort to replace potassium deficits, is usually adequate to control the metabolic acidosis. The exact prognosis of the entity is not completely known because cases have not as yet been treated for adequate periods. It is certain that the disease is only slowly progressive, renal function remaining apparently unchanged for long periods. The main hazard in the well-controlled patient is progressive renal damage from fibrosis secondary to nephrocalcinosis and to pyelonephritis resistant to treatment.

Respiratory Acidosis

General Considerations

Respiratory acidosis is a disorder characterized by an increase in CO_2 tension and sometimes by a decrease in blood pH. This disorder reflects an imbalance between CO_2 production from metabolism and CO_2 excretion by the lungs. The accumulation of carbon dioxide will lead to an increase in the carbonic acid concentration of the ECF (and also of the ICF). Since CO_2 production from metabolism does not change significantly under most circumstances, being in the order of 13,000–15,000 millimol/day, the usual mechanism by which CO_2 tension increases is related to decreased excretion of CO_2 via the lung. If the excretion of CO_2 is less than the daily metabolic production, CO_2 accumulation will occur within body fluids. As the CO_2 tension increases, a new balance may be reestablished such that all of the metabolic CO_2 produced will now be excreted via the lungs but only at levels of CO_2 tension, which are higher than those seen in normal individuals. As the blood CO_2 tension rises, the amount of dissolved CO_2 increases and shifts the equilibrium reaction to favor the production of H_2CO_3; $CO_2 + H_2O \rightleftarrows H_2CO_3$. Since this increased acid participates in the body buffer system controlling pH, the net result of accumulation of CO_2 will be the generation of carbonic acid and hence a fall in blood pH.

As in any other disturbance of acid-base balance the first line of defense in respiratory acidosis is the chemical reaction by which the increased H_2CO_3 resulting from an increase in the arterial pressure of CO_2 is buffered to mitigate a marked fall in pH. The buffering is related mainly to buffers other than the bicarbonate-carbonic acid pair (particularly protein, phosphate, etc.) and occurs mainly in the intracellular compartment. The second line of defense relates to the role of the kidney in respiratory acidosis. As intracellular pH falls, presumably as a consequence of increased carbonic acid within cells, the renal tubular cells increase hydrogen ion secretion, which in turn generates new bicarbonate.

In the initial phases of respiratory acidosis, the increased pCO_2 is a stimulus for the generation and secretion of hydrogen ions. Increased excretion of titratable acid and particularly ammonium will result in the de novo generation of bicarbonate. Thus, during the period of adaptation to hypercapnia (respiratory acidosis), there is an increased urinary excretion of ammonium and chloride, which leads to an increase in plasma bicarbonate and a decrease in plasma chloride concentration. When a "steady-state" hypercapnia is reached, excretion of ammonium will return to normal, and the excess hydrogen secreted will be utilized to reabsorb the greater amount of bicarbonate filtered. This persistent increased hydrogen ion secretion, therefore, will maintain the plasma bicarbonate concentrations at levels greater than normal, a mechanism that would tend to increase the numerator of the Henderson-Hasselbalch equation and hence prevent marked shifts in blood pH. The only effective way of restoring the acid-base disorder to normal is the correction of defective ventilation. In the final analysis, only the restoration of ventilation to normal will result in the disappearance of the acid-base disorder that characterizes respiratory acidosis.

Clinical Features and Systemic Effects of Respiratory Acidosis

From a clinical point of view, respiratory acidosis can be divided into two major categories: acute and chronic. In acute respiratory acidosis, caused by a marked and sudden decrease in the excretion of CO_2 with a primary elevation of pCO_2, only the buffering defenses have time to be utilized. This is the picture seen in the first 24 hours following a marked decrease in the ability of the lung to excrete CO_2. Although compensation (involving renal mechanisms) may not occur during this initial period, there is, in effect, an increase in plasma bicarbonate as a result of the buffering of carbonic acid by other buffer systems of the organism. Thus, in acute respiratory acidosis, plasma bicarbonate increases but very seldom to levels above 30 mEq/liter. The acute onset of hypercapnia is usually accompanied by hypoxemia, which may dominate the clinical manifestations. The patient may present with signs or symptoms of acute respiratory distress with marked restlessness, tachypnea, and marked dyspnea. As the process progresses, other manifestations may occur, including fatigue, weakness, confusion, occasional hyperactivity, even manic periods and headache. With high levels of pCO_2, semicoma and coma occur.

The physical signs observed include tremor, asterixis like that of hepatic coma, weakness, incoordination, occasional cranial nerve signs, papilledema and retinal hemorrhages, and frequently abnormal pyramidal tract signs. Tendon reflexes are most often decreased or absent. Other eye signs noted in these patients (chemosis, edema and cyanosis of the conjuctiva, dilated dark retinal veins, and abnormal arborization of the macular area) probably result from hypoxia and other factors.

Coma begins at various levels of pCO_2 from 70 to 100 mm Hg, depending on arterial pH and on the rapidity of elevation of pCO_2. (Acute elevations of pCO_2 would likely produce coma at levels of 70 to 80 mm Hg.) Within minutes of pCO_2 increases in blood, the cerebrospinal fluid pCO_2 rises with lowering of pH. Measurements of brain intracellular pH have shown similar rapid changes in pH as expected from the rapid penetration of CO_2 into the intracellular space. There is an increase in cerebrospinal fluid pressure, since CO_2 retention produces vasodilation with increased cerebral blood flow. It has been postulated that the main reason for the increase in cerebrospinal fluid pressure is related to vasodilatation. Other mechanisms, however, are possible, and the role of CO_2 in cerebrospinal fluid formation has not been completely characterized. The syndrome of pseudotumor cerebri with increased cerebrospinal fluid pressure and papilledema is produced on occasion by respiratory acidosis. The picture may be quite deceptive, since in addition to marked papilledema with increased retinal venous engorgement, a variety of neurological signs may sometimes be found. The key is, of course, recognition of the pulmonary problem and of the marked pCO_2 elevation. Control of pCO_2 usually produces prompt regression of the neurological signs. Occasionally, however, some patients show a slow clearing of neurological findings, even when pCO_2 is brought down rapidly, especially if coma has been prolonged or severe.

Although arrythmias are not common in clinical respiratory acidosis, there is some suggestion that in special clinical circumstances arrythmias can occur. Although cardiac output usually rises with CO_2 inhalation, cardiac activity may be affected adversely by high levels of pCO_2. The increase in pCO_2 produces a vasoconstriction of the pulmonary circulation with marked vasodilation in vessels of most other areas.

Cerebral, renal, extremity, and coronary flows have been shown to increase. CO_2 apparently produces vasoconstriction of the splanchnic vascular bed. The rise in pCO_2 may also affect airway resistance (bronchoconstriction). However, the findings in this respect are somewhat conflicting. The metabolic effects of pCO_2 elevation are not well understood. Severe interference with normal metabolism is believed to be present, especially in the central nervous system, particularly as a result of changes in intracellular pH. Autonomic reactions may be altered in several ways by respiratory acidosis. A rise in epinephrine and norepinephrine has been noted in the blood of humans during inhalation of 7% to 14% CO_2. During severe acidosis, the responses of pulse and blood pressure to injected catecholamines are altered.

Patients with chronic respiratory acidosis have few if any signs or symptoms related directly to hypercapnia. The signs and symptoms of the chronic pulmonary disease, with or without cor pulmonale, usually predominate.

Laboratory Findings in Respiratory Acidosis

The arterial blood is characterized by a marked increase in the partial pressure of pCO_2 and sometimes a moderately elevated plasma bicarbonate. As mentioned previously, in acute respiratory acidosis, plasma bicarbonate rarely exceeds 30 millimol/liter; however in chronic compensated respiratory acidosis levels of bicarbonate may be as high as 40 millimol/liter. Usually the partial pressure of oxygen is decreased. Plasma reveals an increase in total CO_2 content usually with normal concentrations of sodium and potassium, although with chronic acidosis there is a marked decrease in plasma chloride. Urine pH under most circumstances is acid in respiratory acidosis.

Differential Diagnosis of Respiratory Acidosis

The causes of respiratory acidosis are summarized in Table 16-2 and discussed below.

Table 16-2

Differential Diagnosis of Respiratory Acidosis

I. Acute respiratory acidosis
    A. Airway obstruction
        1. Aspiration (vomit, food)
        2. Foreign body
        3. Severe bronchospasm
        4. Laryngeal edema
    B. Suppression of the respiratory center—hypnotics, sedatives, other drugs
    C. Hypoventilation due to muscular or neuromuscular disorders
        1. Myasthenia gravis
        2. Brain stem injury or high cord injury
        3. Guillain-Barré syndrome
        4. Botulism
        5. Hypokalemia
    D. Disease of the lung or thoracic wall
        1. Flail chest
        2. Pneumothorax
        3. Pneumonia
        4. Smoke inhalation
        5. Severe cardiogenic pulmonary edema
        6. Massive pulmonary embolization
II. Chronic respiratory acidosis
    A. Lung disease
        1. Progressive lung disease associated with chronic obstructive emphysema and chronic bronchitis
        2. End-stage interstitial lung disease
    B. Neuromuscular abnormalities
        1. Poliomyelitis
        2. Diaphragmatic paralysis
        3. Myasthenia gravis
    C. Chronic suppression of the respiratory center
        1. Chronic use of narcotics
    D. Obesity with a decrease in alveolar ventilation (pickwickian syndrome)
    E. Primary or idiopathic alveolar hypoventilation

I. Acute Respiratory Acidosis

A. Airway Obstruction

The causes of airway obstruction may be grouped as endomural, intramural, and extramural. Endomural causes include bronchial secretions and aspirated foreign bodies; intramural causes include benign and malignant neoplasms, edema, and fibrous strictures; extramural causes result mainly from enlargement of lymph nodes and other structures, with airway compression. The effects of obstruction vary according to its location and whether it is complete or partial.

Laryngeal obstruction may be caused by laryngeal spasm, carcinoma, partial paralysis of the vocal cords, or collapse of the cartilaginous elements of the larynx as in rheumatoid arthritis or polycondritis.

Tracheal obstruction is uncommon. Foreign bodies either impact in the larynx or descend beyond the bifurcation. External compression of the trachea may occur from goiter, thymic tumors, or neoplastic lymph nodes. Such pressures initially cause an irritating, nonproductive cough that may progress to severe obstruction with stridor.

Localized bronchial obstruction does not cause interference with resting air flow unless it is severe; it is more likely to cause infection distally by interfering with mucus flow. When obstruction is nearly complete, overdistention of the distal lung tissue (obstructive emphysema) may occur; complete obstruction results in atelectasis.

B. Suppression of the Respiratory Center

Barbiturates, opiate derivatives (morphine, etc.), and tranquilizers, as well as other drugs, may cause depression of the respiratory center. Under these conditions, inadequate response of the center to increases in pCO_2 retention may occur with development of respiratory acidosis. A careful history may reveal the administration or use of some of the drugs mentioned above.

C. Hypoventilation Due to Muscular or Neuromuscular Disorders

Neurological or muscular disease may cause either peripheral or central respiratory failure. Peripheral respiratory failure results when the skeletal musculature of the diaphragm, chest wall, abdomen, and neck become so weakened that the chest bellows cannot move sufficient air to ventilate the lungs. Potential causes of peripheral respiratory failure include (1) diseases of respiratory muscles such as progressive muscular dystrophy, myotonic muscular dystrophy, polymyositis; (2) diseases and disorders of the myoneural junction: myasthenia gravis, botulism, anticholinesterase poisons (parathione, DFP), hypersensitivity to curare in patients with pseudomyasthenia (malignancy); (3) peripheral neuropathies: Guillain-Barré syndrome, diphtheria, acute intermittent porphyria; (4) anterior horn cell diseases: poliomyelitis, amyotrophic lateral sclerosis; (5) lesions of the spinal conducting pathways: high cervical trauma, acute myelitis, high spinal compression, or malignancy.

The symptoms and manifestations of peripheral respiratory failure depend partly upon which muscles are affected first. Patients suffering progressive paralysis of the chest wall or abdomen may have few symptoms until their diaphragms are involved, at which time no respiratory reserves are left. On the other hand, patients whose diaphragms are paralyzed initially may feel breathless almost immediately. It should be remembered that patients with acute peripheral respiratory failure almost never becomes anoxemic or hypocarbic until ready to collapse, so that therapy, to be effective, must be started before cyanosis appears or abnormalities really appear in blood gases. Central respiratory failure results when the respiratory integrating neurons in the medulla oblongata become damaged or diseased. Common causes include *infections* (encephalitis, encephalitic poliomyelitis, disseminated encephalomyelitis), *trauma*, *brain stem hemorrhage*, or *neoplasm* and craniovertebral abnormalities. Central respiratory failure produces defects in the respiratory rate and rhythm, and symptoms usually evolve through progressive stages. Patients may report that it is impossible to sleep or that they must concentrate on the breathing act. The breathing pattern may be frankly irregular. Respiratory sensitivity to CO_2 is reduced, and anoxia and CO_2 retention develop unless treatment is instituted.

D. Diseases of the Lung or Thoracic Wall

Respiratory failure of a certain degree may occur with diseases of the chest wall in which the muscles of respiration become ineffective, such as in flail chest. A history of previous injury to the chest wall may be helpful in the differential diagnosis. Acute development of pneumothorax or severe pneumonia may also impair the exchange of CO_2 and lead to acute respiratory acidosis. Other causes include pulmonary edema and massive pulmonary embolism. Electrocardiographic changes, chest x-rays, and physical examination, with a careful examination of heart and lungs, are essential to differential diagnosis.

II. Chronic Respiratory Acidosis

A. Lung Disease

Chronic obstructive lung disease embraces a number of clinical syndromes of varying etiology and pathology with a common feature of increased hindrance to the flow of air out of the lungs as a result of an intrapulmonary pathologic condition. In some, air flow obstruction is intermittent, and the clinical presentation is one of asthma; in others, air flow obstruction is continuous, often associated with chronic bronchitis or emphysema or both, and the clinical presentation varies, depending upon the degree to which the pulmonary condition results in disturbance of pulmonary and circulatory function.

Typically, the patient with chronic airway obstruction is a male cigarette smoker between 50 and 60 years old who may or may not have a long history of chronic bronchitis with recurrent winter bronchitis. Cardinal symptoms are breathlessness on exertion, often with wheezing, which is most severe in the morning, and associated with a sensation of tightness; and intolerance on sudden exposure to cold air or smoky atmospheres, which induce coughing, tightness, and breathlessness. There is often orthopnea along with shortness of breath on stooping.

B. and C. Neuromuscular Abnormalities and Chronic Suppression of the Respiratory Center

These conditions have been considered above.

D. Cardiorespiratory Failure of Extreme Obesity

Cardiorespiratory failure has been described in association with extreme obesity, the average weight being approximately 325 pounds. The similarity in appearance and behavior of these patients to the description of the fat boy, Joe, in Dickens' *Pickwick Papers* has led to this association being termed the pickwickian syndrome. Prominent cyanosis, tachycardia, raised central venous pressure with cardiac dilatation, functional tricuspid incompetence, hepatomegaly and peripheral edema may be observed.

E. Primary or Idiopathic Alveolar Hypoventilation

This term denotes a rare clinical syndrome occurring in patients with normal pulmonary and thoracic cage mechanics in whom the primary abnormality is alveolar hypoventilation. The syndrome is characterized by symptoms of headache, drowsiness or somnolence, exertional dyspnea, and signs of cyanosis and congestive heart failure. It is a rare disease first described in 1955, and since then, fewer than 30 cases have been reported. The majority of patients have been males between the ages of 30 and 50. Symptoms have usually been present for many years, but occasionally the presentation has been more acute, usually in response to a respiratory infection. The causes of this syndrome are not known. Resistance to breathing and respiratory muscular power are essentially normal, which distinguishes it from hypoventilation occurring in chronic bronchitis, in neuromuscular disorders, in skeletal abnormalities of the thorax, and the like.

Clinical Problem

A 45-year-old man was first seen in February 1972 at Barnes Hospital with a 2-year history of progressive easy fatigability, headache, and somnolence. During that period, he had been admitted to another hospital several times and treated with radioactive phosphorus (^{32}P) and repeated phlebotomies.

In 1967, he had been admitted elsewhere for pericarditis, and at the time physical examination revealed a somnolent well-developed man of normal weight. The patient was plethoric and cyanotic. There was a loud second pulmonic sound. Blood pressure was 135/65, the pulse was 74 beats per minute and regular, the liver was palpable about two finger breadths below the costal margin, and there was a positive hepatojugular reflex. The spleen was not palpable. Neurological examination was within normal limits. The hematocrit was 49%.

In 1972, the hematocrit was 56%, with a hemoglobin value of 17 gm% and a WBC of 6200. BUN level was 20 mg%, and plasma uric acid level was 4.6 mg%. Urinalysis did not reveal any abnormalities, and most of the serum electrolytes were normal. His pCO_2, however, was 76 mm Hg, with a total CO_2 content of 37, and his blood pH was 7.32. Funduscopic examination showed only venous distention; electrocardiogram showed evidence of right axis deviation and an incomplete right bundle branch block. Chest x-rays revealed prominent pulmonary vasculature but no evidence of primary lung disease. Cardiac catheterization revealed the following: pressures (in millimeters of mercury) were: right atrium, 13/7; right ventricle, 32/5; pulmonary artery, 32/20; wedge pressure, 14/9; brachial artery, 110/80; oxygen saturation was 72 in the right atrium, 75 in the right ventricle, and 74 in the pulmonary artery. Cardiac output was 7.62 liters. The pulmonary function tests revealed the following: inspiratory capacity, 3200 ml; excretory residual volume, 880 ml; vital capacity, 4100 ml (104% of predicted); tidal vital capacity (% in 3 seconds) 98%; residual volume, 1550 ml; tidal volume, 570 ml; minute volume, 4000 ml/min; estimated dead space, 150 ml; alveolar ventilation, 2900 ml/min (1500/m^2); maximal breathing capacity, 129 liter/min (105% of predicted); respiratory rate, 10 per minute. No cardiac or vascular shunt was demonstrated. Arterial O_2 saturation was low (82%) at rest and normal (100%) after exercise. A rise in the arterial O_2 saturation to a normal level was also achieved by inhalation of oxygen for 25 minutes. In addition, 2 minutes of voluntary hyperventilation lowered the pCO_2 from 68 to 50, caused a rise in pO_2 and in arterial pH. These changes indicated the improbability of marked alveolar capillary diffusion impairment. Oxygen inhalation intensified the alveolar hypoventilation already present.

Questions

1. What is the explanation for the increase in total carbon dioxide in plasma?
2. What are the most common causes of respiratory acidosis?

3. What would be the acid-base effects and clinical consequences of decreasing the pCO_2 to normal (by mechanical ventilation) in a patient with respiratory acidosis?

Discussion

Intracardiac pressures and pulmonary vascular resistance were within normal limits or slightly increased. The results of the pulmonary function tests indicated the presence of alveolar hypoventilation. The alveolar ventilation was 1.5 liters/min/m^2 instead of the mean normal value of 2–2.5 liters/min/m^2. This was apparently due to the slow respiratory rate (10 per minute); tidal volume and dead space were within normal limits. Vital capacity was normal, as was the timed vital capacity and residual volume. These findings ruled out pulmonary emphysema or other pulmonary obstructive disease. Noteworthy was the presence of hypoventilation in the presence of potent chemical stimuli of respiration; namely, increased arterial pCO_2, hypoxia, and low arterial pH.

The most characteristic clinical findings in the present case were polycythemia, cyanosis, and CNS symptoms of respiratory acidosis. A remarkable decrease and irregularity in the respiratory rate, especially during sleep, were also observed. The absence of splenomegaly, leukocytosis, the thrombocytosis and the normal alkaline phosphatase of leukocytes make a diagnosis of primary polycythemia unlikely.

In respect to secondary polycythemia, the patient's history, the findings of physical examination, the absence of cardiac and pulmonary symptoms at the onset of illness, the result of the hemodynamic studies, and the correction of anoxemia by O_2 inhalation, rule out the presence of a right-to-left shunt (including a pulmonary venous-to-arterial shunt).

Impairment of diffusion is also ruled out because of the CO_2 retention and the low pH in the absence of pulmonary emphysema or other pulmonary disease. The pulmonary function studies demonstrated the presence of alveolar hypoventilation. Alveolar hypoventilation may occur in association with a variety of diseases, but each of the know etiologies can be ruled out in the present case. The values obtained for the mechanics of breathing and lung volumes exclude obstructive pulmonary disease particularly pulmonary emphysema. In addition, when a patient with hypoventilation secondary to parenchymal pulmonary diseases is hyperventilated, hyperventilation is very limited and accompanied by discomfort, which was absent in our patient. The disappearance of anoxemia by voluntary hyperventilation excludes contributory diseases of the spinal cord, motor nerves and respiratory muscles. The cardiopulmonary syndrome of obesity is somewhat similar, but this patient was of normal weight.

In the present case the administration of oxygen was accompanied by a decrease in alveolar ventilation. Such a response occurs in chronic respiratory acidosis, in which the respiratory center is less than normally sensitive to the increased pCO_2, and the principal chemical stimulus to respiration is hypoxemia. Correction of hypoxemia by the administration of oxygen may further decrease alveolar ventilation, cause greater elevations of pCO_2, and further depress pH. This patient presumably represents a case of alveolar hyperventilation where no organic basis for the disease in any system is found.

This variety of alveolar ventilation constitutes a syndrome whose course has been ascribed by deduction to abnormalities of the medullary respiratory center (although no definite histological changes have yet been found in previous published cases). However, in three patients there was a history of encephalitis and another one had been subjected to insulin shock. This entity has been designated primary alveolar hypoventilation, more precisely alveolar hypoventilation due to disturbance of the function of the respiratory center of unknown etiology. In this syndrome the clinical picture is dominated by cyanosis and secondary polycythemia despite normal heart, lungs, and chest bellows. The cyanosis becomes more intense during exercise but is relieved by hyperventilation or by breathing enriched oxygen mixtures. During exercise the strikingly cyanotic patient remains free of respiratory distress. The prime chemical abnormality in the arterial blood is an increase in pCO_2. Despite a compensatory elevation in plasma bicarbonate, there is usually a decrease in blood pH. These findings are characteristic of respiratory acidosis.

Metabolic Alkalosis

General Considerations

Metabolic alkalosis results when the net loss of hydrogen from the extracellular space exceeds the entry of hydrogen into this space or when base is gained in excess of its rate of excretion. The hallmark of metabolic alkalosis is an increase in blood pH characterized by a primary increase in the concentration of plasma bicarbonate. The increase in plasma bicarbonate concentration may occur because of (1) net loss of hydrogen from the extracellular space, (2) net addition of bicarbonate or its precursors to the extracellular space, or (3) loss of ECF containing chloride in a concentration greater than bicarbonate. Therefore, metabolic alkalosis results from abnormal loss of acid or excessive retention of base or both.

Normally, uncomplicated metabolic alkalosis is short-lived because the kidneys promptly excrete the excess bicarbonate. In established metabolic alkalosis two major mechanisms should be considered: the phase or events responsible for the development of metabolic alkalosis (i.e., the generation of such an acid-base disorder) and the elements that allow this disorder to persist (i.e., the maintenance of metabolic alkalosis). In the final analysis the maintenance of metabolic alkalosis concerns the inability of the kidney to excrete bicarbonate. The kidney under normal circumstances has the ability to excrete excess bicarbonate rapidly and will restore plasma bicarbonate to normal after the generation of metabolic alkalosis unless other factors are present that constrain this ability. These constraints are critical to the maintenance of metabolic alkalosis. The factors that affect the renal tubular reabsorption of bicarbonate include the volume status of the ECF, the levels of plasma and intracellular potassium, and the mineralocorticoid levels in plasma.

The initial differential diagnosis of metabolic alkalosis relates to its generation. Was it due to a net loss of hydrogen ions from the ECF, to the net addition of bicarbonate or its precursors to the ECF, or the external loss of a fluid containing chloride in greater concentration and bicarbonate in a lesser concentration than the ECF? Hydrogen can be lost from the ECF via the gastrointestinal tract, the kidneys, or into the cells. If this loss of hydrogen is greater than the net access of acid from the diet and catabolism, plasma bicarbonate concentrations will rise. Secretion of hydrochloric acid by the stomach results in the generation of bicarbonate, which finds its way into the extracellular space. Increased losses of hydrochloric acid from the stomach, for example, as a result of gastric drainage or vomiting, will result in increased generation of bicarbonate and may result in metabolic alkalosis. The kidney also secretes hydrogen, thus generating new bicarbonate that is added to body stores. When the process of hydrogen secretion is accelerated in such a way that it exceeds the need to reclaim filtered bicarbonate and excrete the daily acid load, the plasma bicarbonate will rise above the normal range. This situation probably occurs in hyperaldosteronism, where the excess mineralocorticoid hormones obligate increased reabsorption of sodium in the distal nephron with continued secretion of hydrogen and generation of new bicarbonate, which will play a role in the generation of metabolic alkalosis. Metabolic alkalosis can also be generated as a consequence of potassium loss from the body. Under these conditions, as extracellular potassium decreases, potassium will leave cells in exchange for hydrogen so that intracellular potassium shifts occur as hydrogen enters the cells, and metabolic alkalosis with a rise in plasma bicarbonate will occur in the extracellular space.

The administration of bicarbonate or organic compounds capable of generating bicarbonate, such as acetate, lactate, and citrate, at a rate greater than that of daily acid production will lead to a rise in plasma bicarbonate. In the presence of normal renal function the excess bicarbonate will be eliminated, and the metabolic alkalosis will be only modest. Under certain conditions fluid may be lost from the extracellular space in which the concentration of chloride is greater than that of bicarbonate. This may occur, for example, with the use of certain diuretics that induce sodium and chloride losses without bicarbonate losses and in certain gastrointestinal diseases characterized by diarrhea of high chloride content.

Clinical Features and Systemic Effects of Metabolic Alkalosis

There are no specific symptoms or signs that point to the diagnosis of metabolic alkalosis. The disorder should be looked for in patients with a history of vomiting, surgery and gastric drainage, diuretic therapy, muscle cramps and weakness, and hypertension (primary hyperaldosteronism). Physical examination may reveal the presence of neuromuscular irritability such as tetany or hyperactive reflexes. These signs will be more pronounced if hypocalcemia is an accompanying feature, since ionized calcium decreases as the pH rises.

Laboratory Findings

Laboratory findings reveal an elevated blood pH, an increased plasma bicarbonate, and an increased arterial pCO_2. The pCO_2 elevation, however, very seldom exceeds values of 50 mm Hg. This is not surprising, since alveolar hypoventilation required to elevate arterial CO_2 tension (pCO_2) also would reduce arterial oxygen tension. The combination of increased pCO_2 and reduced oxygen tension in arterial blood would stimulate the chemoreceptors, thereby tending to restore ventilation and blood gases toward normal. Several recent reports have described occasional patients with metabolic alkalosis associated with marked hypercapnia (CO_2 retention) that could not be ascribed to accompanying pulmonary disease or neuromuscular weaknesses. It was concluded, therefore, that the elevated pCO_2, in some instances in excess of 75 mm Hg, was the consequence of alveolar hypoventilation caused by compensatory depression of the respiratory center. The factors governing the degree of respiratory compensation are obscure. Cerebrospinal fluid pH has been proposed as the major regulatory mechanism. The fact that hypercapnia tends to be a feature of metabolic alkalosis only in the absence of hypokalemia suggests that the intracellular pH of the respiratory center may play a critical role. Presumably, potassium deficiency, by promoting intracellular acidosis, might stimulate the respiratory center and thereby prevent hypercapnia. It is important, therefore, to recognize that significant hypercapnia need not be attributed to CNS or pulmonary disease, particularly in patients with metabolic alkalosis with no potassium deficiency.

The serum electrolyte pattern of patients with metabolic alkalosis is characterized by an elevated total CO_2 content, hypochloremia, and almost invariably hypokalemia. The hypokalemia is related to several factors. Renal loss of potassium, however, is the predominant event and is due in part to accelerated distal potassium secretion. Initially, both hydrogen and potassium secretion are enhanced, but as significant potassium depletion develops the renal secretion of potassium decreases to variable extent. Hypokalemia is almost universally present in metabolic alkalosis. Volume depletion in certain states of metabolic alkalosis may lead to elevations of BUN levels and creatinine concentrations. The hematocrit reading may also increase as a result of hemoconcentration. The anion gap may be increased by as much as 5–6 millimol/liter due in part to elevations of lactic acid concentrations and in part to increased concentrations of undefined anions. However, this change has no diagnostic significance as is the case in metabolic acidosis.

Changes in urine pH do not help in the differential diagnosis. However, they are of interest. The urine pH may be acid (so-called paradoxical aciduria) during steady-state conditions when the renal tubular capacity for bicarbonate reabsorption has been stimulated sufficiently to reclaim all of the filtered bicarbonate. On the other hand, the urine pH may be alkaline during periods immediately following increments in plasma bicarbonate when tubular mechanisms have not been adjusted to a degree sufficient to reclaim all of the filtered bicarbonate.

The concentration of chloride in the urine may be used as an important tool in the differential diagnosis of the conditions underlying metabolic alkalosis. It may serve to distinguish between metabolic alkalosis that is accompanied by volume expansion mainly related to pathological conditions of the adrenal gland and metabolic alkalosis that courses with volume depletion mainly related to loss of fluid as through vomiting, use of diuretics, and the like. A spot urine chloride of less than 10 mEq/liter suggests that the kidney is avidly reabsorbing sodium and chloride at all sites in the tubule. A spot urine chloride concentration greater than 20 mEq/liter in the presence of metabolic alkalosis indicates that neither ECF volume depletion nor chloride availability is a critical factor in the maintenance of such metabolic alkalosis and points to a diagnosis of excess mineralocorticoid activity as the cause of the metabolic alkalosis. The only word of caution in analyzing chloride concentrations relates to those patients who have received diuretics 24 to 48 hours preceding such a spot analysis of urine. In such patients the validity of the above assumptions is open to question.

Differential Diagnosis of Metabolic Alkalosis

Most of the conditions responsible for the development of metabolic alkalosis are listed in Table 16-3. From a clinical point of view, it is helpful to divide metabolic alkalosis into two major categories: those characterized by ECF volume contraction, usually with mineralocorticoid excess present, and those characterized by ECF volume expansion, usually the result of excessive mineralocorticoid secretion. This latter group is characterized

Table 16-3

Differential Diagnosis of Metabolic Alkalosis

- I. ECF volume contraction (urinary Cl < 10 mEq/liter)
  - A. Gastrointestinal loss of H^+
    1. Vomiting, gastric drainage
    2. Villous adenoma of the colon
    3. Diarrhea with high chloride content
  - B. Rental loss of H^+
    1. Diuretic therapy—current or remote
    2. Laxative abuse
  - C. Other
    1. Bartter's syndrome
    2. Cystic fibrosis
- II. ECF volume expansion with mineralocorticoid excess (urinary Cl > 20 mEq/liter)
  - A. Primary or secondary aldosteronism
  - B. Cushing's syndrome
  - C. Licorice abuse
  - D. Liddle's syndrome
- III. Excessive bicarbonate loads
  - A. Excessive intake of HCO_3 or alkalinizing salts
    1. The milk-alkali syndrome
  - B. Conversion of accumulated or administered organic acids (lactate, acetate) to bicarbonate
  - C. Glucose-induced alkalosis during fasting
  - D. Posthypercapnic state

almost consistently by the presence of hypertension. This hypertension may be accompanied by high levels of renin and aldosterones, but it might be hypertension with low renin and high aldosterone levels or even low renin and low aldosterone levels where other mineralocorticoids may play a primary role in the expansion of the ECF and increased excretion of potassium and hydrogen via the kidney. Patients with ECF volume contraction, with the possible exception of Bartter's syndrome, are characterized by low chloride concentrations in their urine (usually below 10 mEq/liter). In the volume-expanded group, urinary chloride concentrations are usually in excess of 20 mEq/liter.

I. Metabolic Alkalosis Characterized by Volume Contraction and Mineralocorticoid Excess

A. Loss of Hydrogen via the Gastrointestinal Tract

1. Vomiting or Gastric Drainage

Excessive loss of acid gastric juice as a result of vomiting or gastric suction will result in the development of metabolic alkalosis. Hydrogen ions that enter the gastric lumen are produced in the parietal cells of the gastric mucosa and then transported into the lumen of the stomach. The loss of hydrogen ions via vomiting or continued gastric aspiration will result in an increased rate of secretion of new hydrogen ions. The source of these protons is carbonic acid derived from CO_2 and water within the parietal cells. Hence, the increased rate of secretion of hydrogen ions will be associated with an increased rate of bicarbonate ion synthesis. These bicarbonate ions will enter the gastric venous circulation and then the systemic circulation and favor the development of metabolic alkalosis.

Initially, the alkalosis and the increase in plasma bicarbonate will result in a marked diuresis and excessive losses of potassium in the urine. As chloride depletion occurs, ECF volume is contracted, and hypokalemia develops. The necessary mechanisms for the maintenance of acid-base balance operate if hydrochloric acid is not lost to the exterior as is the case under normal conditions. Normally, the excess bicarbonate generated from the secretion of hydrochloric acid is probably buffered internally by hydrogen ions secreted into the bloodstream as the consequence of bicarbonate secretion in the pancreatic juice, and an internal balance will occur. This balance will be disrupted when vomiting or gastric suction occurs. It should be remembered that the hypokalemia of vomiting results mainly from excessive potassium losses via the kidney and not from potassium losses through vomiting, since potassium content of gastric juice is usually low, on the order of 5–10 mEq/liter.

2. Villous Adenoma of the Colon

A certain number of patients have been described in whom a villous adenoma was responsible for diarrhea characterized by high concentrations of protein, sodium, potassium, and chloride. In these patients, metabolic alkalosis with hypokalemia may result from the loss of chloride in a concentration greater than its plasma concentration and from the resulting volume depletion with secondary mineralocorticoid excess.

3. Diarrhea with High Chloride Content

Darrow and Gamble and their associates described a syndrome termed congenital alkalosis and diarrhea beginning at birth. The syndrome is characterized by watery diarrhea in which stool chloride is higher than stool sodium plus potassium and in which an acid stool, metabolic alkalosis, and a chloride-free urine are present. The primary defect in this entity was postulated to be an inability of the gastrointestinal tract to absorb chloride, which then acted as an osmotic agent causing diarrhea. The diarrhea, in turn, is responsible for potassium deficiency and cell potassium depletion.

B. Renal Loss of Hydrogen

1. Diuretic Therapy

Apart from losses of hydrogen via the gastrointestinal tract, diuretic administration is a common cause of ECF volume contraction with mineralocorticoid excess. If the diuretic is given to a normotensive subject or one whose hypertension has been corrected by treatment, the patient may display high levels of renin and aldosterone. In this instance, the hyperaldosteronism results from diuretic-induced negative sodium balance and volume contraction. Ordinarily, this should result in very little urinary excretion of sodium and chloride. However, chronic diuretic administration may successfully inhibit sodium chloride reabsorption, even during volume contraction. The resulting distal delivery of sodium salts in the presence of hyperaldosteronism accelerates potassium and hydrogen loss, predisposing to the development of hypokalemic alkalosis. If the urine is examined after the cessation of diuretic action, it may contain little potassium or sodium and, therefore, may lead to an impression of extrarenal generation of hypokalemic alkalosis. If the urine is examined in the presence of diuretic action, it may contain large amounts of sodium, potassium, and chloride, a pattern suggestive of the renal generation of hypokalemic alkalosis. It is therefore mandatory to define the state of diuretic action, either current or remote, in any evaluation of the renal or extrarenal generation of hypokalemic alkalosis.

Perhaps the most common cause of hypokalemic alkalosis as a result of volume contraction is diuretic administration to edematous patients in whom reduction in effective arterial blood volume stimulates secondary hyperaldosteronism while the diuretic administration promotes distal delivery of sodium salts. Some hypertensive patients do not become normotensive on diuretic therapy. Nevertheless, successful diuresis may lead to high levels of renin and aldosterone with resultant hypokalemic alkalosis. This combination of findings may simulate certain forms of metabolic alkalosis with volume expansion. A history of previous or current diuretic administration may help in the differential diagnosis.

C. Other Causes

1. Bartter's Syndrome

Bartter's syndrome is a disorder characterized by juxtaglomerular hyperplasia, very high plasma renin levels, with normal or low blood pressure and secondary hyperaldosteronism with hypokalemic alkalosis. Recent studies indicate that renal prostaglandin synthesis and urinary prostaglandin excretion are markedly increased. Treatment of such patients with inhibitors of prostaglandin synthetase, such as aspirin or indomethacin, may result in a reversal of many of the abnormalities. Volume contraction is probably secondary to salt wasting and in some way mediated by increased renal levels of prostaglandins. The patients are resistant to the pressor action of angiotensin. In the normal steady state, these patients are volume contracted, probably as a result of salt wasting. The renin-angiotensin-aldosterone system is presumably activated by chronic volume contraction and the high levels of renal prostaglandins, the latter being responsible for the salt-wasting state, with continuous delivery of sodium salts to the distal nephron and development of hypokalemic alkalosis.

2. Cystic Fibrosis

This is a generalized disorder of exocrine and sweat glands. Malabsorption from deficiency of pancreatic enzymes is the leading problem in childhood. Chronic pulmonary infection, emphysema, bronchitis, pulmonary fibrosis, and cor pulmonale constitute the major problems seen later in childhood and adolescence. A defect in the control of excretion of electrolytes in sweat, specifically an excess of sodium and chloride, is an important feature of the disease. Several cases of children with cystic fibrosis have been reported in which metabolic alkalosis has occurred, presumably as a result of a marked loss of chloride in excess of bicarbonate in sweat; combined with a low-salt diet and ECF volume contraction, this results in the generation of and appropriate setting for the maintenance of metabolic alkalosis.

II. Metabolic Alkalosis Characterized by Extracellular Fluid Volume Expansion and Mineralocorticoid Excess

A. Primary or Secondary Aldosteronism

The disorders in this group have a number of features in common. Different stimuli may be responsible for the excessive mineralocorticoid activity. This activity may be caused by aldosterone, the hypersecretion of which may result from increased renin-angiotensin activity. *Renal artery stenosis, accelerated or malignant hypertension,* and *intrarenal vascular disease* are well-recognized causes of secondary nonedematous aldosteronism and at times may be associated with hypokalemic alkalosis. Under these conditions, plasma renin activity is high, and hypertension is present.

High levels of aldosterone also may be seen in the presence of suppressed plasma renin. *Primary aldosteronism* due to an *adrenal tumor (adenoma)* is the best delineated syndrome. In rare instances, an *adrenal carcinoma* may secrete continuously excessive amounts of aldosterone along with hydrocortisone and at times deoxycorticosterone. The aldosteronism of *bilateral adrenal hyperplasia* results in a clinical syndrome identical to primary aldosteronism due to an adenoma. The only difference is the absence of any neoplasm at surgery and the failure of bilateral adrenalectomy to relieve the hypertension. Hyperaldosteronism that is suppressible by dexamethasone administration apparently represents an adrenogenital syndrome in which there is excessive aldosterone secretion suppressed by the administration of dexamethasone.

B. Cushing's Syndrome

A series of patients may exhibit evidence of excessive mineralocorticoid activity attributable to compounds other than aldosterone. In pituitary ACTH-producing tumors or primary adrenal hyperplasia or tumors, there may be an increase in glucocorticoid and related corticosteroid production. High levels of hydrocortisone may be responsible for major mineralocorticoid effects. Cushing's syndrome, due to exogenous administration of hydrocortisone or ACTH, or such endogenous disorders as adrenal adenoma, bilateral adrenal hyperplasia, and especially extra-adrenal tumors producing ACTH-like hormones may be associated with hypokalemic alkalosis, hypertension, and low renin and low aldosterone levels.

Deoxycorticosterone seems to be the principal mineralocorticoid in two types of adrenogenital syndrome. In 17-α-hydroxylase deficiency, the block to hydrocortisone synthesis is associated with high levels of corticosterone and deoxycorticosterone, as well as the absence of adrenal androgens and estrogens. In addition to hypokalemic alkalosis and hypertension, these patients display evidence of a failure of secondary sexual development of puberty, with amenorrhea and hypogonadism in girls and ambiguous genitalia in boys. In -11-hydroxylase deficiency, the block to hydrocortisone synthesis results in excessive secretion of androgens with virilization and excessive mineralocorticoid activity due to deoxycorticosterone. Deoxycorticosterone has also been shown to be secreted in large amounts by certain adrenal tumors.

C. Excess Licorice Intake

The active priniciple of licorice, glycyrrhizic acid, resembles aldosterone in its chemical structure and possesses similar activity. It has been associated in certain patients with a syndrome of mineralocorticoid excess closely simulating hyperaldosteronism.

D. Liddle's Syndrome

Liddle and his associates have reported a syndrome in which there is an intrinsic increase in distal sodium reabsorption resulting in hypokalemic alkalosis and hypertension but low levels of renin and aldosterone.

In the syndromes of volume expansion with mineralocorticoid excess, as long as dietary salt intake is normal the delivery of sodium salts to the distal segments of the nephron will be plentiful. This is a particularly characteristic feature of this disorder and differs from the pattern of sodium retention in the edematous states, such as cirrhosis with ascites, congestive heart failure, and nephrotic syndrome. In these latter disorders, there is also mineralocorticoid excess that persists in the face of dietary salt intake. Because of a disturbance in Starling's forces in the circulation, the retained salt and water are sequestered in the interstitial spaces or behind the failing left ventricle, so that there is no expansion of effective arterial blood volume. Sodium reabsorption in proximal segments may be increased. As long as the patient is untreated, distal delivery of sodium tends to be low.

By contrast, it should be remembered that in patients with primary mineralocorticoid excess, extracellular volume expansion occurs, suppressing proximal reabsorption and allowing a continuous and abundant supply of sodium chloride to the distal tubule. Mineralocorticoid excess plus dietary salt intake result in volume expansion with a gain of 2 or 3 liters of body fluids (a gain in body weight of 2–3 kg). This increase in weight is not unrelenting, since an "escape" type of phenomenon occurs, so that balance is restored but at the expense of an expanded ECF volume.

Edema very seldom, if ever, occurs under conditions of primary mineralocorticoid excess. There is continued distal delivery of sodium chloride which, in the presence of mineralocorticoid excess, results in losses of potassium with development of hypokalemia, potassium deficiency and the generation of metabolic alkalosis. Most of these patients have impaired urinary concentrating ability and polyuria with hypernatremia.

III. Excessive Bicarbonate Loads

A. Excessive Intake of Bicarbonate or Alkalinizing Salts

It is extremely difficult to produce metabolic alkalosis in individuals with normal renal function by the simple administration of sodium bicarbonate. Amounts as high as 140 gm of sodium bicarbonate given daily to normal subjects may result in only slight elevation in the serum concentration of bicarbonate. The striking capacity of the kidney to excrete sodium bicarbonate is due to an apparent limiting Tm or transport maximum for bicarbonate reabsorption. The steady-state serum concentration of bicarbonate of 26 mEq/liter in humans is close to the threshold for bicarbonate, and the apparent Tm for bicarbonate (28 mEq/liter per GFR) is also close to these figures, so that small elevations in serum concentrations quickly exceed the threshold and are rapidly excreted into the urine. Second, the administration of sodium bicarbonate tends to expand ECF volume, which in turn decreases bicarbonate reabsorption in the proximal and distal tubule. Even in patients with some degree of renal insufficiency the ability to excrete bicarbonate is well preserved. Patients with renal failure tend to excrete sodium bicarbonate more rapidly than equivalent amounts of sodium chloride. In addition, in advanced renal failure the bicarbonate threshold and the Tm for bicarbonate are depressed, conditions that favor the excretion of bicarbonate via the kidney. Administration of sodium bicarbonate in renal failure therefore usually does not result in the generation of metabolic alkalosis. If, however, concomitant deterioration of the circulation exists in such a fashion that administration of sodium salts cannot expand effective arterial blood volume, alkalosis may result.

1. The Milk-Alkali Syndrome

This syndrome may occur in patients treated for peptic ulcer disease or gastric distress with a combination of milk ingestion and absorbable alkali. The syndrome is characterized by alkalosis, hypercalcemia without hypercalcuria, calcinosis (especially band keratopathy), and severe renal insufficiency with azotemia. The mechanism of production of metabolic alkalosis probably relates to increased alkali ingestion with impaired renal bicarbonate excretion due to decreased glomerular filtration. Other factors may also play a role. Hypercalcemia apparently accelerates bicarbonate reabsorption by a direct effect on the renal tubules. It may also do so by decreasing the levels of circulating parathyroid hormone. Hyperphosphatemia, which occurs in the milk-alkali syndrome, may also enhance bicarbonate reabsorption, perhaps through an effect on renal intracellular pH. Hypokalemia, which is a frequent concomitant finding in this syndrome, tends to maintain the metabolic alkalosis.

B. Conversion of Accumulated or Administered Organic Acids to Bicarbonate

Metabolic alkalosis may occasionally occur during the recession of an acute metabolic acidosis. The usual setting is that of a metabolic acidosis with a high production of metabolizable acid such as lactate or ketoacids. These acids have the potential of being reconverted to bicarbonate once the metabolic derangement has subsided. For example, patients in shock with lactic acidosis may, once the circulatory collapse is corrected, reutilize the excess lactate into sodium bicarbonate, and a rebound type of metabolic alkalosis may occur. Acids such as lactate and ketoacids have been termed "potential bicarbonate" in the sense that, unlike the acids that accumulate in uremic acidosis or hyperchloremic acidosis, they may be metabolically converted to bicarbonate without the intervention of the kidney. During acidosis, large amounts of bicarbonate also are administered. The reversal of the primary condition responsible for the acidosis and accumulation of organic acids with potential bicarbonate generation may result in severe metabolic alkalosis. Some degree of metabolic alkalosis can also be observed in patients undergoing dialysis where acetate or lactate are used as organic acids. Prolonged use of solutions containing acetate or lactate, especially during peritoneal dialysis, may result in excessive generation of bicarbonate from these organic acids and hence in metabolic alkalosis.

C. Glucose-Induced Alkalosis During Fasting

The mechanisms responsible for the alkalosis and salt retention that develop during starvation upon the resumption of food intake are not completely understood. These effects of refeeding are more pronounced when glucose is the substance administered. In obese patients the period of starvation is usually characterized by a mild metabolic acidosis, presumably ketonemic in nature, with an increased anion gap and sodium, potassium, and chloride retention. Despite metabolic acidosis the bicarbonate Tm, as measured by bicarbonate titration studies, may be increased. During glucose refeeding, a frank metabolic alkalosis associated with a further increase in the apparent bicarbonate Tm occurs in obese patients, and further sodium retention may result in edema. The factors responsible for increasing bicarbonate reabsorptive capactiy during fasting and its further augmentation during glucose refeeding have not been identified. Neither potassium deficiency nor reduced effective arterial blood volume can be implicated in the enhanced bicarbonate reabsorptive capacity. It is possible that metabolism of ketone bodies to bicarbonate when glucose is fed would result in an increase in plasma bicarbone. Why this phenomenon does not restore bicarbonate concentrations to normal rather than to levels higher than normal is not known.

D. Posthypercapnic State

This state develops when the hypercapnia (CO_2 retention) of respiratory acidosis is corrected rapidly in a setting in which the kidney is stimulated to reabsorb sodium and hence to reclaim bicarbonate. One factor that is important in determining the retention of bicarbonate after hypercapnia has been corrected is salt balance. It has been shown in experimental animals on a salt-free diet that the abrupt removal from an atmosphere high in CO_2 did not result in a fall in serum bicarbonate levels to the normal range. A respiratory acidosis in patients with chronic pulmonary disease can be converted acutely by mechanical ventilation into a metabolic alkalosis. This problem can be avoided by maneuvers that tend to increase salt and bicarbonate excretion via the kidney. However, in patients with lung disease, congestive heart failure, and a tendency to retain salt, a posthypercapnic state may result in profound metabolic alkalosis. Caution is therefore indicated when a rapid correction of a chronic state of hypercapnia is undertaken. Obviously, salt restriction or edema-forming states will perpetuate the alkalosis by increasing sodium and hence bicarbonate reabsorption.

Clinical Problem

A 51-year-old female nurse was admitted to Barnes Hospital for evaluation of arthralgias and was found to have a total carbon dioxide content in plasma of greater than 40 mEq/liter. Her medical history dated back to 1959 when she sought medical help for arthralgias and fever. No specific diagnosis was made. She was treated with steroids and analgesics for 8 years, but osteoporosis developed, and the steroids were discontinued. She was then maintained on analgesics and antiarthritic medication (indomethacin) until 1975, when she was noted to have progressively decreasing renal function. Renal evaluation showed bilateral cortical scarring on IVP, and renal biopsy was performed. The biopsy showed interstitital nephritis that was thought to be due to her analgesic abuse, and her previous medications were discontinued.

She did well until April 1976, when she began to experience bilateral ankle arthralgias for which she was hospitalized at Barnes in July of 1976. On that admission, she was asymptomatic from her renal disease. Her creatinine level was 5 mg/dl; Na^+, 134 mEq/liter; K+, 3.7 mEq/liter; Cl, 71 mEq/liter; and total CO_2, 40 mEq/liter. BUN level was 43 mg/dl. For unknown reasons, no further workup to evaluate the laboratory abnormalities was conducted, and she was discharged.

She was re-admitted in January 1977. On admission, she complained of anorexia with a weight loss of 25 pounds, fatigue, and weakness. She denied vomiting or the use of diuretics or alkalinizing agents. Past history was remarkable for old peptic ulcer disease. Her medications included diazepam, acetaminophen, and aluminum hydroxide for an elevated serum phosphate level. Physical examination revealed a thin, elderly-appearing woman in no distress, with a blood pressure of 110/68 in the recumbent position and 80/60 standing; pulse rate was 72 beats per minute and regular; respirations were 12 per minute; and temperature was 37.8° C. Mucous membranes were dry. Chest and cardiac examinations were within normal limits. There was demonstrable muscle weakness on all four extremities and she had bilateral ankle pain on movement. Chest radiographs and electrocardiogram were interpreted as normal. Laboratory data on admission showed: Na^+, 138 mEq/liter; K+, 3.3 mEq/liter; Cl, 67 mEq/liter; and total CO_2, 40 mEq/liter. BUN level was 70 mg/dl, with a creatinine clearance of 18 ml/min. Because of hypokalemia and increased plasma CO_2 levels, a workup for hyperaldosteronism was undertaken. The patient was placed on 40 mg P.O. Lasix q.i.d., with 120 mEq P.O. of KCl for a 3-day volume depletion program. At the end of this period, the Na^+ was 135 mEq/liter; K+, 2.4 mEq/ liter; Cl, 60 mEq/liter; and total CO_2, 40 mEq/liter.

The patient had orthostatic hypotension and was symptomatic. She was then volume-repleted with 1.5 liter of half normal saline containing 40 mEq/liter of KCl. She was continued on her oral KCl supplements and begun on 12 gm/day salt diet. At the end of 3 days she had ankle edema, a Na^+ of 142 mEq/liter; K+, 3.6 mEq/liter; Cl, 85 mEq/liter; and total CO_2, 40 mEq/liter. Serum BUN level was 44 mg/dl; arterial blood gases were pH 7.54, pCO_2 54, pO_2 58 mm Hg; and calculated HCO_3^- was 40 mEq/liter. On January 31, 1977, her plasma electrolytes were as follows: Cl, 83 mEq/liter, CO_2, 39.1 mEq/liter; K, 3.2 mEq/liter; Na, 138 mEq/liter; creatinine, 2.7 mg/dl; and glucose, 78 mg/dl.

Urine chloride was less than 10 mEq/liter, and urine potassium was 55 mEq/liter. Plasma renin was 21 ng/ml/hr (normal y 3.0 ng/ml/hr) and 28.8 ng/ml/hr. Plasma aldosterone was 22.3 ng/dl during volume loading and presence of edema.

Questions

1. What is the most likely diagnosis?
2. What is the importance of finding low chloride excretion values in the evaluation of metabolic alkalosis?
3. Can you name five causes of metabolic alkalosis?

Discussion

The presence of an elevated plasma bicarbonate level and a pH of 7.54 establish the diagnosis of metabolic alkalosis in this patient. The rise in pCO_2 presumably reflects a compensatory pulmonary mechanism (hypoventilation) designed to increase the concentration of carbonic acid and prevent any further increases in blood pH. Presumably as a consequence of hypoventilation, there was also a decrease in the partial pressure of oxygen. A negative history of vomiting and diarrhea tends to eliminate gastrointestinal losses of hydrogen as a cause of the metabolic alkalosis in this case. Diuretic therapy is a consideration; however, the patient denied use of diuretics or laxative abuse. Most of the entities characterized by ECF volume expansion and mineralocorticoid excess as well as metabolic alkalosis are accompanied by hypertension. Primary or secondary aldosteronism and Cushing's syndrome can be excluded in this case because of the lack of hypertension and the lack of other manifestations that accompany Cushing's syndrome for example. In addition, the urinary chloride measured on at least two occasions was found to be less than 10 mEq/liter. Under most conditions, when ECF volume is expanded and mineralocorticoid excess exists, urinary chloride exceeds 20 mEq/liter. On the other hand the values for plasma renin and plasma aldosterone were found to be markedly elevated. Hence, we are dealing with a patient in whom urinary chloride is low, less than 10 mEq/liter, and at the same time, the levels of plasma aldosterone and renin are elevated. This would suggest secondary aldosteronism. The absence of symptoms or signs of congestive heart failure, nephrotic syndrome, or hepatic disease would tend to exclude these entities as possible causes of secondary aldosteronism.

The most likely diagnosis in this case is that of Bartter's syndrome. This disorder is characterized by juxtaglomerular hyperplasia with very high plasma renins with normal or low blood pressures, as was the case in this patient, and secondary aldosteronism with hypokalemic alkalosis. It is of interest that this patient was treated for a long period of time with inhibitors of prostaglandin synthesis such as aspirin and indomethacin. This treatment may have suppressed evidence of the disease, since recent evidence indicates that renal prostaglandin synthesis and urinary excretion of prostaglandin are markedly increased in Bartter's syndrome. It has been suggested that the initial defect is an increased production of renal prostaglandins that leads to an excessive excretion of salt and water via the kidney, resulting in continous delivery of sodium salts to the distal nephron and the development of hypokalemic alkalosis. Salt losses will result in volume contraction with secondary stimulation of renin release and aldosterone production, which further contributes to the development of hypokalemic alkalosis. Renal prostaglandins may also stimulate renin release directly. In some patients treated with inhibitors of prostaglandin synthesis, such as indomethacin, an almost complete reversal of the whole symptom complex of Bartter's has been achieved. Bartter's syndrome is also one of the entities characterized by high levels of aldosterone and renin, in which urinary chloride tends to be low.

In summary, this case seem to represent an example of an adult patient with Bartter's syndrome. Excessive renal prostaglandin synthesis may lead to excessive urinary losses of salt and water, which result in volume depletion and secondary production of renin and aldosterone, resulting in secondary hyperaldosteronism. This, in turn, would lead to the development of hypokalemia and metabolic alkalosis.

Respiratory Alkalosis

General Considerations

In respiratory alkalosis, there is an increase in alveolar ventilation leading to an increased excretion of CO_2. This is attended by a decrease in pCO_2, a decrease in carbonic acid concentration, and a decrease in hydrogen ion concentration (a rise in blood pH). Since the production of CO_2 from metabolism is usually constant, a negative CO_2 balance can only be achieved through increased alveolar ventilation. Hyperventilation can result from two main processes: (1) increased neurochemical stimulation of ventilation via the respiratory center, and (2) hyperventilation iatrogenically produced by assisted or controlled mechanical ventilation.

As in any other acid-base disturbances, body buffers constitute the initial line of defense in respiratory alkalosis. To maintain blood pH within normal limits, as H_2CO_3 or arterial pCO_2 decreases, the plasma bicarbonate must also be decreased. Release of hydrogen from body buffers may accomplish this by reducing plasma bicarbonate through the following reaction: H^+-anion + cation-bicarbonate = cation + anion + water + CO_2. Most of this hydrogen originates in intracellular buffers.

Changes in cellular metabolism also contribute by increasing the production of lactic acid and probably other organic acids. Buffering as pCO_2 is decreased, occurs within minutes, and a steady state may persist for as long as 2 hours. However, the quantitative change in plasma bicarbonate is not great, and blood pH usually will rise significantly. In general, plasma bicarbonate levels will fall by approximately 2.5 millimol/liter for each decrement of 10 mm Hg in arterial pCO_2 below normal. Although plasma bicarbonate levels may be decreased to values as low as 15 mEq/liter at arterial pCO_2's of 15 mm Hg, one should suspect that at plasma bicarbonates lower than 18 millimol/liter the process is more likely related to metabolic acidosis than to acute respiratory alkalosis.

The second line of defense in respiratory alkalosis occurs at the level of the kidney. The kidneys respond to the rise in pH by diminishing the rate of hydrogen ion secretion into the tubular fluid, and this leads to a bicarbonate diuresis that tends to restore pH toward normal. The process can also be accomplished by reducing the generation of new bicarbonate that serves to replace that consumed in the daily buffering of the metabolic hydrogen load. Initially, the kidney apparently decreases the excretion of ammonium so as to decrease the generation of new bicarbonate rather than decreasing the reabsorption of filtered bicarbonate. As the excretion of the cation, NH_4, decreases, there would be either a decreased excretion of an anion or increased excretion of another cation in order to maintain electroneutrality. In experimental animals, it has been shown that sodium or potassium excretion increases as NH_4 excretion decreases. After a new steady state is reached, excretion of these electrolytes returns to normal. The process of renal adaptation to respiratory alkalosis occurs rapidly and is probably complete within 24 hours.

The third or corrective phase of defense against respiratory alkalosis depends on the total reversal of the causes responsible for the hyperventilation that, in turn, maintains the negative CO_2 balance. This can be accomplished either by removal of the neurochemical stimulus to the respiratory center or by modification or cessation of the assisted ventilation resulting in the abnormality.

Clinical Features and Systemic Effects of Respiratory Alkalosis

Respiratory alkalosis may be manifested by symptoms and signs referable to neuromuscular irritability. Patients may complain of paresthesias located around the perioral region and the extremities. Muscle cramps may be present, and tinnitus may occur. Tetany and seizures may occur in some patients, and an increase in deep tendon reflexes may be observed. Marked alkalosis in seriously ill patients, especially those on digitalis, may result in cardiac arrhythmias that are difficult to manage.

Respiratory alkalosis causes vasoconstriction of the cerebral circulation with a reduction in blood flow to the brain and potentially deleterious effects. Respiratory alkalosis produces a fall in blood pressure and reduced pulmonary vascular resistance with increased pulmonary flow and an increase in cardiac output. The occurrence of abnormal electrocardiograms in hypocapnia has been repeatedly reported. The changes occur acutely upon reduction in pCO_2 and can be rapidly reversed by restoration of pCO_2. Flattening or inversion of ST segments or T waves or both is the change that has been most often described. Alterations in the QRS complex have been occasionally noted but are apparently rare. It has been proposed that myocardial ischemia resulting from impaired release of oxygen from hemoglobin due to the shift in the hemoglobin oxygen dissociation curve in hypocapnia is the mechanism responsible for the electrocardiographic abnormalities. Electrocardiographic changes produced by hyperventilation are important clinically because patients with hypocapnia may present with symptoms suggestive of myocardial disease. Inability to concentrate, anxiety, and reduced psychomotor performance with increased irritability are also consistent findings in hypocapnia. The occurrence of vertigo and syncope is well known and explained on the basis of reduced cerebral blood flow. Clinical observations that hypocapnia may precipitate an attack of petit or grand mal epilepsy led to studies of electroencephalographic patterns in hypocapnia. Abnormal electroencephalographic tracings showing an increase in the number of slow, high-voltage waves have been observed in experimental animals and in normal human subjects as well as in epileptics. The occurrence of a "typical" epileptic electroencephalographic pattern in patients known to have epilepsy and whose tracing between the attacks was normal has led to the routine use of the "hyperventilation EEG" in clinical practice. In animal experiments, the reduction in pCO_2 has been reported to result in decreased tissue glycogen content, and hypocapnia has been suggested as an important contributory factor to the mechanism responsible for the acceleration of erythropoiesis due to reduced pCO_2.

Laboratory Findings in Respiratory Alkalosis

The hallmark of respiratory alkalosis is a decrease in the carbon dioxide tension of body fluids (a decrease in pCO_2). As a consequence, there may be an elevated arterial pH and a decrease in plasma bicarbonate as a compensatory mechanism. The serum electrolyte levels remain within normal limits unless another disorder is also present. Urine pH is not usually helpful in the differential diagnosis, and it usually remains in the acid side. A rise in blood concentration of lactic and pyruvic acids in response to the reduction in pCO_2 has been repeatedly observed. The development of a bicarbonate deficit in the presence of a simultaneous rise in lactic and pyruvic acid should be kept in mind in this disorder, since it may be confused with the findings seen in metabolic acidosis with an increased anion gap.

Differential Diagnosis of Respiratory Alkalosis

Hyperventilation and respiratory alkalosis have been observed in the following clinical states:

1. Alcoholic intoxication, delirium tremens
2. Anemia due to any cause
3. General anesthesia, with assisted respiration
4. Gram-negative sepsis
5. Beri-beri
6. Central nervous system disease
7. Congestive heart failure
8. Congenital cyanotic heart disease
9. 2, 4-Dinitrophenol intoxication
10. Exercise
11. Extracorporeal circulation
12. Fever
13. High altitude residency
14. Hyperventilation syndrome
15. Cirrhosis of the liver
16. Paraldehyde intoxication
17. Pulmonary fibrosis (alveolar capillary block)
18. Early phases of salicylate intoxication
19. Thyrotoxicosis
20. Mechanical hyperventilation

Many of these entities cause an increase in ventilation by central stimulation of the medullary respiratory center as in anxiety, fever, and salicylate intoxication or mechanical irritation of the brain due to trauma or tumors. Stimulation of the peripheral pathways to the medullary respiratory center occur in pulmonary-thoracic disorders that cause hypoxemia with relatively unimpaired CO_2 transport, in high altitude hypoxemia and in disorders that decrease lung compliance without necessarily causing hypoxemia. Mechanical ventilation may produce respiratory alkalosis if the rate and tidal volume are set so that pulmonary excretion of CO_2 is allowed to exceed CO_2 production. However, increased minute ventilation is often necessary in order to deliver adequate quantities of oxygen to patients with severe pulmonary insufficiency. Some of these entities are discussed below.

Hepatic Cirrhosis and Hepatic Coma

With one exception, all recent reviews on hepatic coma consider respiratory alkalosis to be the typical acid-base disturbance in this disorder. However, in addition to respiratory alkalosis, other acid-base disturbances may be encountered in hepatic disease, and mixed respiratory alkalosis and metabolic acidosis may be observed. The mechanisms responsible for respiratory alkalosis in hepatic cirrhosis are not known, although increased pulmonary shunting, hyponatremia, and increased blood ammonia levels have been implicated.

Salicylate Intoxication

Hyperventilation is the outstanding clinical sign in salicylate intoxication. The characteristic course of the associated disturbance in acid-base balance is an early respiratory alkalosis followed by a late metabolic acidosis (see section on metabolic acidosis). The hyperventilation and consequential respiratory alkalosis probably results from a direct stimulating effect of salicylates on the respiratory center. The metabolic acidosis occurs late in the course of salicylate intoxication and probably relates to the metabolism of salicylate to acids capable of donating hydrogen and the effects of salicylate on carbohydrate, resulting in the accumulation of organic acids. The decrease in serum bicarbonate produced by the initial phases of respiratory alkalosis contributes markedly to the development of subsequent metabolic acidosis.

Exercise

Hyperventilation in response to muscular exercise, especially in untrained subjects, is well known and considered to be a reflex mechanism, the exact pathway of which is not clear. Investigation of bicarbonate concentration in severe exercise indicates a progressive bicarbonate deficit concomitant with a reduction in pCO_2. It is difficult to distinguish between respiratory alkalosis and metabolic acidosis as the initial event, since increases in lactic acid occur frequently with severe muscular exercise.

Fever

A pathological rise in body temperature or an increase in environmental temperature precipitates hyperventilation. Although at first the occurrence of respiratory alkalosis was questioned on the assumption that the increased CO_2 production would offset the increased elimination, reduction in pCO_2 severe enough to result in tetany has been described. The exact mechanism responsible for this hyperventilation is unknown. It is reasonable to assume, however, that it is a homeostatic reflex mechanism mediated through the temperature control center. This assumption is based on the well-known role of the lungs or, more specifically, that of the respiratory tract mucosa in the regulation of body temperature.

Congestive Heart Failure

Respiratory alkalosis in various stages of compensation has been observed in patients with chronic congestive heart failure. A rise in blood lactate is known to occur in these patients and has been generally ascribed to hypoxia. However, normal blood lactate and pyruvate levels have been found in patients with decompensated heart failure secondary to severe obstructive pulmonary emphysema, oxygen insaturation, and high pCO_2.

The Hyperventilation Syndrome

The clinical importance of the hyperventilation syndrome is its recognition, since the presenting complaints are multiple, nonspecific, and quite often mimic an organic illness. The following is probably an incomplete list of some of the various presenting complaints that have been reported in the hyperventilation syndrome; the order in which these are listed does not necessarily correspond to the exact frequency of occurrence:

1. Severe precordial chest pain, including sensation of tightness around the chest and precordial palpitations
2. Dyspnea
3. Attacks of weeping and a state of depression
4. Experience of fear and panic; loss of voice
5. Giddiness and lightheadedness, dizziness, syncope
6. Weakness and excessive fatigue

7. Blurred vision
8. Nausea and vomiting
9. Tingling and paresthesias in the upper and lower extremities
10. Sensation of cold extremities
11. Muscle cramps and muscle tightness
12. Emotional excitement and anxiety states
13. Profuse sweating or sweating of hands
14. Diarrhea or constipation; epigastric or lower abdominal cramps
15. Flushing of the face and dryness of the throat

General Anesthesia with Assisted Ventilation

The progression of respiratory alkalosis to metabolic acidosis in patients under general anesthesia and assisted respiration has been reported. A rise in lactic acid concentration accounts for most of the bicarbonate deficit that occurs.

Acute Alcohol Intoxication or Delirium Tremens

Respiratory alkalosis in various stages of compensation has been a consistent finding in certain laboratories in patients with acute alcohol intoxication and in various stages of delirium tremens. In the presence of compensation for respiratory alkalosis, lactate and pyruvate concentrations were found to be elevated.

Clinical Problem

A 42-year-old woman was admitted to the hospital on December 28, 1975 in a semicomatose state 4 days following head and chest trauma incurred in an automobile accident. Following the accident, she had been disoriented, restless, incoherent, and her temperature had fluctuated between 38° and 39.5° C. On admission, after transfer from another hospital, her blood pressure was 100/68; temperature, 38.2°; pulse rate, 80 beats per minute; and respirations, 18 per minute. She was agitated and disoriented but responded to pain. There was a rather large ecchymosis on the anterior chest wall and sutured lacerations on the forehead and right cheek. There were no localizing neurological signs. X-rays of the skull and chest failed to reveal any fractures or abnormalities.

On admission, her laboratory data were as follows: BUN, 18 mg%; pH, 7.37, with a bicarbonate of 23 mEq/liter and a pCO_2 of 35 mm Hg; sodium, 140 mEq/liter; and chloride, 104 mEq/liter. The following day during the nursing shift of 7 A.M. to 3 P.M., her respiratory rate was recorded as 20 per minute, with little change over the next 12 hours. However, the following day, her respiratory rate increased to 30–40 per minute, and her temperature rose to 39.3° C. Later that day, during the nursing shift of 3 P.M. to 11 P.M., it was noted that her respiratory rate was 40–60 per minute. Blood gases were obtained about 10:30 P.M. that day and revealed the following: bicarbonate, 18 mEq/liter; pCO_2, 22 mm Hg; pO_2, 105 mm Hg; pH, 7.49; sodium, 140 mEq/liter; chloride, 112 mEq/liter; potassium level had decreased from 4.2 on admission to 3.4 mEq/liter at this time. A urinalysis performed on the third day of hospitalization when her pH was 7.49 and her potassium level was 3.4 mEq/liter revealed a urine pH of 6, negative for formed elements, glucose, and protein. The day before, the patient had had some vomiting and some diarrhea and was moderately dehydrated.

Her plasma proteins and hemoglobin level had increased by about .6 gm and 1.2 gm%, respectively. Over the next 12 hours, her respiratory rate and temperature decreased, and on the third day of hospitalization, her respiratory rate oscillated between 25 and 30 per minute. A blood culture, obtained on the second hospital day, later revealed the presence of gram-negative organisms and a regimen of broad-spectrum antibiotics was started. Over the next 2 days, her temperature fell to 37.2° C, her respirations were 16–20 per minute, and her plasma bicarbonate level rose. Values for blood gases obtained 3 days later revealed a pCO_2 of 40 mm Hg, a bicarbonate of 25, and a pH of 7.41.

Questions

1. What is the nature of the acid-base disturbance in this patient? Why?
2. What are some of the common causes of respiratory alkalosis in clinical practice?

Discussion

In this patient, presumably either head trauma, fever, and/or a gram-negative septicemia resulted in stimulation of the respiratory center and the development of hyperventilation. This promoted an excessive excretion of CO_2 via the lung and resulted in a decrement of pCO_2 and the concentration of carbonic acid in the ECF. This would lead to an increase in the ratio of bicarbonate to carbonic acid and hence to a marked elevation of blood pH. The compensatory mechanism would involve increased excretion of bicarbonate via the kidney. This would explain the decreased plasma bicarbonate that was observed concomitantly with the decrease in pCO_2. The values obtained are somewhat suggestive of metabolic acidosis, that is, a decreased bicarbonate with a fall in pCO_2, the latter representing a compensatory respiratory adjustment to metabolic acidosis. However, the fact that the pH rose toward the alkaline side while the plasma potassium level decreased strongly suggests that the patient under discussion had respiratory alkalosis rather than metabolic acidosis. It should also be pointed out that when a urinalysis was performed the patient was excreting a urine with a pH of 6 despite systemic alkalosis. This occurred in a setting in which some degree of dehydration was evident, as suggested by the history of vomiting and diarrhea and the increase in plasma proteins and hemoglobin concentrations. However, despite this degree of dehydration and contraction of the ECF volume, the concentration of potassium in serum was at the lower limit of normal. The findings of a history of vomiting and diarrhea plus relatively decreased plasma concentrations of potassium imply some degree of potassium depletion. Under these conditions, even in the presence of systemic alkalosis, as intracellular potassium decreases, a relative acidosis may occur intracellularly, and the pH of the urine may remain on the acid side. Volume depletion plus the fall in serum bicarbonate would also prevent any increased delivery of bicarbonate beyond the proximal tubule, despite decreased pCO_2 values. Intracellular potassium depletion plus volume contraction would lead to the so-called paradoxical aciduria seen in certain alkalotic states.

The patient was treated with potassium chloride in addition to several liters of isotonic saline and dextrose in water in an effort to rehydrate her. After this was accomplished, the patient was clinically improved, her state of hydration appeared normal, the concentration of hemoglobin and plasma proteins had fallen to its original level, and the urine then became slightly alkaline. At the same time the hyperventilation subsided, the fever decreased with antibiotic therapy, and a reversal occurred toward nearly normal concentrations of total carbon dioxide and pCO_2 values in serum. This case illustrates the importance of obtaining pH measurements in the evaluation of acid-base disorders and illustrates the compensatory mechanisms that occur in patients with respiratory alkalosis.

Mixed Acid-Base Disturbances

The entities described, metabolic acidosis, metabolic alkalosis, respiratory acidosis, and respiratory alkalosis, represent simple acid-base disturbances. They denote the presence of one primary process and its appropriate physiologic response (see Table 16-4). A mixed acid-base disturbance refers to the coexistence of two or more primary processes. Since these processes may have either additive or nullifying effects on plasma pH, mixed acid-base disturbances may produce dramatically extreme deviations of hydrogen concentration or disarmingly minor or undetectable deviations.

The coexistence of two or more simple acid-base disturbances is quite common in hospitalized patients. The presence of a mixed acid-base disturbance is frequently suspected from a careful analysis of the acid-base values. When the magnitude of the secondary change in pCO_2 or bicarbonate concentrations (in metabolic and respiratory disorders, respectively) is inappropriate with respect to the magnitude of the initiating process, the presence of a mixed disturbance should be considered (see Table 16-5). Even when a seemingly appropriate relationship exists between an initiating disturbance and an anticipated secondary response, such a relationship may merely be the fortuitous consequence of a dual or even a triple acid-base abnormality. To avoid this diagnostic pitfall, clues to the presence of complicating acid-base disturbances should be sought from a close examination of other laboratory data and particularly from the patient's history.

The following is a discussion of frequently encountered examples of mixed acid-base disturbances. Chronic respiratory acidosis may coexist with metabolic alkalosis, particularly in patients with pulmonary insufficiency and cor pulmonale who are treated with diuretics and a low-salt diet. This disturbance can emerge when hypercapnia of low standing is partially corrected by mechanical ventilation or by other means.

Table 16-4

Summary of Laboratory Findings in Acid-Base Disorders

	pH	pCO_2	(HCO_3^-)
Metabolic acidosis	↓	↓	↓
Metabolic alkalosis	↑	↑	↑
Respiratory acidosis	↓	↑	↑
Respiratory alkalosis	↑	↓	↓

Table 16-5

Usual Magnitude of Compensatory Mechanism in Acid-Base Disorders

Metabolic acidosis	pCO_2 should decrease by 1.0–1.5 mm Hg for every 1 mEq/liter fall in HCO_3^-
Metabolic alkalosis	pCO_2 should increase by 0.5–1.0 mm Hg for every 1 mEq/liter rise in HCO_3^-
Acute respiratory acidosis	HCO_3^- concentration increases but seldom above 30 mEq/liter
Chronic respiratory acidosis	HCO_3^- concentration should increase by 4 mEq/liter for every 10 mm Hg rise in pCO_2
Respiratory alkalosis	HCO_3^- concentration should decrease by 2.5 mEq/liter for every 10 mm Hg fall in pCO_2; HCO_3^- seldom falls below 16–18 mEq/liter

A combination of chronic respiratory acidosis and acute respiratory acidosis may be seen in patients with moderately severe CO_2 retention caused by chronic obstructive lung disease who experience a sudden worsening of pulmonary function as a result of the use of hypnotics or sedatives capable of depressing the respiratory center as a result of correction by their hypoxia by oxygen therapy or acute infections such as acute pneumonitis.

Metabolic acidosis plus acute respiratory acidosis is common in patients with acute cardiopulmonary arrest and results from lactic acidosis (triggered by poor tissue perfusion) and CO_2 retention. A similar picture may be seen in patients with severe, acute pulmonary edema. Extreme degrees of fall in plasma pH may be seen under these conditions.

Respiratory alkalosis converting later into metabolic acidosis is typified by patients with salicylate intoxication and reflects the independent effects of the salicylate molecule on ventilation and cellular metabolism. Patients with gram-negative sepsis may also have this combination, since lactic acidosis or renal failure or both are common complications and may appear in conjunction with primary hyperventilation.

References

Brackett, M. C., Jr., et al. "Acid-base response to chronic hypercapnia in man." N. Engl. J. Med. *280:* 124, 1969.

Bricker, N. S., and Klahr, S. "Treatment of disorders of acid-base metabolism." Modern Treatment *5:* 635, 1968.

Cohen, J. J., and Schwartz, W. B. "Evaluation of acid-base equilibrium in pulmonary insufficiency." Am. J. Med. *41:* 163, 1966.

Edelmann, C. M., Jr. "Renal tubular acidosis." Kidney *4:* 1, 1971.

Eichenholz, A. "Respiratory alkalosis." Arch. Intern. Med. *116:* 699, 1965.

Emmett, M., and Narins, R. G. "Clinical use of the anion gap." Medicine *56:* 38, 1977.

Felig, P. "Diabetic ketoacidosis." N. Engl. J. Med. *290:* 1360, 1974.

Hill, J. B. "Salicylate intoxication." N. Engl. J. Med. *288:* 1110, 1973.

Kassirer, J. P. "Serious acid-base disorders." N. Engl. J. Med. *291:* 773–776, 1974.

Kassirer, J. P., and Schwartz, W. B. "The response of normal man to selective depletion of hydrochloric acid. Factors in the genesis of persistent gastric alkalosis." Am. J. Med. *40:* 10, 1966.

Kurtzman, N. A., White, M. G., and Rogers, P. W. "Pathophysiology of metabolic alkalosis." Arch. Intern. Med. *131:* 702, 1973.

Makoff, D. L. "Acid-base metabolism. "*In:* Clinical Disorders of Fluid and Electrolyte Metabolism, 2nd ed., M. H. Maxwell and C. R. Kleeman (eds.). McGraw-Hill, New York, pp. 297–346, 1972.

Mazzara, J. T., Ayres, S. M., and Grace, W. J. "Extreme hypocapnia in the critically ill patient." Am. J. Med. *56:* 450, 1974.

McCurdy, D. K. "Mixed metabolic respiratory acid-base disturbances: Diagnosis and treatment. Chest *62* (suppl 2): 355–445, 1972.

Neff, T. A., and Petty, T. L. "Tolerance and survival in severe chronic hypercapnia." Arch. Intern. Med. *129:* 591, 1972.

Oliva, P. V. "Lactic acidosis." Am. J. Med. *48:* 209, 1970.

Robin, E. D. "Abnormalities of acid-base regulation in chronic pulmonary disease with special reference to hypercapnia and extracellular alkalosis." N. Engl. J. Med. *268:* 917, 1963.

Sebastian, A., McSherry, E., and Morris, R. C. "Metabolic acidosis with special reference to the renal acidosis." *In:* The Kidney, Brenner and Rector (eds.). W. B. Saunders, Philadelphia, 1976.

Seldin, D. W. "Metabolic alkalosis." *In:* The Kidney, Brenner and Rector (eds.). W. B. Saunders, Philadelphia, 1976.

Index